# HOLISTIC APPROACHES FOR WOMEN'S SUSTAINABLE HEALTH

## Volume 1

*Foundations, Innovations, Challenges, and Management*

**Holistic Approaches for Women's Sustainable Health, 4-volume set**
ISBN: 978-1-77964-170-0 (hbk)

**Volume 1: Foundations, Innovations, Challenges, and Management**
ISBN: 978-1-77964-162-5 (hbk)
ISBN: 978-1-77964-163-2 (ebk)

**Volume 2: Advancements, Socioeconomic Impacts, and Innovative Strategies**
ISBN: 978-1-77964-164-9 (hbk)
ISBN: 978-1-77964-165-6 (ebk)

**Volume 3: Herbs, Spices, Phytochemicals, and Cereals: Body Care, Cancer Prevention, and Hormonal Health**
ISBN: 978-1-77964-166-3 (hbk)
ISBN: 978-1-77964-167-0 (ebk)

**Volume 4: Benefits of Vegetables and Medicinal Plants and Trees**
ISBN: 978-1-77964-168-7 (hbk)
ISBN: 978-1-77964-169-4 (ebk)

# HOLISTIC APPROACHES FOR WOMEN'S SUSTAINABLE HEALTH

## Volume 1

*Foundations, Innovations, Challenges, and Management*

**Megh R. Goyal, PhD**
**Anamika Chauhan, PhD**
**Junaid Ahmad Malik, PhD**
*Editors*

AAP | APPLE ACADEMIC PRESS

First edition published 2027

**Apple Academic Press Inc.**
1265 Goldenrod Circle, NE,
Palm Bay, FL 32905 USA

760 Laurentian Drive, Unit 19,
Burlington, ON L7N 0A4, Canada

**CRC Press**
2385 NW Executive Center Drive,
Suite 320, Boca Raton FL 33431

4 Park Square, Milton Park,
Abingdon, Oxon, OX14 4RN UK



**Library and Archives Canada Cataloguing in Publication**

Title: Holistic approaches for women's sustainable health / Megh R. Goyal, PhD, Anamika Chauhan, PhD, Junaid Ahmad Malik, PhD, editors.
Names: Goyal, Megh R., editor | Cauhāna, Anāmikā, 1985- editor. | Malik, Junaid Ahmad, 1987- editor
Description: First edition. | Includes bibliographical references and indexes. | Content: Volume 1: Foundations, innovations, challenges, and management.
Identifiers: Canadiana (print) 20260181994 | Canadiana (ebook) 20260182001 | ISBN 9781779641700 (set) | ISBN 9781779641625 (v. 1 ; hardcover) ISBN 9781779641632 (v. 1 ; ebook)
Subjects: LCSH: Women—Health and hygiene. | LCSH: Holistic medicine.
Classification: LCC RA778 .H65 2026 | DDC 613/.04244—dc23

**Library of Congress Cataloging-in-Publication Data**

CIP data on file with US Library of Congress

ISBN: 978-1-77964-162-5 (hbk)
ISBN: 978-1-77964-163-2 (ebk)
DOI: 10.1201/9781779641632

# Dedication

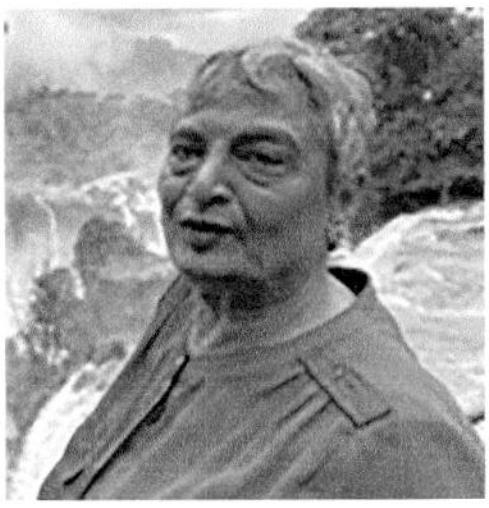

In the sacred verses of Proverbs 31, we find a timeless ode to the essence of womanhood—a testament to strength, wisdom, and compassion. It is within these words that we uncover the embodiment of virtues celebrated in the life of Subhadra Devi Goyal—a remarkable woman whose journey resonates with the noblest qualities of a daughter, wife, mother, pastor, and social worker.

From her earliest days, Subhadra Devi Goyal has exemplified the profound bond of filial love and respect. Her reverence for family, her unwavering support, and her tender care stand as a testament to the enduring legacy of familial ties.

In the sacred covenant of marriage, Subhadra Devi Goyal has shown boundless strength and unwavering commitment. Her partnership with her beloved spouse is marked by resilience, mutual respect, and a shared journey toward growth and understanding.

As a mother, Subhadra's love knows no bounds. Her nurturing embrace, her guiding hand, and her boundless affection shape the lives of her three children, instilling in them the values of integrity, empathy, compassion, and love for God, others, country, and nature.

In her role as a pastor, Subhadra serves as a beacon of light and hope for her congregation and community. Her wisdom, her faith, and her compassionate guidance inspire others to seek solace, understanding, and spiritual growth.

As a social worker, Subhadra's heart knows no bounds. Her selfless service, her tireless advocacy, and her unwavering commitment to justice uplift the marginalized, empower the oppressed, and transform communities with love, compassion, and dedication.

In recognition of her exemplary life, filled with service, devotion, and unwavering faith, we dedicate this book to Subhadra Devi Goyal—a living embodiment of the timeless wisdom of Proverbs 31. May her legacy continue to inspire and uplift all, who are touched by her remarkable spirit!

# About the Editors

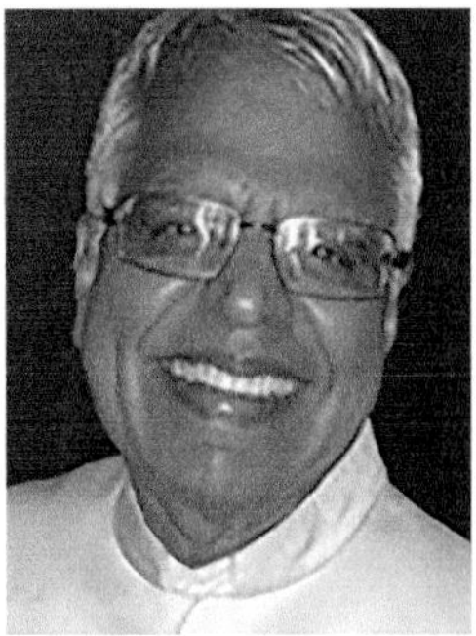

**Megh R. Goyal, PhD**
*Retired Professor in Agricultural and Biomedical Engineering, University of Puerto Rico, Mayaguez Campus; Senior Acquisitions Editor, Biomedical Engineering and Agricultural Science, Apple Academic Press, Inc.*

**Megh R. Goyal, PhD, PE,** is, at present, a Retired Professor in Agricultural and Biomedical Engineering from the General Engineering Department in the College of Engineering at the University of Puerto Rico—Mayaguez Campus (UPRM); and Senior Acquisitions Editor and Senior Technical Editor-in-Chief in Agricultural and Biomedical Engineering for Apple Academic Press, Inc.

He received his BSc degree in engineering from Punjab Agricultural University, Ludhiana, India; his MSc and PhD degrees from the Ohio State University, Columbus; his Master of Divinity degree from Puerto Rico Evangelical Seminary, Hato Rey, Puerto Rico, USA.

Since 1971, he has worked as Soil Conservation Inspector (1971); Research Assistant at Haryana Agricultural University (1972–1975) and the Ohio State University (1975–1979); Research Agricultural Engineer/Professor at the Department of Agricultural Engineering of UPRM (1979–1997); and Professor (Agricultural and Biomedical Engineering) at UPRM (1997–2012). He spent one-year sabbatical leave in 2002–2003 at Biomedical Engineering Department, Florida International University, Miami, USA.

He was the first agricultural engineer to receive the professional license in Agricultural Engineering in 1986 from the College of Engineers and Surveyors of Puerto Rico. On September 16, 2005, he was proclaimed as "Father of Irrigation Engineering in Puerto Rico for the twentieth century" by the American Society of Agricultural and Biological Engineers, Puerto Rico Section, for his pioneer work on micro-irrigation, evapotranspiration, agroclimatology, and soil and water engineering.

During his professional career of 52 years, he has received awards such as: Scientist of the Year, Blue Ribbon Extension Award, Research Paper Award, Nolan Mitchell Young Extension Worker Award, Agricultural Engineer of the Year, Citations by Mayors of Juana Diaz and Ponce, Membership Grand Prize for ASAE Campaign, Felix Castro Rodriguez Academic Excellence, Rashtrya Ratan Award and Bharat Excellence Award and Gold Medal, Domingo Marrero Navarro Prize, Adopted son of Moca, Irrigation Protagonist of UPRM, Man of Drip Irrigation by Mayor of Municipalities of Mayaguez/Caguas/Ponce and Senate/Secretary of Agriculture of ELA, Puerto Rico.

The Water Technology Centre of Tamil Nadu Agricultural University in Coimbatore, India recognized Dr. Goyal as one of the experts "who rendered meritorious service for the development of micro-irrigation sector in India" by bestowing *Award of Outstanding Contribution in Micro Irrigation*. This award was presented to Dr. Goyal during the inaugural session of the National Congress on "New Challenges and Advances in Sustainable Micro Irrigation" on March 1, 2017, held at Tamil Nadu Agricultural University.

At Annual Meeting on August 01, 2018 in Detroit, MI, ASABE bestowed on him Netafim Microirrigation Award for his unselfish contribution. VDGOOD Professional Association of India awarded Lifetime Achievement Award at 12th Annual Meeting on Engineering, Science and Medicine that was held on 20–21 of November of 2020 in Visakhapatnam, India.

He has authored more than 200 journal articles and more than 150 books including: *Elements of Agroclimatology (Spanish)* by UNISARC, Colombia; two *Bibliographies on Drip Irrigation.* Apple Academic Press, Inc. (AAP) has published his books, namely: *Management of Drip/Trickle or Micro Irrigation,* and *Evapotranspiration: Principles and Applications for Water Management,* 10-volume set on *Research Advances in Sustainable Micro Irrigation.* During 2016–2025, AAP will be publishing book volumes on emerging technologies/issues/challenges under book series, *Innovations and Challenges in Micro Irrigation, and Innovations in Agricultural & Biological Engineering.*

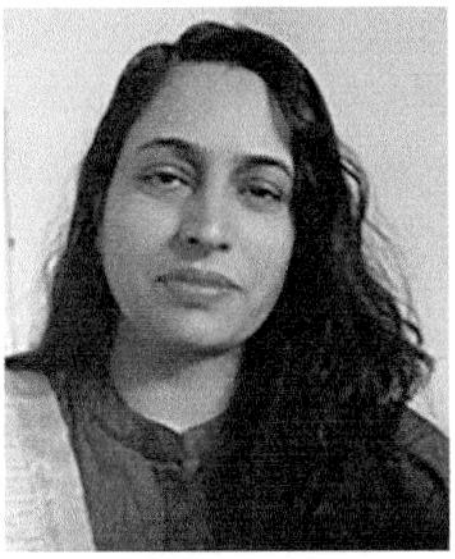

**Anamika Chauhan, PhD**
*Chaman Lal Mahavidhyalya Haridwar (Sri Dev Suman University, Tehri, Uttarakhand), Haridwar, Uttarakhand, India*

**Anamika Chauhan, PhD,** is an accomplished academician who holds a master's degree and a PhD from HNB Garhwal Srinagar, Central University, Uttarakhand, India. In addition to her impressive academic credentials, she boasts master's degrees in English and Education, showcasing the breadth of her intellectual pursuits.

Furthermore, Dr. Chauhan has proven her academic prowess by successfully qualifying for UGC-NET, USET, and MPhil. Her dedication and excellence in the field have earned her the prestigious "Young Scientist Award" from the *Uttarakhand State Council for Science and Technology* and the esteemed "Teacher's Excellence Award" from Motherhood University in Uttarakhand. Notably, she was also recognized with the distinguished "Dr. Sarvepalli Radhakrishnan Global Educator Award-2022" by the International Council for Education, Research, and Training Delhi, India and Teacher of the Year 2023 by the Government of Uttarakhand, India.

Dr. Chauhan's contributions extend beyond accolades, as she holds a patent for her groundbreaking work on "Gold Nanoparticles with *Albizia lebbeck* (L.) Benth Leaves Extract for Dermal Cancer." This patent exemplifies her commitment to advancing scientific knowledge in the field.

Her involvement in academia is not only recognized through awards and patents but is also evident in her role as a valuable member of the Board of Studies at the University. Dr. Chauhan's commitment to academic excellence is further underscored by her lifetime memberships in esteemed organizations, including the Indian Science Congress Association Kolkata, Scientific and Technical Research Association (STRA), and Home Science Association of India.

A prolific researcher, Dr. Chauhan has authored numerous research papers published in peer-reviewed national and international journals. Additionally, she has contributed to academia through the publication of eight edited books and a textbook. Her intellectual engagement extends to active participation in workshops and conferences, further showcasing her dedication to the dissemination of knowledge.

Dr. Chauhan's research interests span a wide spectrum, encompassing critical areas such as the food and nutrition, human health, and social issues. Her multifaceted expertise and commitment to advancing knowledge make her a distinguished figure in the academic community.

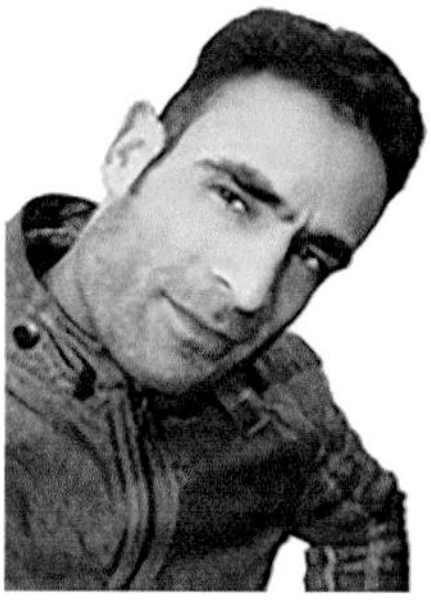

**Junaid A. Malik, PhD**
*Lecturer, Department of Zoology, Government Degree College, Kulgam, Kashmir (J&K), India*

**Junaid A. Malik, PhD,** received BSc (2008) in Science from the University of Kashmir, Srinagar, J&K; MSc (2010) in Zoology from Barkatullah University, Bhopal, Madhya Pradesh; and PhD (2015) in Zoology from the same university. He completed his BEd program in 2017 from the University of Kashmir, Srinagar, J&K. He started his career as Lecturer in the School Education Department, Government of J&K for two years. Dr. Malik is now working as a Lecturer in the Department of Zoology, Government Degree College, Bijbehara, Kashmir (J&K), and is actively involved in teaching and research activities. He has more than eight years of research experience. His areas of interest are ecology, soil macrofauna, wildlife biology, conservation biology, etc.

Dr. Malik has published more than 20 research papers in various national and international peer-reviewed journals. He has authored 4 books, 33 book chapters, edited 16 books, and more than 10 popular editorial articles. He is also serving as editor and reviewer of several journals. He has participated in several state, national, and international conferences, seminars, workshops, and symposia and more than 20 conference papers are to his credit. He is a life member of SBBS (Society for Bioinformatics and Biological Sciences).

# Contents

# Contributors

**Syed Abeera Andrabi**
Jamia Hamdard University, New Delhi, India

**Akhil Arun**
Department of Pharmacy Practice, Amrita School of Pharmacy, Amrita Vishwa Vidyapeetham, AIMS Health Sciences Campus, AIMS Ponekkara, Kerala, India

**Ishwar Basavan**
Jawaharlal Nehru Medical College, Belagavi, Karnataka, India_

**Saqib Bashir**
Government Degree College Hajin Bandipora, Kashmir, Jammu and Kashmir, India

**Tahmina Begum**
Avanthi Institute of Pharmaceutical Sciences, Gunthapalli, Abdullahpurmet, Hyderabad, Telangana, India

**Nitish Bhatia**
Department of Pharmacology, Faculty of Pharmacy, Vishwakarma University, Laxmi Nagar, Kondhwa Budruk, Pune, Maharashtra, India

**Anamika Chauhan**
Chaman Lal Mahavidhyalya Haridwar (Sri Dev Suman University, Tehri, Uttarakhand), Haridwar, Uttarakhand, India

**Maitrayee Ghosh**
Department of Pharmacy, C. V. Raman Global University, Bidyanagar, Mahura, Janla, Bhubaneswar, Odisha, India

**Pitam Ghosh**
Bengal College of Pharmaceutical Technology, Dubrajpur, West Bengal, India

**V. Gopinath**
Department of Physical Education, Annamalai University, Annamalai Nagar, Chidambaram, Tamil Nadu, India

**Megh R. Goyal**
Apple Academic Press Inc., USA

**Showkeen Bilal Ahmad Gul**
Government College of Education, Srinagar, Kashmir, Jammu and Kashmir, India

**Chitra Gunasekar**
Department of Medical Surgical Nursing, Sri Manakula Vinayagar Nursing College, Pondicherry

**Faisal Susleh Hayyat**
Government Degree College for Women, Zakura, Srinagar, Kashmir, Jammu and Kashmir, India

**Anushri Jadhav**
Department of Pharmaceutical Sciences, School of Health Sciences and Technology, Dr. Vishwanath Karad MIT World Peace University, Kothrud, Pune, Maharashtra India

**Seeham Jaleel**
Government Medical College Baramulla, Baramulla, Kashmir, Jammu and Kashmir, India

**Tasleema Jan**
School of Education & Behavioral Sciences, University of Kashmir, Hazratbal Srinagar, Kashmir, Jammu and Kashmir, India

**Junaid Ahmad Malik**
Government Degree College, Kulgam, Jammu and Kashmir, India

**Javid Manzoor**
Department of Environmental Sciences, JJT University, Jhunjhunu, Rajasthan, India

**Himel Mondal**
All India Institute of Medical Sciences, Deoghar, Jharkhand, India

**Shaikat Mondal**
Raiganj Government Medical College and Hospital, Raiganj, West Bengal, India

**Muhammad Muzzamil**
Health Services Academy, Chak Shahzad, Islamabad Capital Territory, Pakistan

**Maryam Nisa**
Health Services Academy, Chak Shahzad, Islamabad Capital Territory, Pakistan

**Urooj Nissar**
Government Medical College Baramulla, Baramulla, Kashmir, Jammu and Kashmir, India

**Surjabha Pal**
Jawaharlal Nehru Medical College, Belagavi, Karnataka, India

**Vijayapandi Pandy**
Department of Pharmaceutical Sciences, School of Health Sciences and Technology, Dr. Vishwanath Karad MIT World Peace University, Kothrud, Pune, Maharashtra, India

**Sowndariya Perumal**
Department of Medical Surgical Nursing, Kasturba Gandhi Nursing College, SBV University, Pondicherry, India

**Heena Qadir**
Department of Sociology, Government Degree College, Awantipora, Jammu and Kashmir, India

**Debajyoti Roy**
Department of Pharmacy, C. V. Raman Global University, Bidyanagar, Mahura, Janla, Bhubaneswar, Odisha, India

**Sumana Saha**
College of Nursing, R.G. Kar Medical College and Hospital, Kolkata, West Bengal, India

**Rahul Saxena**
Department of Biochemistry, School of Allied Health Sciences, Sharda University, Greater Noida, Uttar Pradesh, India

**Suyash Saxena**
Department of Biochemistry, Sharda School of Allied Health Sciences, Sharda University, Greater Noida, Uttar Pradesh, India

**Mohammad Muzamil Shah**
Department of Physical Education, School of Education, Central University of Kashmir, Ganderbal, Jammu and Kashmir, India

**Ajit Pal Singh**
Department of Medical Lab Technology Sharda School of Allied Health Sciences, Sharda University, Greater Noida, Uttar Pradesh, India

**Ufaq Sumera**
Noncommunicable Disease Department of Health, Government of Jammu and Kashmir, India

**N. L. Swathi**
Department of Pharmacy Practice, Sri Venkateswara College of Pharmacy, Jawaharlal Nehru Technological University, Anantapur, Ananthapuramu, Andhra Pradesh, India

**Khursheed Ahmad Wani**
Department of Environmental Sciences, Government Degree College, Thindim, Kreeri, Baramulla, Jammu & Kashmir, India

# Abbreviations

| | |
|---|---|
| 5 HT | 5-hydroxy tryptamine |
| ACOG | American College of Obstetricians and Gynaecologists |
| AD | Alzheimer's disease, |
| ADHD | attention deficit hyperactivity disorder |
| AI | artificial intelligence |
| AMP | adenosine monophosphate |
| ANC | antenatal care |
| APH | ante partum hemorrhage |
| ART | assisted reproductive technology |
| ART | antiretroviral |
| ARVs | antiretroviral drugs |
| ATAC-seq | assay for transposase-accessible chromatin with sequencing |
| BDNF | brain derived neurotrophic factor |
| BMI | body–mass index |
| BMPs | bone morphogenetic proteins |
| CAG | cytosine-adenine-guanine |
| CAM | complementary and alternative medicine |
| cAMP | cyclic adenosine monophosphate, |
| Cas9 | crispr-associated protein 9 |
| CBAs | carbamates |
| CBT | cognitive behavioral therapy |
| CD 8 and 16 | cluster of differentiation 8 and 16 |
| CD38 | cyclic ADP ribose hydrolase |
| CDC | centers for disease control and prevention |
| CGRP | calcitonin gene-related peptide |
| ChIP-seq | chromatin immunoprecipitation sequencing |
| CIN | cervical intraepithelial neoplasia |
| CL | conventional laparoscopy |
| CNS | central nervous system |
| COVID | coronavirus |
| COVID-19 | coronavirus-2019 |
| *CREB* | camp response element-binding protein |
| CRH | corticotropin-releasing hormone |
| CRISPR | clustered regularly interspaced palindromic repeats |
| CS | cesarean section |
| CSD | cortical spreading depression |

| | |
|---|---|
| CT | computed tomography |
| D&C | dilatation and curettage |
| D&E | dilatation and evacuation |
| *DA* | *dopamine* |
| DAG | diacylglycerol |
| DALYs | disability-adjusted life-years |
| DBCA | drug-based cellular assay |
| DDT | dichlorodiphenyltrichloroethane |
| DHA | docosahexaenoic acid |
| DSD | decreased sexual desire |
| EBP | evidence-based practice |
| ECT | electroconvulsive therapy |
| EGFR | epidermal growth factor receptor |
| EMS | endometriosis |
| ENDS | electronic nicotine delivery systems |
| EPA | eicosapentaenoic acid |
| EpiLCs | epiblast-like cells |
| ER β | estrogen receptor β |
| ERK2 | extracellular signal regulated kinase 2 |
| ESC | embryonic stem cells |
| FAS | fetal alcohol syndrome |
| FASD | fetal alcohol spectrum disorder |
| FMEA | failure mode and effects analysis |
| fMRI | functional magnetic resonance imaging |
| FOBT | fecal occult blood testing |
| GABA | gamma amino butyric acid |
| GAD | generalized anxiety disorder |
| GDP | gross domestic product |
| GMCs | general medical conditions |
| HD | hypothalamic dysfunction |
| HD | Huntington's disease |
| HER | electronic health record |
| hESCs | human embryonic stem cells |
| HIPAA | health insurance portability and accountability act |
| HIV | human immunodeficiency virus |
| HLD | high level disinfection |
| HPA | hypothalamic pituitary adrenal axis |
| HPE | holoprosencephaly |
| HPL | hyperprolactinemia |
| HPV | human papillomavirus |
| HRT | hormone replacement therapy |
| HSG | hysterosalpingography |

| | |
|---|---|
| ICPD | international conference on population and development |
| IP3 | inositol triphosphate |
| iPSCs | induced pluripotent stem cells |
| IUCD | intrauterine contraceptive device |
| IV | intravenous |
| IVF | in vitro fertilization |
| LBW | low birth weight |
| LMICs | low- or middle-income country |
| MAOIs | monoamine oxidase inhibitors |
| MAPK | mitogen activated protein kinase |
| MAT | medication-assisted treatment |
| MBCT | mindfulness-based cognitive therapy |
| MBI | mindfulness-based interventions |
| MBSR | mindfulness-based stress reduction |
| MEK2 | mitogen activated protein kinase 2 |
| MICP | migraine interactive care plan |
| ML | machine learning |
| MOUD | medications for opioid use disorder study |
| MRI | magnetic resonance imaging |
| MS | menopausal symptoms |
| MTCT | mother-to-child transmission |
| Myd88 | myeloid differentiation primary response 88 |
| NAS | neonatal abstinence syndrome |
| NF-κB | nuclear factor kappa B |
| NICU | neonatal intensive care unit |
| NLP | natural language processing |
| NOWS | neonatal opioid withdrawal syndrome |
| OCs | organochlorines |
| OHCs | online health communities |
| OPD | out-patient department |
| Ops | organophosphates |
| OPS | osteoporosis |
| OTC | over-the-counter |
| OXTR | oxytocin receptor |
| PAP smear | papanicolaou smear test |
| PCOS | polycystic ovarian syndrome |
| PCPs | primary care physicians |
| PCR | polymerase chain reaction |
| PD | Parkinson's disease |
| PID | polyphenol-induced disease |
| PID | pelvic inflammatory disease |
| PKA | *protein kinase A* |

| | |
|---|---|
| PLC | phospholipase C |
| PMS | premenstrual syndrome |
| POD | polypeptide disorder |
| PPH | post-partum hemorrhage |
| PTSD | post-traumatic stress disorder |
| PYRs | pyrethroids |
| RALP | robot assisted laparoscopic prostatectomy |
| RAS | robotic-assisted surgery |
| RAS | reticular activating system |
| RBCs | red blood cells |
| RCTs | randomized controlled trials |
| RLRS | real-life risk simulation |
| RNA | ribonucleic acid |
| SDG | sustainable development goals |
| SIDS | sudden infant death syndrome |
| s-IgA | salivary immunoglobulin A |
| SNRIs | serotonin and noradrenaline reuptake inhibitors |
| SOD | superoxide dismutase |
| SOL | space occupying lesion |
| SSA | sub-Saharan Africa |
| SSRIs | selective serotonin reuptake inhibitor |
| STD | sexually transmitted disease |
| STI | sexually transmitted infection |
| TAU | treatment as usual |
| TCAs | tricyclic antidepressants |
| tDCS | transcranial direct current stimulation |
| TLR4 | toll-like receptor |
| tMS | transcranial magnetic stimulation |
| TQM | total quality management |
| TRD | treatment-resistant depression |
| UNGASS | special session of the united nations general assembly |
| VVF | vesico vaginal fistula |
| WHI | women's health initiative |
| WHO | World Health Organization |
| WITS | women and newborns transmission study |

# Preface

In a world where women's health issues often remain shrouded in mystery or approached with fragmented solutions, there arises an urgent need for a comprehensive and holistic perspective. *Holistic Approaches for Women's Sustainable Health* is a four-volume set that is a culmination of extensive research, practical insights, and a heartfelt commitment to empowering women to achieve their optimal health and well-being. The book delves deep into the labyrinth of women's health conditions. From the cradle to the golden years, women encounter a unique set of challenges that demand thoughtful understanding and proactive management.

*Volume 1: Foundations, Innovations, Challenges, and Management* explores these challenges with a keen eye on medical science, offering accessible explanations and evidence-based strategies for women and their healthcare providers. Our aim is to equip readers with the knowledge they need to make informed decisions about their health, with an emphasis on prevention, diagnosis, and treatment.

In our modern healthcare landscape, there is a growing recognition that true wellness extends beyond the purely physical. Embracing a holistic approach, we journey into the second aim exploring the mind-body-spirit connection. This book delves into the profound impact of nutrition, exercise, stress management, mindfulness, and complementary therapies on women's health. By integrating these holistic approaches, we aim to empower women to not only recover from illness but to thrive in every aspect of their lives. The book also extends the conversation beyond the individual and into the broader healthcare ecosystem. We acknowledge that women's health is not solely an individual responsibility but a collective effort that encompasses healthcare professionals, policymakers, and society as a whole.

Lastly, we scrutinize the systems and structures that shape women's healthcare experiences, and we advocate for improvements and reforms that prioritize women's well-being. We also provide guidance on navigating the healthcare system, accessing support networks, and advocating for one's own health.

In *Holistic Approaches for Women's Sustainable Health, Volume 1: Foundations, Innovations, Challenges, and Management,* our mission is to break down the barriers that have long hindered women from achieving their full health potential. We are driven by the belief that every woman deserves not just a life free from illness, but a life enriched by vitality, purpose, and joy. As we embark on this journey through the intricate tapestry of women's health, we encourage you, the reader, to be an active participant in your own well-being. We hope this book serves as a trusted companion, offering insights, tools, and inspiration to help you navigate the complex terrain of female health with confidence and resilience. The entire 4-volume set consists of:

**Holistic Approaches for Women's Sustainable Health**

**Volume 1: Foundations, Innovations, Challenges, and Management**

**Volume 2: Advancements, Socioeconomic Impacts, and Innovative Strategies**

**Volume 3: Herbs, Spices, Phytochemicals, and Cereals: Body Care, Cancer Prevention, and Hormonal Health**

**Volume 4: Benefits of Vegetables, Medicinal Plants, and Trees**

Ultimately, this 4-volume set is a celebration of the strength, resilience, and boundless potential of women. It is a call to action, a source of knowledge, and a testament to the transformative power of holistic healthcare. Together, let us embark on a journey toward a future where women's health is embraced, understood, and elevated to its rightful place of honor.

# PART I

# FOUNDATIONS OF HOLISTIC FEMALE HEALTH

CHAPTER 1

# Holistic Approaches for Women's Sustainable Health: An Introduction

FAISAL SUALEH HAYYAT,* V. GOPINATH, and
SHOWKEEN BILAL AHMAD GUL

*Corresponding author

## ABSTRACT

This chapter provides a comprehensive scientific exploration of women's health, examining the intricate interplay of physical, mental, and emotional dimensions. From holistic approaches to reproductive care, preventive measures, and cultural considerations, evidence-based insights are integrated to elucidate the complexities inherent in women's well-being. Discussions encompass the scientific foundations of complementary therapies, the impact of cultural diversity, and strategies for addressing barriers to healthcare access. Rooted in scientific principles, this chapter serves as a call to action for the integration of evidence-based strategies into healthcare practices, policies, and community engagement, promoting a paradigm shift toward personalized, equitable, and culturally competent care for women globally.

## 1.1 INTRODUCTION

In recent years, the paradigm of healthcare has evolved beyond the conventional reductionist approach to embrace a more comprehensive and integrative perspective. The significance of holistic approaches in

Holistic Approaches for Women's Sustainable Health, Volume 1: Foundations, Innovations, Challenges, and Management. Megh R. Goyal, Anamika Chauhan, and Junaid Ahmad Malik (Eds)


DOI: 10.1201/9781779641632-2

women's health has garnered increasing attention within the scientific community [6]. This chapter aims to delve into the intricate interplay of physiological, psychological, and social factors that collectively influence women's well-being. Central to this exploration is the concept of holistic health, an approach rooted in scientific principles that recognizes the intricate interconnectedness of various facets of an individual's life. Holistic health, as applied to women's well-being, is a paradigm that considers the entirety of an individual—encompassing physical, mental, emotional, social, and spiritual dimensions. This comprehensive approach acknowledges that the multifaceted nature of women's health cannot be adequately addressed by isolating specific symptoms or physiological systems. Instead, it posits that a woman's health is profoundly influenced by her lifestyle, environment, and unique circumstances, emphasizing the need for personalized and targeted interventions.

The relevance of holistic health to sustainable well-being is underscored by its capacity to transcend mere symptom management, directing attention toward preventive strategies and long-term health maintenance. By recognizing the dynamic interrelationships between different aspects of health, holistic approaches empower women with the knowledge and tools necessary to actively participate in their healthcare decisions. Scientifically, sustainable well-being is contingent upon the delicate equilibrium among biological, psychological, and social determinants. Holistic health interventions, when grounded in evidence-based practices, contribute to the cultivation of this equilibrium [9]. Moreover, the emphasis on preventive measures, informed by scientific insights into lifestyle and behavioral factors, positions holistic approaches as instrumental in averting health disparities and fostering enduring well-being throughout a woman's lifespan [28].

As we embark on an in-depth exploration of holistic approaches for sustainable women's health, this chapter seeks to bridge the gap between scientific understanding and practical application. By synthesizing empirical evidence and acknowledging the complexity of women's health, this chapter aims to provide a comprehensive scientific foundation for the integration of holistic practices into contemporary healthcare paradigms, ultimately advancing the discourse on sustainable well-being for women.

## 1.2 FOUNDATIONS OF HOLISTIC WOMEN'S HEALTH

The intricate tapestry of women's health is woven from a complex interplay of physiological, psychological, emotional, and social determinants, each thread influencing the other in a dynamic and interconnected manner. From a scientific standpoint, comprehending the holistic nature of women's health necessitates an exploration of how these multifaceted dimensions converge to shape overall well-being. Physically, the biological underpinnings of women's health are intricately linked with mental and emotional states. Neuroendocrine pathways, immune responses, and genetic predispositions interact with cognitive and emotional processes, collectively influencing the body's homeostasis [1].

The physiological manifestations of stress, for instance, underscore the tangible links between mental and physical health. Chronic stress can induce alterations in immune function, hormonal balance, and cardiovascular health, underscoring the inextricable connection between the mind and body. Emotionally, the psychological well-being of women is intertwined with their physical and mental states. Psychosocial factors, such as stressors, traumas, and life events, contribute to emotional responses that, in turn, impact neurological and hormonal pathways. Neurotransmitter regulation, including serotonin and dopamine pathways, connects emotional experiences to physiological processes, highlighting the integral relationship between mental and emotional dimensions [34].

Social factors further amplify the complexity of women's health, exerting both direct and indirect influences. Social support networks, community engagement, and socioeconomic determinants collectively contribute to the social fabric that envelops women's health. Social isolation, economic disparities, and cultural contexts profoundly shape health behaviors and outcomes, establishing a nexus between social dynamics and overall well-being. Lifestyle factors emerge as pivotal contributors to women's health, encapsulating dietary choices, physical activity, sleep patterns, and substance use. Scientific evidence robustly affirms the profound impact of lifestyle on physiological and psychological health. Dietary habits, for instance, influence hormonal regulation, immune function, and metabolic processes, thereby exerting direct implications on physical health. Simultaneously, lifestyle choices significantly impact mental and emotional well-being, with physical activity demonstrating neuroprotective and mood-regulating effects [32].

The amalgamation of these dimensions elucidates the holistic framework through which women's health should be comprehended. Scientifically, the bidirectional relationships among physical, mental, emotional, and social aspects underscore the need for an integrative approach that transcends reductionist perspectives. As we navigate the scientific terrain of holistic approaches for sustainable women's health, it is imperative to acknowledge and unravel the intricacies of this interconnectedness, offering a comprehensive understanding that forms the foundation for effective and nuanced healthcare interventions [25].

## 1.3 NUTRITION AND WOMEN'S HEALTH

The pivotal role of nutrition in women's health extends beyond mere sustenance, profoundly impacting hormonal balance and reproductive health. A nuanced examination of the relationship between dietary patterns and physiological processes reveals the intricate interplay that underscores the significance of a balanced diet in promoting optimal hormonal function throughout various life stages. Scientifically, a balanced diet serves as a cornerstone for hormonal equilibrium by supplying essential nutrients that contribute to the synthesis and regulation of key hormones. Macronutrients such as proteins, fats, and carbohydrates play pivotal roles in hormonal production and transportation. A deficiency or excess of these macronutrients can disrupt hormonal balance, impacting reproductive cycles, fertility, and overall endocrine function. Micronutrients, encompassing vitamins and minerals, emerge as critical contributors to women's hormonal health. For instance, vitamin D is intricately linked to reproductive function, with deficiencies associated with menstrual irregularities and compromised fertility. The role of vitamin B, particularly folate, is paramount in preconception and pregnancy, influencing embryonic development and preventing neural tube defects [14].

The significance of omega-3 fatty acids, specifically docosahexaenoic acid and eicosapentaenoic acid, extends to reproductive health by supporting fetal brain development during pregnancy. Antioxidant-rich nutrients, including vitamins C and E, safeguard reproductive tissues from oxidative stress, thereby preserving fertility and hormonal balance. Different life stages warrant distinct nutritional considerations, with adolescence, pregnancy, lactation, and menopause representing critical periods. During adolescence, adequate intake of calcium and vitamin D is crucial for bone health and the establishment of hormonal patterns. Pregnancy demands heightened requirements for iron, folic acid, and other micronutrients to support fetal growth and development. Lactation necessitates sustained nutrient intake to facilitate breastfeeding and maternal recovery. Menopausal transitions underscore the importance of maintaining bone health through sufficient calcium and vitamin D intake, while phytoestrogen-rich foods may offer support in mitigating hormonal fluctuations. A balanced diet serves as a linchpin in promoting hormonal balance and reproductive health in women. The intricate interplay of macronutrients and micronutrients underscores the necessity of a nuanced dietary approach tailored to specific life stages. Scientific understanding of these nutritional intricacies forms the basis for informed dietary recommendations that aim to optimize women's health and hormonal well-being across the continuum of life [3].

## 1.4 PHYSICAL ACTIVITY AND WELLNESS

The exploration of the benefits of regular exercise constitutes a fundamental facet in the pursuit of comprehensive women's health. Scientific inquiry into the physiological, psychological, and metabolic responses to physical activity reveals a multifaceted spectrum of advantages, encompassing cardiovascular health, weight management, and mental well-being.

### *1.4.1 CARDIOVASCULAR HEALTH*

From a cardiovascular perspective, regular exercise induces a cascade of adaptive responses that fortify the cardiovascular system. Aerobic activities, such as brisk walking, running, or cycling, enhance cardiac output, promote vascular elasticity, and contribute to optimal blood pressure regulation. These adaptations collectively reduce the risk of cardiovascular diseases, including hypertension, atherosclerosis, and myocardial infarction. The scientifically established link between regular exercise and improved cardiovascular health underscores its role as a cornerstone in preventive healthcare strategies for women [15].

### 1.4.2 WEIGHT MANAGEMENT

In the realm of weight management, the thermogenic effects of exercise extend beyond the immediate caloric expenditure. Regular physical activity augments basal metabolic rate, promoting the utilization of stored energy reserves and facilitating weight loss or maintenance. Additionally, resistance training contributes to the development of lean muscle mass, further enhancing metabolic efficiency. Scientific evidence consistently supports the role of exercise, when integrated into a holistic approach, as a pivotal factor in sustainable weight management for women [4].

### 1.4.3 MENTAL WELL-BEING

The impact of exercise on mental well-being is underscored by its profound effects on neurotransmitter regulation, neuroplasticity, and stress response systems. Scientifically, aerobic exercise stimulates the release of endorphins, neurotransmitters associated with mood elevation and stress reduction. Furthermore, regular physical activity has been shown to enhance cognitive function, alleviate symptoms of anxiety and depression, and mitigate the risk of neurodegenerative disorders. The intricate neurobiological mechanisms linking exercise to mental well-being position it as a potent modality for promoting mental resilience and emotional balance [17].

### 1.4.4 PRACTICAL INTEGRATION INTO DAILY LIFE

Practical tips for integrating physical activity into daily life are rooted in scientific principles that emphasize consistency, variety, and individualization. Scientific evidence supports the efficacy of incorporating short bouts of activity throughout the day, such as taking brisk walks, using stairs, or engaging in brief strength exercises. Structured exercise programs, tailored to individual preferences and fitness levels, offer sustainable approaches to fostering a physically active lifestyle.

Additionally, scientific insights into the importance of social and environmental factors suggest that incorporating physical activity into social interactions or choosing outdoor settings can enhance adherence and overall well-being. The prescription of exercise as a personalized and integrative component of women's health aligns with evidence-based practices that acknowledge the dynamic interplay of biological, psychological, and social determinants. The scientific exploration of the benefits of regular exercise for cardiovascular health, weight management, and mental well-being underscores its indispensable role in promoting comprehensive women's health. Practical tips grounded in scientific evidence facilitate the seamless integration of physical activity into daily life, empowering women with actionable strategies to optimize their health across multiple dimensions [13].

## 1.5 MENTAL AND EMOTIONAL WELL-BEING

The examination of the impact of mental health on overall wellness reveals a profound interconnectedness between cognitive, emotional, and physiological dimensions. Scientific scrutiny of mental health underscores its pivotal role in shaping an individual's overall well-being. Within this context, strategies for stress management, mindfulness, and fostering mental resilience emerge as crucial components of a comprehensive approach to women's health. Scientifically, mental health exerts pervasive influences on physiological processes, immune function, and inflammatory responses. Psychoneuro-immunological pathways underscore the intricate connections between mental states and physical health outcomes. Stress, anxiety, and depression, when chronic or severe, have been associated with increased susceptibility to infectious diseases, compromised immune responses, and heightened inflammation—all of which contribute to a diminished state of overall wellness. Furthermore, the neurobiological implications of mental health extend to the cardiovascular system, endocrine regulation, and neural plasticity. Chronic stress, for instance, can elevate cortisol levels, contributing to metabolic dysregulation, weight gain, and cardiovascular risk. Thus, a nuanced understanding of mental health as a foundational element in the holistic framework of overall wellness necessitates the integration of strategies that address cognitive and emotional well-being [7].

Scientifically informed strategies for stress management encompass evidence-based interventions that modulate the body's stress response systems. Cognitive-behavioral techniques, relaxation exercises, and mindfulness practices have demonstrated efficacy in reducing stress hormones, improving mood, and enhancing overall mental well-being. The scientific basis for these strategies lies in their capacity to influence neuroendocrine pathways, neurotransmitter release, and autonomic nervous system balance. The scientific exploration of mindfulness reveals its transformative effects on mental health. Mindfulness practices, rooted in contemplative traditions, have been shown to induce neuroplastic changes in the brain, fostering resilience and emotional regulation. Scientific studies consistently support the benefits of mindfulness in alleviating symptoms of anxiety, depression, and chronic stress, emphasizing its role in promoting mental well-being [27].

The scientific understanding of mental resilience highlights its dynamic nature, shaped by genetic predispositions, environmental factors, and individual coping mechanisms. Evidence-based interventions, such as cognitive-behavioral therapy, resilience training, and positive psychology, offer scientifically grounded approaches to enhancing mental resilience. These strategies aim to bolster adaptive coping mechanisms, modify cognitive patterns, and promote a proactive mindset, contributing to sustained mental well-being. The scientific exploration of the impact of mental health on overall wellness elucidates the critical need for integrative strategies in women's health. The scientific foundations of stress management, mindfulness, and fostering mental resilience underscore their relevance as evidence-based components of a comprehensive approach to mental well-being. As we navigate the scientific landscape of mental health in the context of women's wellness, these strategies emerge as instrumental tools in optimizing mental health across the spectrum of cognitive, emotional, and physiological dimensions [23].

## 1.6 REPRODUCTIVE HEALTH AND FAMILY PLANNING

An in-depth discussion on comprehensive reproductive care unveils the intricate array of considerations essential to women's health across different life stages. Scientific exploration into family planning, prenatal care, and menopause provides a robust foundation for understanding and addressing the unique reproductive health challenges women may encounter. This discussion encompasses evidence-based solutions grounded in scientific principles, contributing to the formulation of comprehensive strategies for women's reproductive well-being. Scientifically, family planning is a dynamic domain encompassing contraceptive methods, fertility awareness, and reproductive health education. Contraceptive options, ranging from hormonal methods to barrier devices, are founded on rigorous research into safety, efficacy, and individual suitability. Fertility awareness methods, rooted in menstrual cycle tracking, leverage scientific insights into ovulation and conception probabilities, empowering women with natural family planning choices. Reproductive health education, a cornerstone of family planning, draws upon scientific understanding to provide accurate information about contraception, sexually transmitted infections, and reproductive anatomy. The integration of evidence-based family planning strategies into women's health initiatives contributes to informed decision-making, personalized care, and reproductive autonomy [19].

The scientific underpinnings of prenatal care center on optimizing maternal and fetal outcomes through comprehensive monitoring and intervention strategies. Evidence-based guidelines delineate prenatal care schedules, nutritional recommendations, and screening protocols, reflecting a synthesis of research findings on maternal–fetal health. Scientific advancements in prenatal diagnostics, including ultrasound imaging and genetic testing, enhance the early detection of fetal anomalies and maternal health risks. Moreover, nutritional guidance draws on scientific knowledge to ensure optimal maternal and fetal development, addressing critical factors such as folic acid supplementation, iron intake, and dietary diversity [24].

Scientific exploration of menopause elucidates the physiological transitions and hormonal fluctuations that characterize this life stage. Evidence-based interventions for managing menopausal symptoms include hormone replacement therapy, cognitive-behavioral approaches, and lifestyle modifications. Scientific studies inform the risks and benefits of hormone therapy, enabling personalized decision-making in collaboration with healthcare providers. The impact of menopause on bone health, cardiovascular risk, and mental well-being underscores the importance of comprehensive care. Scientifically guided strategies for maintaining bone density, cardiovascular health, and emotional balance during menopause are integral components of women's health initiatives [21].

Reproductive health challenges, including infertility, reproductive disorders, and complications during pregnancy, necessitate evidence-based solutions. Scientifically informed interventions may include assisted reproductive technologies, medical treatments, and surgical interventions, all tailored to address specific reproductive health challenges. Research-driven preventive measures and early interventions contribute to improved outcomes in managing common reproductive health issues. An in-depth discussion on comprehensive reproductive care, grounded in scientific principles, encompasses family planning, prenatal care, and menopause. The scientific foundations of these reproductive health domains contribute to the development of evidence-based strategies that empower women with informed choices, optimize maternal and fetal outcomes, and address challenges across the reproductive lifespan. Integrating these insights into women's healthcare frameworks ensures a holistic and scientifically sound approach to reproductive well-being [16].

## 1.7 PREVENTIVE HEALTHCARE FOR WOMEN

An overview of regular check-ups, screenings, and vaccinations constitutes a fundamental pillar in the proactive management of women's health, underlining the significance of early detection and prevention. Scientifically grounded preventive healthcare measures are pivotal in mitigating the risk of common women's health issues, fostering optimal well-being across the lifespan. Scientifically, regular check-ups form the bedrock of preventive healthcare, enabling healthcare providers to monitor key health indicators, assess risk factors, and detect emerging health issues at their earliest stages. Routine physical examinations, blood pressure assessments, and measurements of vital signs contribute to the systematic evaluation of overall health. These check-ups provide an opportunity for open communication between patients and healthcare professionals, facilitating the identification of symptoms and risk factors that may warrant further investigation [2].

Evidence-based screenings play a pivotal role in the early detection of specific health conditions, guiding timely interventions and personalized care plans. Mammography, Pap smears, and pelvic examinations, for instance, are integral components of women's health screenings, aimed at identifying early signs of breast and cervical cancers. Scientific guidelines dictate the frequency and timing of screenings, ensuring a targeted and evidence-based approach that aligns with individual risk profiles and age-related considerations. Moreover, screenings for metabolic conditions, such as cholesterol levels and blood glucose, contribute to the prevention and management of cardiovascular and metabolic disorders. Bone density screenings aid in the early detection of osteoporosis, allowing for proactive measures to maintain bone health [22].

Scientifically validated vaccinations play a crucial role in preventing infectious diseases that may disproportionately affect women. Vaccines against human papillomavirus protect against cervical cancer, while vaccinations against influenza and pneumonia reduce the risk of respiratory infections. The development of vaccines is rooted in rigorous scientific research, ensuring safety, efficacy, and long-term immunity against specific pathogens. The scientific rationale underlying early detection and prevention lies in the principle that timely interventions can mitigate the severity and progression of health issues. Early detection of cancers, for example, often allows for less invasive treatment options and higher chances of successful outcomes. Preventive measures, including vaccinations and lifestyle interventions, are grounded in research demonstrating their efficacy in reducing the incidence of preventable diseases. Moreover, preventive healthcare contributes to the reduction of healthcare costs by minimizing the burden of advanced and potentially more complicated medical conditions. By emphasizing regular check-ups, screenings, and vaccinations, healthcare systems can shift the focus from reactive care to proactive health maintenance, aligning with evidence-based practices that prioritize overall well-being. The overview of regular check-ups, screenings, and vaccinations for women's health is deeply rooted in scientific principles, emphasizing the importance of early detection and prevention. Evidence-based healthcare strategies ensure a systematic and personalized approach, empowering women to take proactive measures that contribute to their long-term health and well-being [11].

## 1.8 EDUCATION AND EMPOWERMENT

The role of education in empowering women to make informed health decisions is paramount and grounded in scientific principles. Education serves as a catalyst for knowledge acquisition, fostering an understanding of the intricate facets of women's health. Scientifically informed information dissemination, encompassing women's health issues and available resources, represents a dynamic and integral component of this educational paradigm. Scientifically, education equips women with the foundational knowledge needed to comprehend the physiological, psychological, and social determinants influencing their health. It empowers them to decipher complex medical information, critically evaluate healthcare interventions, and actively engage in shared decision-making with healthcare providers. Moreover, educational initiatives are instrumental in cultivating health literacy—an individual's ability to obtain, comprehend, and apply health information—which is associated with improved health outcomes. The dissemination of scientifically accurate information on women's health issues is crucial for fostering awareness and promoting evidence-based decision-making. Information on reproductive health, preventive measures, lifestyle choices, and disease management equips women with the tools to navigate their healthcare journeys. Scientifically validated resources contribute to the cultivation of a robust knowledge base, ensuring that women can access and utilize information that aligns with the latest advancements in medical research and healthcare practices [10].

Furthermore, education serves as a catalyst for dismantling barriers to healthcare access, addressing disparities in health outcomes, and promoting equity in women's health. Scientific insights into the social determinants of health underscore the importance of educational interventions in mitigating factors such as socioeconomic status, cultural influences, and systemic biases that may impact women's access to healthcare information and resources. The dynamic interplay between education, information dissemination, and women's health underscores the necessity of a continuous and integrative approach. This involves utilizing evidence-based educational strategies to enhance health literacy, leveraging scientific communication principles to disseminate information effectively, and fostering a collaborative environment where women are active participants in their healthcare decisions. The scientific rationale for emphasizing the role of education in women's health is rooted in its capacity to empower individuals with knowledge, enhance health literacy, and foster informed decision-making. The continuous dissemination of scientifically accurate information ensures that women are equipped to navigate the complexities of their health, make informed choices, and actively participate in the promotion of their overall well-being [31].

## 1.9 SOCIAL SUPPORT AND COMMUNITY ENGAGEMENT

The importance of social connections for mental and emotional well-being is deeply embedded in scientific understanding, reflecting the intricate interplay between social dynamics and psychological states. Scientifically, the role of social connections in influencing mental and emotional well-being is substantiated by research across disciplines such as psychology, neuroscience, and sociology. The imperative to build support networks and foster community engagement emerges as a scientifically grounded strategy for promoting sustainable mental and emotional health. Social connections serve as vital buffers against stress, adversity, and emotional distress. The neurobiological underpinnings of social support involve the release of oxytocin and endorphins, neurotransmitters associated with bonding and mood regulation. Scientific studies consistently demonstrate that individuals with robust social networks exhibit lower levels of stress hormones, improved emotional resilience, and enhanced mental well-being [29].

Furthermore, the psychological constructs of social support, including emotional, instrumental, and informational support, contribute to adaptive coping mechanisms and mitigate the impact of life challenges. Scientific inquiry into the social determinants of mental health highlights the profound influence of social connections on risk and resilience factors, emphasizing the importance of community ties in shaping emotional states. Building support networks and engaging with communities align with evidence-based strategies for sustaining mental and emotional well-being. Scientifically, interventions that promote social connections have been shown to reduce the risk of mental health disorders, enhance emotional regulation, and contribute to overall psychological resilience. Participating in community activities, cultivating interpersonal relationships, and establishing a sense of belonging have demonstrated positive effects on mental health outcomes. Moreover, the scientific exploration of the "social brain" underscores the evolutionary significance of social connections in human well-being. From an evolutionary perspective, humans are inherently social beings, and social interactions have played a crucial role in survival and adaptation. This biological predisposition to seek social connections and engage with communities reinforces the fundamental importance of social ties for mental and emotional flourishing [29].

The emphasis on the importance of social connections for mental and emotional well-being is grounded in a wealth of scientific evidence. Building support networks and fostering community engagement are integral components of evidence-based approaches to promoting sustainable mental health. By recognizing the scientific underpinnings of social dynamics and their impact on psychological states, interventions can be designed to enhance social connections, fortify emotional resilience, and contribute to the enduring well-being of individuals.

## 1.10 HOLISTIC THERAPIES AND INTEGRATIVE MEDICINE

The overview of complementary therapies, including acupuncture, herbal medicine, and yoga, involves a scientific exploration of their evidence-based benefits and considerations for their integration into holistic healthcare paradigms. Scientifically, these complementary therapies have been subject to rigorous research to elucidate their physiological mechanisms, therapeutic effects, and potential contributions to overall well-being. Acupuncture, rooted in traditional Chinese medicine, involves the insertion of thin needles into specific points on the body to stimulate energy flow. Scientific studies on acupuncture have revealed its effects on modulating neural pathways, releasing endorphins, and influencing neurotransmitter levels. Evidence supports its efficacy in pain management, stress reduction, and improvements in conditions such as chronic pain, migraines, and musculoskeletal disorders. Herbal medicine encompasses the use of plant-based substances for therapeutic purposes. Scientific investigations into herbal remedies involve the identification of bioactive compounds and their mechanisms of action. Evidence-based benefits of herbal medicine include anti-inflammatory, antioxidant, and immune-modulating effects. Certain herbs have demonstrated efficacy in conditions such as anxiety, insomnia, and digestive disorders. However, considerations for standardized formulations, dosage, and potential interactions underscore the importance of a scientifically informed approach to herbal medicine [26].

Yoga, an ancient practice that combines physical postures, breath control, and meditation, has gained recognition for its holistic health benefits. Scientific studies on yoga indicate its impact on stress reduction, improvements in mental health, and enhancements in physical flexibility and strength. The physiological effects of yoga include regulation of the autonomic nervous system, modulation of stress hormones, and alterations in brain activity patterns. The integration of holistic therapies into healthcare necessitates careful consideration of scientific evidence, individualized patient needs, and collaborative approaches. Scientifically informed considerations include assessing the safety and efficacy of complementary therapies through systematic reviews and meta-analyses. Understanding the physiological mechanisms and potential interactions with conventional treatments is paramount in ensuring a cohesive and evidence-based approach to healthcare [33].

Moreover, the integration of complementary therapies underscores the importance of collaboration between healthcare providers and practitioners of holistic modalities. Interdisciplinary communication ensures a comprehensive understanding of patients' health profiles, aligning complementary therapies with conventional treatments for optimal outcomes. Scientific evidence also supports the importance of individualized care, recognizing that responses to complementary therapies may vary among individuals. Personalized treatment plans, based on thorough assessments and consideration of scientific evidence, contribute to the integration of complementary therapies into holistic healthcare frameworks. The overview of complementary therapies such as acupuncture, herbal medicine, and yoga is intricately tied to scientific exploration. Evidence-based insights into their benefits and considerations for integration emphasize the importance of a holistic and informed approach to healthcare. By bridging the gap between traditional practices and scientific understanding, these complementary therapies can contribute meaningfully to holistic healthcare paradigms [12].

## 1.11 CULTURAL SENSITIVITY IN WOMEN'S HEALTHCARE

The recognition of cultural diversity in healthcare is grounded in scientific principles that acknowledge the profound impact of cultural backgrounds and beliefs on health outcomes. Scientifically, cultural competence in healthcare is essential for ensuring equitable, effective, and patient-centered care. Tailoring healthcare approaches to respect cultural diversity involves a comprehensive understanding of the scientific underpinnings of how cultural factors influence health behaviors, treatment adherence, and overall well-being. Scientific research underscores the importance of cultural competence—a healthcare provider's ability to understand, communicate with, and effectively treat individuals from diverse cultural backgrounds. Studies have demonstrated that culturally competent care is associated with improved patient satisfaction, adherence to medical recommendations, and health outcomes. Scientific exploration into cultural competence encompasses the development of skills in cultural awareness, knowledge, and sensitivity, emphasizing the need for health-care providers to continually educate themselves on diverse cultural practices and beliefs [20].

Cultural factors exert significant influence on health-related behaviors, perceptions of illness, and healthcare utilization. Scientific evidence highlights the impact of cultural beliefs on preventive practices, dietary habits, and attitudes toward medical care. For example, cultural beliefs about the causes of illness or the effectiveness of certain treatments can influence an individual's decision to seek healthcare and adhere to prescribed interventions. Recognizing and understanding these cultural nuances is crucial for providing patient-centered care that aligns with individual values and preferences.

Scientifically informed approaches to tailoring healthcare involve adapting communication styles, treatment plans, and healthcare delivery to meet the unique needs of individuals from diverse cultural backgrounds. Research supports the implementation of culturally tailored interventions that consider linguistic preferences, health literacy levels, and cultural norms. Tailoring healthcare approaches extends beyond language proficiency to encompass broader cultural competencies, ensuring that care is respectful, inclusive, and sensitive to diverse belief systems. The scientific discourse on cultural diversity in healthcare aligns with broader discussions on health equity. Health disparities rooted in cultural, socioeconomic, and systemic factors underscore the need for interventions that address the unique challenges faced by diverse populations. Scientific studies advocate for policies and practices that promote inclusivity, reduce cultural barriers to care, and address social determinants of health. The concept of patient-centered care, grounded in scientific principles, emphasizes the active involvement of patients in their healthcare decisions. Recognizing and respecting cultural diversity is integral to patient-centered care, as it acknowledges the importance of individual values, preferences, and experiences. Scientifically, patient-centered approaches contribute to improved communication, shared decision-making, and ultimately, better health outcomes. The recognition of cultural diversity in healthcare is underpinned by scientific principles that emphasize the importance of cultural competence, understanding the influence of cultural factors on health, and tailoring healthcare approaches to respect individual cultural backgrounds and beliefs. This scientific approach contributes to the creation of inclusive healthcare environments that prioritize equity, patient-centered care, and the well-being of diverse populations [18].

## 1.12 ACCESS TO HEALTHCARE AND HEALTH EQUITY

The examination of barriers to healthcare access for women is grounded in scientific principles, shedding light on the multifaceted challenges that hinder equitable healthcare delivery. Scientifically informed strategies for promoting health equity and ensuring universal access involve a comprehensive understanding of these barriers, encompassing socioeconomic, cultural, and systemic factors. Scientific research identifies a spectrum of barriers that impede women's access to healthcare. Socioeconomic factors, including income levels and employment status, influence access to health insurance and out-of-pocket expenses. Geographic disparities, transportation challenges, and the availability of healthcare facilities contribute to spatial barriers. Additionally, cultural and linguistic differences, coupled with systemic issues such as discrimination and bias, further compound challenges to healthcare access. Scientific evidence underscores the interconnectedness of these barriers, recognizing that they often intersect and disproportionately affect marginalized populations. Scientifically informed strategies for promoting health equity involve targeted interventions that address specific barriers and foster inclusive healthcare systems. Research supports the implementation of policies that eliminate financial barriers, such as expanding access to affordable health insurance and reducing out-of-pocket costs. Ensuring geographic accessibility involves strategies like the development of community-based clinics and telehealth options to bridge spatial gaps [30].

Culturally competent care, informed by scientific principles, is pivotal for overcoming linguistic and cultural barriers. Healthcare providers should be equipped with the skills and knowledge needed to engage effectively with diverse populations, recognizing and respecting individual beliefs and practices. Scientifically grounded interventions also address systemic issues by actively working to dismantle discriminatory practices and biases within healthcare systems. Scientific exploration into ensuring universal access emphasizes the need for systemic reforms that transcend individual barriers. Policymakers and healthcare administrators can utilize evidence-based practices to develop and implement policies that prioritize universal access. This may include legislative measures to eliminate discriminatory practices, funding initiatives to support community clinics, and the expansion of public health programs that address preventive care and health education [8].

Moreover, scientific studies underscore the importance of data collection and analysis to identify and monitor healthcare disparities. By employing rigorous research methodologies, policymakers can make informed decisions to address specific barriers and measure the impact of interventions on health equity. Scientifically grounded approaches to data-driven policymaking contribute to evidence-based strategies that drive systemic change. The examination of barriers to healthcare access for women is rooted in scientific principles that inform strategies for promoting health equity and ensuring universal access. By addressing socioeconomic, cultural, and systemic factors through evidence-based interventions, healthcare systems can work toward dismantling barriers and fostering inclusivity. A scientific approach to understanding and overcoming these challenges is essential for creating equitable healthcare environments that prioritize the diverse needs of women and marginalized populations [5].

## 1.13 SUMMARY

In conclusion, this comprehensive exploration of women's health has been guided by a scientific lens, delving into multifaceted dimensions that shape the well-being of women across the lifespan. From the intricate interplay of physical, mental, and emotional aspects to the nuanced considerations of reproductive care, preventive measures, and cultural influences, our scientific inquiry underscores the complexity inherent in women's health. Throughout this chapter, the integration of evidence-based insights has been central to our endeavor. Scientifically grounded discussions have elucidated the importance of holistic approaches, recognizing the interconnectedness of various facets in the pursuit of sustainable well-being. The scientific exploration of complementary therapies, recognition of cultural diversity, and strategies for overcoming barriers to healthcare access contribute to a nuanced understanding of the challenges and opportunities in contemporary women's health. As we navigate the scientific terrain of women's health, it is evident that a holistic, patient-centered approach is essential. From the microscopic intricacies of cellular processes to the macroscopic impact of societal determinants, this chapter has sought to bridge the gap between scientific understanding and practical application. The scientific foundations laid herein provide a robust framework for healthcare practitioners, policymakers, and researchers alike to address the complexities of women's health comprehensively. Moving forward, the integration of scientific principles into healthcare practices, policies, and community engagement is imperative. By leveraging evidence-based strategies, we can foster a paradigm shift toward personalized, equitable, and culturally competent care. This chapter, rooted in scientific exploration, serves as a call to action, urging a collective commitment to advancing the discourse and practices that promote the holistic well-being of women worldwide. May this scientific endeavor catalyze positive change and contribute to the continual evolution of women's health, ensuring that evidence-based principles guide our journey toward improved health outcomes and enduring well-being.

## KEYWORDS

- **mental health**
- **mental well-being**
- **reproductive care**
- **women's health**

## REFERENCES

1. Baheiraei, A., Bakouei, F., Mohammadi, E., Montazeri, A., & Hosseni, M. (2015). The social determinants of health in association with women's health status of reproductive age: A population-based study. *Iranian Journal of Public Health*, *44*(1), 119–129.

2. Becker, N. V., Moniz, M. H., Tipirneni, R., Dalton, V. K., & Ayanian, J. Z. (2021). Utilization of women's preventive health services during the COVID-19 pandemic. *JAMA Health Forum*, *2*(7), e211408.
3. Coletta, J. M., Bell, S. J., & Roman, A. S. (2010). Omega-3 fatty acids and pregnancy. *Rev Obstet Gynecol*, *3*(4), 163–171.
4. Cox, C. E. (2017). Role of physical activity for weight loss and weight maintenance. *Diabetes Spectrum*, *30*(3), 157–160.
5. Dye, B. A., Duran, D. G., Murray, D. M., Creswell, J. W., Richard, P., Farhat, T., Breen, N., & Engelgau, M. M. (2019). The importance of evaluating health disparities research. *American Journal of Public Health*, *109*(S1), S34–s40.
6. Fiandaca, M. S., Mapstone, M., Connors, E., Jacobson, M., Monuki, E. S., Malik, S., Macciardi, F., & Federoff, H. J. (2017). Systems healthcare: A holistic paradigm for tomorrow. *BMC Systems Biology*, *11*(1), 142–144.
7. General, U. S. (2001). *Mental Health: Culture, Race, and Ethnicity.* A supplement to mental health: A report of the Surgeon General. US Department of Health and Human Services: Rockville, MD.
8. Handtke, O., Schilgen, B., & Mösko, M. (2019). Culturally competent healthcare - A scoping review of strategies implemented in healthcare organizations and a model of culturally competent healthcare provision. *PLoS One*, *14*(7), e0219971.
9. Jasemi, M., Valizadeh, L., Zamanzadeh, V., & Keogh, B. (2017). A concept analysis of holistic care by hybrid model. *Indian Journal of Palliative Care*, *23*(1), 71–80.
10. Jaysawal, N., & Saha, S. (2023). Role of education in women empowerment. *International Journal of Applied Research*, *9*(4), 08–13.
11. Kaarthigeyan, K. (2012). Cervical cancer in India and HPV vaccination. *Indian Journal of Medical Paediatric Oncology*, *33*(1), 7–12.
12. Kalariya, Y., Kumar, A., Ullah, A., Umair, A., Neha, F. N. U., Madhurita, F. N. U., Varagantiwar, V., Jaffari, S. M. I. A., Ahmad, A., Aman, M., & Sapna, F.N.U. (2023). Integrative medicine approaches: Bridging the gap between conventional and renal complementary therapies. *Cureus*, *15*(9), e46033.
13. Kohl III, H. W., & Cook, H. D. (2013). *Educating the Student Body: Taking Physical Activity and Physical Education to School* (p. 488). Committee on Physical Activity and Physical Education in the School Environment, National Academies Press: United States.
14. Marshall, N. E., Abrams, B., Barbour, L. A., Catalano, P., Christian, P., Friedman, J. E., Hay Jr, W.W., Hernandez, T.L., Krebs, N.F., Oken, E., & Purnell, J.Q., (2022). The importance of nutrition in pregnancy and lactation: Lifelong consequences. *American Journal of Obstetrics and Gynecology*, *226*(5), 607–632.
15. Nystoriak, M. A., & Bhatnagar, A. (2018). Cardiovascular effects and benefits of exercise. *Frontiers in Cardiovascular Medicine*, *5*, e408204.
16. Ombelet, W. (2013). The Walking Egg Project: Universal access to infertility care - from dream to reality. *Facts Views and Vision ObGyn*, *5*(2), 161–175.
17. Ren, J., & Xiao, H. (2023). Exercise for mental well-being: Exploring neurobiological advances and intervention effects in depression. *Life*, *13*(7), 1505.
18. Ricci, L., Villegente, J., Loyal, D., Ayav, C., Kivits, J., & Rat, A. C. (2022). Tailored patient therapeutic educational interventions: A patient-centered communication model. *Health Expect*, *25*(1), 276–289.

19. Sadik, N. (1997). Reproductive health/family planning and the health of infants, girls, and women. *Indian Journal Pediatrics*, *64*(6), 739–744.
20. Saha, S., Beach, M. C., & Cooper, L. A. (2008). Patient centeredness, cultural competence, and healthcare quality. *Journal of National Medical Association*, *100*(11), 1275–1285.
21. Santoro, N., Epperson, C. N., & Mathews, S. B. (2015). Menopausal symptoms and their management. *Endocrinology and Metabolism Clinics* (*North America*), *44*(3), 497–515.
22. Selvin, E., & Brett, K. M. (2003). Breast and cervical cancer screening: Sociodemographic predictors among White, Black, and Hispanic women. *American Journal of Public Health*, *93*(4), 618–623.
23. Shrivastava, A., & Desousa, A. (2016). Resilience: A psychobiological construct for psychiatric disorders. *Indian Journal of Psychiatry*, *58*(1), 38–43.
24. Staff, I. O. M. (1900). *Prenatal Care: Reaching Mothers, Reaching Infants*. National Academies Press: United States.
25. Stoewen, D. L. (2017). Dimensions of wellness: Change your habits, change your life. *The Canadian Veterinary Journal*, *58*(8), 861–862.
26. Tabish, S. A. (2008). Complementary and alternative healthcare: Is it evidence-based? *International Journal of Health Sciences* (*Qassim*), *2*(1), v–ix.
27. Toussaint, L., Nguyen, Q. A., Roettger, C., Dixon, K., Offenbächer, M., Kohls, N., Hirsch, J., & Sirois, F. (2021). Effectiveness of progressive muscle relaxation, deep breathing, and guided imagery in promoting psychological and physiological states of relaxation. *Evidence-Based Complementary and Alternative Medicine*, *2021*, 5924040.
28. Tulchinsky, T. H., & Varavikova, E. A. (2014). Expanding the concept of public health. *The New Public Health*, *2014*, 43–90.
29. Umberson, D., & Karas Montez, J. (2010). Social relationships and health: A flashpoint for health policy. *Journal of Health and Social Behavior*, *51*(1_suppl), S54–S66.
30. Vohra-Gupta, S., Petruzzi, L., Jones, C., & Cubbin, C. (2023). An intersectional approach to understanding barriers to healthcare for women. *Journal of Community Health*, *48*(1), 89–98.
31. Wakefield, M., Williams, D. R., & Le Menestrel, S. (2021). *The Future of Nursing 2020–2030: Charting a Path to Achieve Health Equity*. National Academy of Medicine, National Academies Press: United States.
32. Walters, V. (2004). The social context of women's health. *BMC Women's Health*, *4*(1), S2–S10.
33. Woodyard, C. (2011). Exploring the therapeutic effects of yoga and its ability to increase quality of life. *International Journal of Yoga*, *4*(2), 49–54.
34. Yaribeygi, H., Panahi, Y., Sahraei, H., Johnston, T. P., & Sahebkar, A. (2017). The impact of stress on body function: A review. *EXCLI Journal*, *16*, 1057–1072.

# CHAPTER 2

# Ethical Considerations in Female Health

HIMEL MONDAL* and SHAIKAT MONDAL

*Corresponding author

## ABSTRACT

Ethics plays a crucial role in female health, serving as a fundamental aspect of responsible and patient-centric healthcare practices. The significance of ethical considerations becomes evident as we explore the various dimensions of women's well-being. Essential concepts such as autonomy and informed consent are general healthcare faces challenges in female healthcare due to multifaceted cultural practices. Reproductive rights, decisions related to family planning, pregnancy, and childbirth, are the major issues in female health in developing countries. There is a substantial influence of cultural and societal factors on reproductive choices. The very next issue is prenatal care and obstetric interventions, delicately balancing maternal well-being with the imperative of preserving autonomy. The ethical perspective expands to include women's participation in crucial areas such as clinical trials, genetic testing, and counseling, emphasizing the need for gender-inclusive research advocacy. Simultaneously, ethical considerations delve into the dimensions of violence against women in healthcare, calling for healthcare professionals to take active roles in supporting victims. This ethical exploration further extends to end-of-life care, illuminating the intricate decisions surrounding female patients. Additionally, it scrutinizes the ethical implications arising from emerging technologies and innovations in female healthcare.

Holistic Approaches for Women's Sustainable Health, Volume 1: Foundations, Innovations, Challenges, and Management. Megh R. Goyal, Anamika Chauhan, and Junaid Ahmad Malik (Eds)


DOI: 10.1201/9781779641632-3

## 2.1 INTRODUCTION

In the ever-evolving landscape of healthcare, ethical considerations in female health emerge as crucial components that not only influence individual well-being but also shape the fabric of our broader society. The significance of ethical considerations in female health becomes evident when we reflect on the diverse challenges that women may encounter throughout their healthcare journey [62]. From the deeply personal decisions surrounding reproductive rights and family planning to the complexities of maternal care and the ethical implications of emerging technologies, a nuanced understanding of ethical principles is paramount. In embracing these principles, we not only ensure the provision of quality healthcare but also contribute to the creation of a healthcare system that is just, equitable, and responsive to the unique needs of women [23].

Moreover, ethical considerations extend beyond immediate healthcare concerns. The ethical framework provides a roadmap for healthcare professionals, policymakers, and society at large to address systemic disparities. This helps to advocate for gender-inclusive research and actively combat violence against women in healthcare settings. By prioritizing ethical values, we lay the groundwork for a healthcare landscape that not only addresses current challenges but also actively shapes a future where the health and well-being of women are central to our collective vision of a better society [8].

This chapter highlights the scope/challenges/issues in ethical considerations for women's health.

## 2.2 ETHICS IN HEALTHCARE

Ethics in healthcare constitutes the fundamental principles and values that can guide healthcare professionals and organizations in their interactions with patients, colleagues, and the broader communities. Table 2.1 enlists the top 10 core concepts for ethics in healthcare [108, 117].

Central to this ethical framework is the principle of beneficence, emphasizing the obligation to act in the best interests of patients, striving to maximize their well-being. Concurrently, the principle of nonmaleficence underscores the imperative not to harm, highlighting the ethical

**TABLE 2.1** Core Concepts of Ethics in Healthcare [108, 117]

| Concepts | Definition |
|---|---|
| Autonomy | The principle that emphasizes individuals' right to make decisions free from any coercion. |
| Beneficence | The responsibility to actively pursue actions that contribute positively to the welfare and betterment of others |
| Confidentiality | The ethical duty is to protect sensitive information and maintain privacy. |
| Cultural competence | Understanding and respecting diverse cultural backgrounds, and adapting approaches to accommodate different beliefs and values. |
| Fidelity | Loyalty and the importance of keeping promises and honoring commitments. |
| Integrity | Consistency between one's actions and ethical principles, acting in alignment with moral values. |
| Justice | Entails ensuring that resources, opportunities, and advantages are shared justly and fairly among all members of a community. |
| Nonmaleficence | The principle of "do no harm," emphasizing the ethical duty to avoid causing harm intentionally. |
| Respect for persons | Recognizing and valuing the inherent dignity and worth of individuals, and treating people with respect. |
| Veracity | The commitment to truthfulness and honesty, avoiding deception or misleading information. |

responsibility to minimize potential risks and adverse effects associated with medical interventions. Autonomy, another cornerstone, is concerned about respecting patients' or research participants' or any persons' right to make informed decisions about their participation in research or obtaining healthcare, promoting shared decision-making and informed consent. Justice remains integral, emphasizing the equitable distribution in fairly manner of healthcare resources, services, and treatments, and addressing disparities to ensure that all individuals receive dignified and unbiased care [50].

The ethical fabric of healthcare extends beyond individual patient interactions to encompass broader societal considerations, involving issues such as public health policies, research integrity, and the allocation of limited resources. Upholding these ethical principles not only fosters trust between healthcare providers and patients but also reinforces the moral foundation of the healthcare profession, ultimately contributing to the delivery of compassionate, effective, and equitable healthcare services [83].

## 2.3 ETHICS IN FEMALE HEALTH

In the multifaceted landscape of healthcare, ethical considerations in the realm of female health hold profound significance, shaping the quality, equity, and effectiveness of medical services provided to women. The major ethical issues [17] related to women's health are summarized in Table 2.2.

**TABLE 2.2** Core Domains of Female Health

| Domain | Ethical Considerations |
|---|---|
| Access to comprehensive healthcare | Equitable access to reproductive health services and healthcare overall.<br>Addressing disparities in healthcare access and outcomes. |
| Assisted reproductive technologies | Ethical use and accessibility of fertility treatments<br>Moral implications of intervening in the reproductive process |
| Cultural sensitivity | Cultural competence in healthcare delivery<br>Respecting diverse cultural beliefs and practices in reproductive health |
| Emerging technologies and innovations | Ethical implications of genetic testing and personalized medicine<br>Balancing benefits with privacy, equity, and safety. |
| End-of-life decisions | Advanced care planning and preserving dignity and autonomy in serious illness. |
| Family planning | Equitable access to contraceptive methods<br>Informed decision-making<br>Respect for choices in planning and spacing pregnancies |
| Gender equity in research | Inclusive and diverse participation in clinical trials and research studies |
| Pregnancy and childbirth | Respectful maternity care<br>Informed consent for medical interventions<br>Addressing disparities in maternal healthcare outcomes |
| Reproductive rights | Autonomy in decision-making<br>Access to safe abortion services<br>Right to choose or refuse contraception |
| Violence against women in healthcare | Active roles of healthcare professionals in supporting victims<br>Ensuring a safe and respectful healthcare environment |

At the core of this importance lays the recognition that female health is not just a medical issue but a complex interconnected relationship of biological, psychological, social, and cultural factors [15, 103]. Ethical considerations act as guiding principles, ensuring that the unique needs, vulnerabilities, and rights of women are appropriately acknowledged and safeguarded within the healthcare framework [39].

Furthermore, ethical considerations serve as a linchpin in fostering a trusting and collaborative relationship between healthcare providers and female patients. Respecting women's autonomy, ensuring informed consent, and promoting shared decision-making are integral components of ethical healthcare practices. By acknowledging and addressing the unique ethical challenges associated with female health, we not only enhance the quality of care but also contribute to a healthcare system that is grounded in principles of fairness, justice, and the overarching goal of improving the health and well-being of all individuals, irrespective of gender [113].

## 2.4 LANDMARK EVENTS AND MILESTONES

Several landmark events and milestones have played a crucial role in shaping ethical discussions in the realm of female health. These moments have contributed to the evolution of ethical principles, influenced healthcare policies, and advanced the establishment of women's rights and autonomy. The following are some key milestones:

1. Introduction of the Birth Control Pill (1960): The approval and widespread use of the birth control pill marked a significant milestone in reproductive rights and ethical considerations in female health. It empowered women to have greater control over their reproductive choices, sparking conversations about autonomy, informed consent, and the societal impact of contraception [114].
2. Declaration of Helsinki (1964, revised in 2013): The Declaration of Helsinki, developed by the World Medical Association, outlines all the ethical principles that should be followed before, during, and after conducting research involving any human as a research participant. Its impact on research ethics has been significant, emphasizing the importance of informed consent, participant safety, and the inclusion of vulnerable populations, including women, in clinical trials [1].

3. Roe v. Wade (1973): The landmark when the Supreme Court of the United States of America took decision to legalize abortion in the United States, recognizing and honoring a woman's right to choose about the outcome of her pregnancy. This ruling ignited ethical discussions surrounding reproductive rights, bodily autonomy, and the role of healthcare providers in supporting women's decisions regarding abortion [63].
4. Women's Health Initiative (WHI) Study (1992): The WHI, a large-scale clinical trial in the United States, aimed to address health issues in postmenopausal women. The study had a profound impact on ethical considerations by highlighting the importance of transparency in research, informed consent, and ongoing monitoring of the ethical implications of clinical trials [94].
5. International Conference on Population and Development (ICPD)—Cairo (1994): The ICPD marked a global shift in addressing women's reproductive wellbeing, related health issues, and rights about making their own decisions. It emphasized the importance of comprehensive sexual and reproductive health services, recognizing the ethical imperative of ensuring women's easy and justifiable access to optimum information, education, and healthcare services [48].
6. Fourth World Conference on Women—Beijing (1995): The Beijing Declaration and Platform for Action emerged from this conference, advocating for women's rights and equality. It influenced ethical discussions by emphasizing the need for gender-sensitive healthcare policies, including access to quality maternal healthcare, family planning, and the prevention of violence against women [110].
7. Patient Protection and Affordable Care Act (2010): The Affordable Care Act in the United States included provisions that expanded women's access to preventive services, maternity care, and contraception. It addressed ethical considerations related to healthcare access and affordability, recognizing women's specific health needs [98].
8. #MeToo Movement (2017): The #MeToo movement shed light on sexual harassment and assault, including within healthcare settings. It sparked discussions on ethical responsibilities in

addressing gender-based violence, advocating for safer healthcare environments, and promoting a culture of respect and accountability [87].

These events and milestones have collectively shaped the ethical landscape in female health, contributing to ongoing discussions about autonomy, reproductive rights, research ethics, and the broader goal of ensuring equitable and comprehensive healthcare for women.

## 2.5 INFORMED CONSENT AND AUTONOMY

### *2.5.1 INFORMED CONSENT*

Informed consent is a vital ethical principle in healthcare that emphasizes the importance of providing patients, including women in various aspects of healthcare, with thorough and comprehensible information on their health issues, accessible treatments, possible advantages, and disadvantages. The significance of informed consent in female healthcare cannot be overstated, particularly in areas such as reproductive health, maternal care, and gynecological interventions [4]. Ensuring informed consent not only respects the autonomy and decision-making capacity of women but also contributes to building trust between healthcare providers and patients [42].

In reproductive health, where choices may profoundly impact a woman's life, informed consent becomes essential. This includes decisions related to contraception methods, fertility treatments, and prenatal testing. Informed consent for female patients involves providing comprehensive information in plain language, being culturally sensitive, and offering opportunities for questions to ensure understanding. It requires verifying voluntariness, assessing capacity, and thorough documentation. The use of a consent form is essential, detailing discussed information, alternatives, and a signed acknowledgment. The process must consider privacy, respecting the patient's cultural background, and fostering an environment that prioritizes the patient's autonomy and comprehension throughout the decision-making process. The major components of informed consent are summarized in Table 2.3 [10, 77, 88].

**TABLE 2.3** Major Components of Informed Consent Process

| Aspect | Description |
|---|---|
| Capacity assessment | Verify the patient's capacity to understand the information, make decisions, and appreciate the consequences, especially in cases where cognitive impairments may be a concern. |
| Comprehensive information | Give thorough details regarding the intended course of therapy, including its goals, any drawbacks, advantages, and available alternatives. |
| Consent form | Utilize a written consent form detailing the discussed information, signed by the patient or their authorized representative, acknowledging their agreement. |
| Cultural sensitivity | Acknowledge and respect the patient's cultural background, adapting communication to align with their beliefs and values. |
| documentation | Clearly document the informed consent process, including details of discussions, the patient's understanding, and any specific conditions or preferences expressed. |
| Ensuring privacy | Conduct the informed consent discussion in a private setting to maintain confidentiality and encourage open communication. |
| Opportunity for questions | Allow ample time for the patient to ask questions and seek clarification, ensuring they have a complete understanding before providing consent. |
| Plain language | Communicate in clear and understandable language, avoiding medical jargon, to ensure the patient fully grasps the information provided. |
| Review of potential alternatives | Discuss alternative treatments, if available, and the potential risks and benefits associated with each, allowing the patient to make a more informed choice. |
| Voluntariness | Ensure the patient's decision to consent is voluntary, free from coercion or pressure, and that they understand they can withdraw their consent at any point. |

However, despite its significance, ensuring informed consent in female healthcare faces challenges, such as (1) One challenge involves the complexity of medical information, particularly in areas with intricate procedures or intricate reproductive technologies; (2) It may be challenging for both healthcare providers and patients to navigate complex information, emphasizing the need for effective communication strategies and tools to enhance understanding [118]; (3) Moreover, cultural and linguistic diversity can pose barriers to obtaining truly informed consent [25]. In multicultural societies, healthcare providers must be attuned to diverse cultural perspectives on healthcare decision-making and adapt their communication styles accordingly. Language barriers may also impede the effective exchange of information, making it essential to provide translation services and culturally sensitive materials; (4) Additionally, power dynamics within the healthcare system can influence the informed consent process; and (5) Women may face challenges in asserting their preferences and understanding their rights, particularly if there is a significant power imbalance or a lack of patient-centered care [84].

Ensuring that the informed consent process is conducted in an environment that respects the patient's autonomy and values is crucial. Addressing these challenges requires ongoing efforts to improve communication skills among healthcare professionals, develop culturally competent approaches to informed consent, and create environments that prioritize patient-centered care. By overcoming these challenges, healthcare providers can uphold the ethical imperative of informed consent in female healthcare, promoting transparency, trust, and collaborative decision-making.

Autonomy and informed consent are perhaps the most important aspects to protect the dignity of individuals seeking medical treatment [55]. Autonomy, in the context of healthcare, encapsulates the fundamental idea that any person has the right to make his/her own decisions about their bodies and medical care. In this context, we would like to share one of our personal experiences.

Around 2008 in Kolkata, there lived a resilient woman named Shanti. She worked tirelessly as a maid, trying to make ends meet for her family back in Patna. One day, she discovered a lump in her breast and grew increasingly worried. Her neighbor and close friend, Radha, noticed Shanti's distress and encouraged her to seek medical help. Together, they embarked on a journey to the local hospital and were advised to get admitted for a surgery. Shanti, being illiterate, faced challenges in understanding the medical procedures. Radha, being a true friend, decided to help her through the process. When it came time for the consent form, Radha stepped up and agreed on behalf of Shanti, who could not sign herself. In the hustle and bustle of the hospital, a well-intentioned postgraduate student quickly explained the procedure to Radha and obtained her consent. Unfortunately, the student, burdened with a hectic schedule, did not delve into the details of the surgery as much as they should have. The day of the operation arrived, and Shanti, a bundle of nerves, found herself in the preoperative room. When the surgeon approached her and explained that they needed to remove one of her breasts, Shanti, in a moment of clarity and concern, hesitated (Figure 2.1).

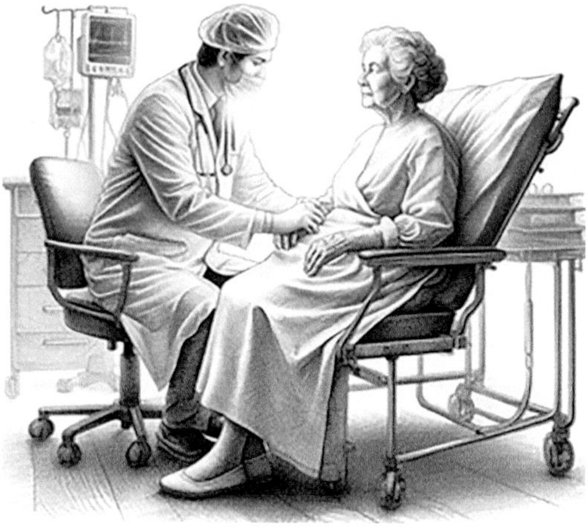

**FIGURE 2.1** A doctor is describing the surgery procedure to a patient who was not informed properly about her surgery.

*Source:* The image was created by Microsoft Copilot on February 15, 2024 with prompt of the authors.

She realized that she needed to consult her husband before proceeding with such a life-altering decision. The news reached the surgical team, and with respect for Shanti's autonomy, the operation was halted. Shanti's courage to speak up about needing her husband's input demonstrated the importance of clear communication and understanding, especially in situations where patients may not fully grasp the implications of medical procedures.

Shanti's story serves as a poignant reminder that every patient, regardless of their background, deserves clear communication, understanding, and respect for their choices in matters of healthcare. The concept of autonomy is particularly pertinent in female health, where decisions related to reproductive choices, interventions, and treatment options often carry profound personal, cultural, and societal implications. Recognizing and fostering autonomy not only empowers patients but also contributes to a more patient-centered and ethically grounded healthcare system [76].

In tandem with autonomy, the principle of informed consent serves as a pillar in ethical research and healthcare practices. Informed consent is a crucial aspect of medical care that requires healthcare providers to furnish patients with detailed and easily comprehensible information regarding various facets of their medical situation. This includes elucidating their current health status, outlining proposed treatment options, discussing potential risks and benefits associated with those treatments, and presenting available alternatives. This ensures that patients are fully aware of their medical circumstances and can make informed decisions about their care in collaboration with their healthcare team. In the preceding story, we have observed how a hurried consent from patients' friend would create a havoc if the surgery would have done without talking to the patients' willingness to undergo the surgery. A transparent communication enables individuals to make well-informed decisions aligned with their values and preferences. By guaranteeing that patients have sufficient information and actively engage in the decision-making process, healthcare providers not only adhere to ethical standards but also foster a relationship built on trust and mutual respect [21].

### *2.5.2 AUTONOMY IN FEMALE HEALTH*

Autonomy in the context of female health decisions is a foundational ethical principle that recognizes and respects a woman's right to make choices regarding her own body, healthcare, and reproductive options [74]. Empowering women with autonomy means recognizing their right to make decisions free from coercion, undue influence, or external pressures. In the context of reproductive health, this extends to choices about contraception, fertility treatments, pregnancy, and childbirth. For example, autonomy asserts that women have the right to decide whether to pursue or decline certain medical interventions, such as cesarean sections or specific prenatal screenings, based on their values, beliefs, and informed preferences [28, 123]. Moreover, autonomy encompasses the right to privacy and confidentiality in healthcare settings, ensuring that women can freely discuss sensitive issues with their healthcare providers without fear of judgment or breaches of confidentiality. This is particularly significant in areas such as sexual and reproductive health, where open and honest communication is vital for making informed decisions.

In ethical healthcare practices, recognizing autonomy involves fostering an environment where women are active participants in their care, engaging in shared decision-making with healthcare professionals. Healthcare providers play a crucial role in facilitating informed discussions, providing comprehensive information, and respecting the diverse perspectives and cultural backgrounds that influence women's healthcare choices. Potential strategies that can be adopted to protect autonomy are summarized in Table 2.4 [46, 76].

**TABLE 2.4** Potential Strategies to Protect Autonomy of Women in Healthcare

| Aspect | Description |
|---|---|
| Advance care planning | Support the patient in making decisions about future healthcare preferences, ensuring their values guide medical choices, especially in critical situations. |
| Advocate for patient's rights | Advocate for the patient's rights within the healthcare system, ensuring their autonomy is respected and protected. |
| Clear communication | Use plain language, actively listen, and encourage the patient to express their concerns, fostering a transparent and open dialogue. |
| Informed consent | Ensure thorough discussions about treatment options, potential risks, and benefits, allowing the patient to make informed decisions about their care. |
| Patient education | Provide understandable information about health conditions and treatment options, empowering the patient to actively participate in decision-making. |
| Privacy and confidentiality | Safeguard the confidentiality of medical information, providing a secure space for the patient to discuss personal details without fear of unwarranted disclosure. |
| Regular check-ins | Maintain ongoing communication, checking in with the patient to assess their understanding, address concerns, and adapt the care plan based on their evolving needs. |
| Respect for cultural values | Recognize and respect the patient's cultural background, considering individual beliefs and practices when tailoring healthcare plans. |
| Shared decision-making | Foster a collaborative approach where healthcare providers and patients work together to make decisions, acknowledging the patient's preferences and input. |
| Support system involvement | Include family or support persons as desired by the patient, ensuring their involvement aligns with the patient's autonomy and wishes. |

A clear and open communication, coupled with respect for cultural values, fosters a patient-centered approach. Protecting privacy and confidentiality provides a secure environment for personal discussions. Advance care planning allows patients to align decisions with their values, while patient education empowers them with understandable information. Advocacy for patient rights, shared decision-making, involvement of support systems, and regular check-ins contribute to a comprehensive strategy, prioritizing and preserving the autonomy of female patients throughout their healthcare experience [34, 115].

## 2.6 REPRODUCTIVE RIGHTS

Reproductive rights, a fundamental component of human rights, encompass the autonomy and freedom individuals have in making decisions about their reproductive lives. These rights are grounded in the principles of dignity, equality, and the recognition that every person should have the ability to control and plan their family, free from discrimination and coercion. The concept of reproductive rights extends far beyond the realm of family planning and contraception; it encompasses the right to access comprehensive reproductive healthcare, make informed choices about fertility, and navigate the various stages of pregnancy and childbirth with dignity and autonomy. As a subject of ongoing global discourse, reproductive rights navigate the delicate intersection of medical ethics, public policy, and the deeply personal choices individuals make regarding their bodies and families [91, 106].

### *2.6.1 CULTURAL AND SOCIETAL ASPECT*

Cultural and societal factors exert a profound effect on individuals' reproductive choices, shaping their attitudes, modifying their beliefs, and influencing practices related to family planning, childbirth, and fertility. The impact of these factors is complex, as cultural norms and societal expectations vary widely across different regions and communities. Understanding how these influences shape reproductive decisions is crucial for promoting culturally sensitive and inclusive healthcare practices. Figure 2.2 encompasses the key ways in which cultural and societal factors impact reproductive choices [27, 29, 102].

Cultural norms often dictate expectations regarding family size, gender roles, and the ideal structure of a family. Societal expectations may influence individuals' decisions regarding the number of children they desire, the spacing between pregnancies, and the roles assigned to men and women in child-rearing. Cultural beliefs about the importance of lineage, extended family structures, and familial responsibilities can significantly influence reproductive choices [7].

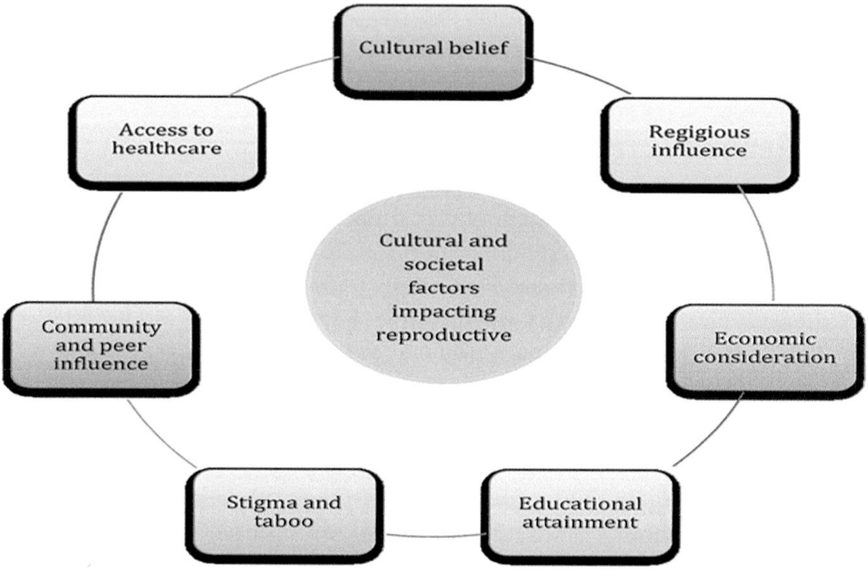


**FIGURE 2.2** Factors influencing the reproductive choices.

*Source:* Authors.

Here, in this context, we would like to share one of our experiences. It was 2011, in a slum area in South Kolkata, we, as a team of healthcare workers, were there to spread awareness about polio vaccination. During the community visit, we met an old man who spoke about his family (Figure 2.3).

His two daughters-in-law have three children only. He expressed worry that without more children, the family might not have additional earning members in the future. Moreover, he touched on the harsh reality of child mortality in the slum. He explained that losing two children to disease would have devastating consequences for the family. Then we explained that polio vaccine would save the children. However, he informed that the vaccine would make the children sterile and in the future they will fail to reproduce!

This experience taught us how cultural beliefs shape reproduction decisions. Along with cultural beliefs, religious beliefs also play a pivotal role in shaping reproductive choices. Different religious traditions may have distinct teachings and perspectives on contraception, fertility treatments, and abortion [99]. Adherence to religious doctrines can impact individuals' decisions and may create ethical dilemmas, particularly when religious teachings conflict with medical recommendations or societal norms. The very next issues are the stigma and taboo in the community.

For example, stigma related to infertility, unplanned pregnancies, or certain contraceptive methods may lead individuals to make choices that align with societal expectations rather than their personal preferences or medical needs. Socioeconomic factors, including financial stability and access to resources, strongly influence reproductive choices [86]. Hence, many of the countries started distributing contraceptives and other reproductive services at the doorstep of people by various means.

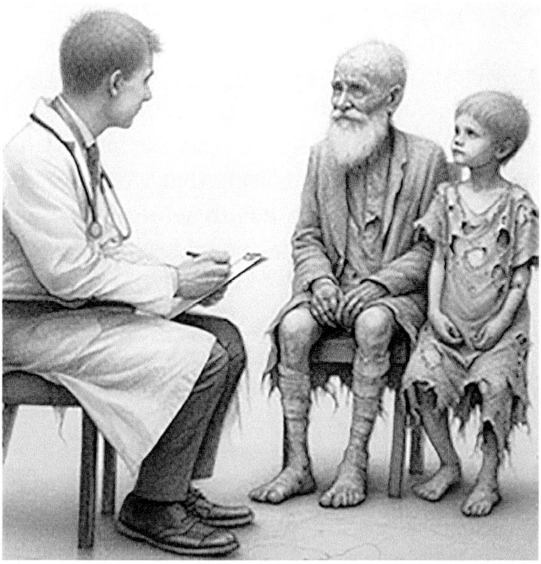

**FIGURE 2.3** A poor man interacting with a doctor and describing that his daughter-in-law is not having more children.

*Source:* The image was created by Microsoft Copilot on February 15, 2024 with prompt of the authors.

Cultural attitudes toward education, particularly for women, can influence reproductive choices. Societal expectations regarding career aspirations, educational attainment, and the timing of family planning may shape decisions about when to have children and the number of children desired. The cultural context of communities and peer groups can significantly impact reproductive choices [92]. In addition, trust in healthcare providers and medicine may impact individuals' access to reproductive healthcare services.

Understanding the interplay of these cultural and societal factors is essential for healthcare providers to offer patient-centered care that respects the diversity of reproductive choices. Culturally sensitive health-care practices involve acknowledging and addressing these influences, fostering open communication, and tailoring reproductive health services to meet the needs of individuals within their cultural context. Additionally, community-based education and awareness initiatives can contribute to dismantling harmful stigmas and promoting informed, empowered reproductive decision-making [12].

### 2.6.2 ETHICS OF REPRODUCTIVE HEALTH

The ethical considerations surrounding reproductive rights and choices for women are complex and multifaceted, encompassing a range of issues related to autonomy, bodily integrity, and societal values. Addressing these considerations is crucial to ensuring that women can make informed decisions about their reproductive health while upholding principles of ethics and justice. Some key ethical considerations and approaches are shown in Figure 2.4 [2, 26, 100].

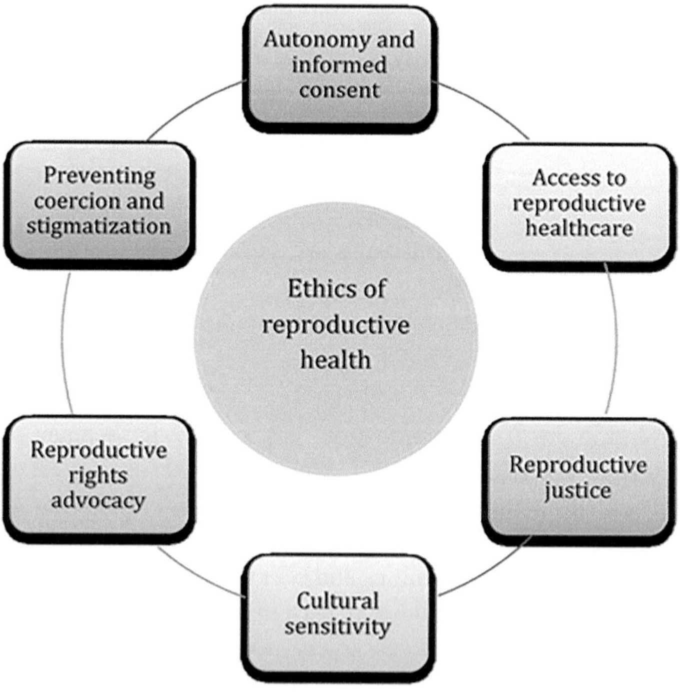


**FIGURE 2.4** Ethical aspects of reproductive health.

Ethical healthcare practices prioritize women's decision about their reproductive health. This involves providing comprehensive information about contraceptive options, fertility treatments, and reproductive technologies. Several governments and nongovernment organizations are working to provide these at a large scale. Healthcare providers should engage in open and honest communication, ensuring that women fully understand the potential risks, benefits, and alternatives before making choices [35, 109]. Ensuring equitable access to reproductive healthcare services is an ethical imperative. Barriers to access, whether due to economic constraints, geographic location, or discriminatory policies, raise ethical concerns. Efforts should be made to eliminate these barriers, promoting universal access to family planning, contraception, and other reproductive health services. Reproductive justice goes beyond individual choices and emphasizes the broader social, economic, and political factors that influence reproductive rights. Hence, recognizing and respecting diverse cultural perspectives on reproductive health is crucial. The healthcare system should involve tailoring discussions and interventions to be culturally sensitive, acknowledging the influence of cultural beliefs on reproductive choices, and fostering an inclusive healthcare environment [6].

Ethical healthcare providers and stakeholders can actively engage in reproductive rights advocacy. This may involve supporting policies that protect and expand reproductive rights, participating in public health campaigns, and collaborating with organizations working toward reproductive justice. Advocacy efforts should prioritize inclusivity, respect for diversity, and the elimination of discriminatory practices. In the advocacy, one of the important aspects is to prevent coercion and stigmatization related to reproductive choices. Healthcare providers should create environments that respect individuals' decisions, free from judgment or pressure. Protecting women's rights to make choices without fear of coercion is fundamental to ethical reproductive healthcare [38].

## 2.7 DISPARITIES IN FEMALE HEALTH

Healthcare disparities, often rooted in social, economic, and systemic inequities, give rise to ethical concerns as they result in unequal access to quality healthcare, differential health outcomes, and perpetuation of societal injustices. Addressing these disparities is a moral imperative, grounded in principles of fairness, justice, and the recognition of every individual's right to equitable health opportunities. Key disparities and their ethical implications are shown in Table 2.5 [43, 45, 101, 111].

**TABLE 2.5** Disparities in Female Health and Its Ethical Implications

| Aspect | Disparity | Ethical Implications |
|---|---|---|
| Access to healthcare services | Unequal access based on income, location, race, and ethnicity. | Denies justice, violates the ethical obligation to provide care for all, irrespective of socioeconomic factors. |
| Cultural competence | Lack of cultural competence hindering culturally sensitive care. | Infringes upon respect for autonomy and dignity, emphasizing the ethical obligation to understand and address cultural nuances. |
| Health information and literacy | Variations in health information and literacy levels. | Ensuring equity requires addressing disparities, promoting informed decision-making and respecting autonomy. |
| Health outcomes | Disproportionate health outcomes among demographic groups. | Raises ethical concerns about fairness and equity, emphasizing the need to address systemic disparities for justice. |
| Implicit bias | Unconscious biases affecting clinical decision-making. | Compromises justice by perpetuating unequal treatment, highlighting the need for ongoing efforts to mitigate bias and ensure equitable care. |
| Quality of care | Variations in care quality due to biases, discrimination, or inadequate resources. | Violates beneficence and non-maleficence principles, undermines the ethical duty to prioritize patient well-being and treat individuals equally. |

Addressing healthcare disparities encompasses a multifaceted approach, with various dimensions revealing challenges and ethical considerations. Unequal access to healthcare services, influenced by income, location, and ethnicity, raises ethical concerns by denying justice and perpetuating health inequities. Concurrently, disparities in the quality of care, driven by biases and inadequate resources, compromise beneficence and non-maleficence principles, demanding a commitment to prioritizing patient well-being regardless of background [68]. Disproportionate health outcomes among demographic groups not only spotlight concerns about fairness and equity but also underscore the ethical imperative to rectify systemic disparities for justice. The lack of cultural competence in healthcare delivery poses ethical challenges by infringing upon the principles of respect for autonomy and dignity. Disparities in health information and literacy further underscore the need for equitable access to knowledge, respecting autonomy, and promoting informed decision-making [33]. Additionally, the impact of implicit bias on clinical decision-making compromises justice, emphasizing the ongoing ethical obligation to mitigate bias and ensure equitable care for all patients. In essence, the interconnected aspects of healthcare disparities underscore the urgent need for systemic changes that prioritize justice, beneficence, non-maleficence, respect for autonomy, and equitable care provision for all individuals [52].

Mitigating healthcare disparities requires a comprehensive and concerted effort across various levels of the healthcare system. Implementing policies that ensure equitable and balanced access to healthcare services that is not influenced by and geographic location, race, or ethnicity, or income, is crucial [122]. Strategies such as expanding community clinics, improving transportation infrastructure, and addressing language barriers can enhance accessibility. Furthermore, promoting cultural competence within healthcare delivery is essential, involving training programs for healthcare professionals to understand and respect diverse cultural backgrounds. Initiatives aimed at improving health literacy, including community education programs and accessible health information [95], play a vital role in empowering individuals to make informed decisions about their health. Additionally, addressing implicit bias through ongoing training and awareness programs can contribute to more equitable clinical decision-making. Collaboration between healthcare providers, policymakers, and community leaders is pivotal to developing and implementing effective strategies that prioritize justice, beneficence, non-maleficence, respect for autonomy, and equal care provision, ultimately working toward a healthcare system that ensures health equity for all [13, 119].

## 2.8 RESEARCH ON FEMALE HEALTH

Female health research is of paramount importance as it addresses the unique physiological, reproductive, and socio-cultural aspects of women's well-being [47]. Understanding and advancing female-specific health knowledge is crucial for improving healthcare outcomes and ensuring equitable access to medical interventions. From reproductive health to chronic diseases, women may experience conditions differently from men, necessitating tailored research initiatives. Comprehensive female health research not only contributes to enhancing preventive measures, diagnostics, and treatment options but also promotes gender-inclusive healthcare policies [89].

By investigating the intricacies of women's health, researchers contribute to a more holistic understanding of the factors influencing women's lives, paving the way for informed medical practices, improved public health interventions, and ultimately, the empowerment of women in healthcare decision-making [37].

Research involving female subjects requires special considerations compared to male subjects due to the unique biological, reproductive, and social factors that characterize women's health. Here are some specific considerations, shown in Figure 2.5 [22, 44, 124].

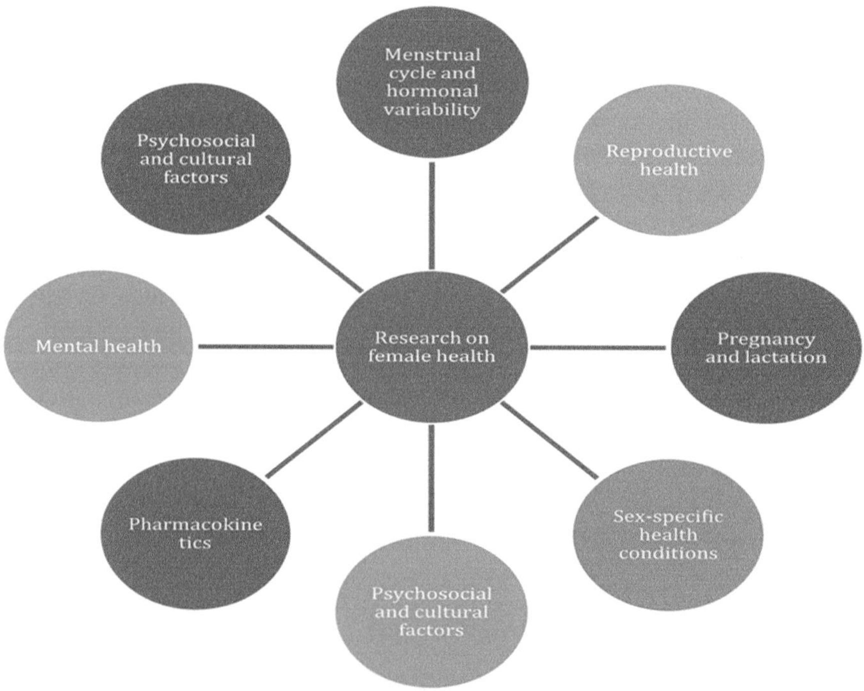


**FIGURE 2.5** Special issues of research on women.

Female participants may experience variations in hormonal levels across the menstrual cycle. Researchers need to consider these fluctuations when designing studies, as they can influence physiological responses to interventions or exposures. Timing research activities to specific phases of the menstrual cycle may be relevant in certain studies. Female participants may be of reproductive age, potentially impacting the research design, especially in studies involving medications, interventions, or exposures that may affect fertility or pregnancy. Ethical considerations regarding pregnancy testing, contraception, and potential risks to fetal health must be carefully addressed [85].

For studies involving pregnant or lactating women, additional ethical considerations come into play. Researchers need to ensure the safety of both the mother and the developing fetus or breastfeeding infant [67]. Special attention should be given to potential risks and benefits, and appropriate measures must be in place to safeguard the well-being of both the mother and child. Certain health conditions, such as breast cancer or gynecological disorders, are exclusive to women. Studies focusing on these conditions need to consider the specific nuances and challenges associated with women's health, including potential psychological, emotional, and social impacts [81]. Women's health research should consider psychosocial and cultural factors that may influence health outcomes. Cultural norms, societal expectations, and gender roles can impact health behaviors, perceptions, and healthcare-seeking patterns, necessitating a nuanced understanding in the research design and interpretation of findings. When investigating drug interventions, researchers need to consider potential sex differences in drug metabolism, efficacy, and side effects. Women may metabolize drugs differently than men due to factors such as body composition, enzyme activity, and hormonal fluctuations, influencing treatment outcomes [75, 97]. Recognizing the intersectionality of women's identities is crucial. Numerous characteristics, such as race, ethnicity, financial class, sexual orientation, and more, influence the lives of women. Researchers must consider how these intersecting identities may contribute to health disparities and tailor interventions or study designs accordingly.

Research involving mental health should consider gender-specific mental health issues, such as postpartum depression, which predominantly affects women. The impact of hormonal changes, societal expectations, and biological factors on mental health outcomes should be explored and addressed in study designs. Given the dynamic nature of women's health across the lifespan, longitudinal and lifecycle approaches are essential. Researchers should consider how health conditions, behaviors, and outcomes evolve over time and how interventions may need to be tailored to different life stages [70, 104].

Hence, conducting research involving female subjects requires a comprehensive understanding of the unique aspects of women's health.

By considering these special considerations, researchers can contribute to the development of more inclusive, effective, and ethical healthcare practices that address the specific needs of women across diverse populations. Safeguarding the rights and well-being of female participants in clinical trials and studies is not only an ethical imperative but also crucial for the advancement of scientific knowledge and the development of healthcare interventions that are safe and effective for diverse populations.

## 2.9 VIOLENCE AGAINST WOMEN

Violence against women profoundly impacts their health across physical, mental, and reproductive dimensions. The immediate consequences often manifest as physical injuries, ranging from bruises to life-threatening trauma. Yet, the repercussions extend far beyond the visible, affecting mental health and causing diseases such as anxiety, sadness, and post-traumatic stress disorder [11]. Chronic conditions, gynecological issues, and obstacles to seeking healthcare further compound the toll. Witnessing violence can adversely affect children's health, perpetuating intergenerational cycles of harm [79]. Social isolation, economic dependence, and mortality risks add layers to the complex web of health consequences. Addressing violence against women necessitates a holistic approach encompassing prevention, intervention, and comprehensive support services to mitigate the profound and often enduring impacts on women's health and well-being [53].

Healthcare professionals play a crucial role in supporting victims of violence, including women who have experienced various forms of abuse. Their role extends beyond providing medical treatment to encompass offering comprehensive care, advocacy, and support to address the physical, emotional, and psychological impact of violence. Healthcare professionals are often the first point of contact for victims of violence seeking medical assistance. They play a critical role in identifying signs and symptoms of abuse through routine screenings and assessments [56, 112].

By recognizing indicators of violence, such as unexplained injuries, chronic pain, or emotional distress, healthcare professionals can initiate conversations with patients about their safety and well-being. Victims of violence often experience significant emotional and psychological trauma. Healthcare professionals, including psychologists, social workers, and counselors, provide essential psychosocial support to help victims cope with the trauma, manage stress, and rebuild their sense of safety and self-esteem. This may involve individual counseling, group therapy, or referral to support services in the community [19, 71].

Healthcare professionals collaborate with victims to develop safety plans that address their immediate safety needs and long-term protection. This may include connecting victims with local shelters, legal advocacy services, or law enforcement agencies to ensure they have access to resources and support to stay safe from further harm [9]. In addition, healthcare professionals advocate for the rights and well-being of victims by providing information about their legal rights, supporting their decision-making autonomy, and empowering them to make informed choices about their safety and recovery. By advocating for victims within the healthcare system and beyond, healthcare professionals contribute to a supportive environment that prioritizes the needs and dignity of survivors. The overall violence mitigation strategies are dependent on female education [24]. By raising awareness and promoting prevention strategies, healthcare professionals contribute to creating a culture of safety and respect that aims to prevent future incidents of violence [120].

In summary, healthcare professionals play a multifaceted role in supporting victims of violence, including women, by providing medical treatment, psychosocial support, safety planning, and referrals to support services, advocacy, empowerment, and education. Their compassionate and comprehensive approach is essential in addressing the complex needs of victims and promoting healing and recovery.

## 2.10 COMPLEMENTARY AND ALTERNATIVE MEDICINE

Complementary and Alternative Medicine (CAM) constitutes a diverse and evolving spectrum of healthcare practices that extend beyond conventional medical approaches. Embracing a holistic philosophy, CAM encompasses a wide array of therapies, ranging from herbal remedies and acupuncture to mind–body practices such as meditation and yoga [66]. This multifaceted approach recognizes the interconnectedness of physical, mental, and emotional well-being, aiming to enhance overall health.

CAM often complements mainstream medicine, offering additional avenues for healing, prevention, and wellness promotion. Rooted in both traditional wisdom and contemporary innovations, CAM reflects a growing interest in individualized, patient-centered care. As individuals seek a more comprehensive understanding of health, the exploration of CAM practices has become increasingly prevalent [93]. This introduction serves as a gateway to delve into the principles, ethical considerations, and potential benefits and challenges associated with the rich tapestry of complementary and alternative medicine in the context of human health.

Although the CAM is deeply rooted in the culture, its application and implication may sometimes face ethical issues as summarized in Table 2.6 [49, 57, 105].

**TABLE 2.6** Ethical Issues of Using Complementary and Alternative Medicine for Women

| Issues | Description |
|---|---|
| Cultural competence | Navigating ethical dilemmas when cultural practices in CAM conflict with established medical standards, requiring cultural competence in healthcare. |
| Economic considerations | Ethical concerns arise when the cost of CAM treatments is not covered by insurance, leading to disparities in healthcare access based on economic status. |
| Endangering public health | Ethical considerations surrounding the promotion of CAM treatments without adequate evidence, posing risks to public health. |
| Informed consent | Ensuring individuals are adequately informed about the risks, benefits, and limitations of CAM treatments to make informed decisions. |
| Integration into conventional care | Ethical challenges in establishing guidelines for the responsible integration of CAM into conventional medical practice, considering evidence, safety, and patient preferences. |
| Interactions with conventional medicine | Addressing ethical concerns when CAM and conventional treatments interact, potentially resulting in adverse effects or hindering treatment effectiveness. |
| Patient autonomy | Balancing patient autonomy with the responsibility to provide sound medical advice when CAM choices conflict with evidence-based conventional medicine. |
| Placebo effect | Disclosing the potential placebo effect of certain CAM interventions while respecting patient beliefs and maintaining transparency. |
| Professional integrity | Ethical challenges for healthcare providers when patients seek CAM treatments conflicting with professional beliefs or lacking sufficient evidence. |
| Safety and efficacy | Ethical concerns regarding the lack of standardized regulation and scientific evidence for many CAM practices, raising questions about safety and efficacy. |

One concern is the adequacy of informed consent, as women may engage in CAM practices without fully understanding the potential risks and benefits, particularly when it comes to skin care. Safety and efficacy of certain CAM interventions in pregnancy, fertility treatments, or hormonal imbalances pose ethical dilemmas due to limited scientific validation. Additionally, cultural competence becomes crucial to ensure respectful and tailored care, considering diverse backgrounds and beliefs surrounding women's health [82]. Economic considerations may also emerge, as access to certain CAM therapies may be influenced by financial status, potentially exacerbating healthcare disparities. Striking a balance between respecting patient autonomy, providing evidence-based care, and acknowledging the potential cultural nuances in women's health becomes imperative to address these ethical challenges associated with the use of CAM [20, 31].

## 2.11 END OF LIFE CARE

End-of-life decisions for women involve complex ethical considerations that require careful attention to individual autonomy, cultural beliefs, and the principles of beneficence and non-maleficence [121]. Healthcare professionals must navigate these considerations with sensitivity and respect for the unique experiences and perspectives of each woman.

Respecting the autonomy of women is a fundamental ethical principle. Healthcare professionals must ensure that women are actively involved in decision-making regarding their end-of-life care. This entails respecting the woman's values, tastes, and wishes as well as giving her clear and thorough information about the options that are available and possible results [3]. Encouraging and facilitating advance care planning is an ethical imperative. Women should be supported in documenting their healthcare preferences, including decisions related to life-sustaining treatments, resuscitation, and other end-of-life interventions. This ensures that healthcare decisions align with the woman's values even if she is unable to communicate her wishes later. Considering the role of family and caregivers is crucial in end-of-life decisions. While respecting the autonomy of the woman, healthcare professionals should also involve and support the woman's chosen support system [65].

Open communication with family members and caregivers ensures that everyone is on the same page regarding the woman's wishes and care plan. Ethical end-of-life care extends beyond the physical aspects to encompass emotional and spiritual support. Healthcare professionals should recognize and address the emotional and spiritual needs of women and their families during this challenging time. Providing access to counseling, chaplaincy services, and other forms of emotional support contributes to holistic end-of-life care [40]. In some situations, end-of-life decisions may need to be made urgently. Ethical crisis decision-making involves balancing the need for timely interventions with respect for the woman's autonomy and values. Healthcare professionals should prioritize communication and collaboration with the woman and her support system during such critical moments [64, 80].

In summary, ethical considerations in end-of-life decisions for women involve respecting autonomy, facilitating advance care planning, being culturally sensitive, providing informed decision-making, ensuring pain management and comfort care, involving family and caregivers, making ethical decisions regarding treatment withdrawal, or withholding, offering emotional and spiritual support, and navigating crisis decision-making with sensitivity. By upholding these ethical principles, healthcare professionals contribute to dignified and compassionate end-of-life care for women [14].

## 2.12 USE OF NEW TECHNOLOGIES IN FEMALE HEALTH CARE

Several new technologies have been emerging in the field of female healthcare, aiming to improve diagnostics, treatment, and overall women's health. Keep in mind that the field is continually evolving, and there may be additional advancements beyond this timeframe. Here are some notable technologies in female healthcare.

- **3D mammography**: Three-dimensional mammography or tomosynthesis is an advanced imaging technology that provides more detailed and layered images of the breast. It can improve the detection of breast abnormalities and reduce false positives, enhancing breast cancer screening [60].
- **Digital health platforms**: Digital health platforms and mobile applications have become increasingly popular in women's

health. These platforms may offer features such as menstrual cycle tracking, fertility monitoring, and personalized health insights. They can empower women to manage their reproductive health and receive information tailored to their individual needs [16, 58].

- **Fertility tracking apps and devices**: Advances in fertility tracking technologies include wearable devices and smartphone apps that help women monitor their menstrual cycles, track ovulation, and identify fertile windows. These tools can assist in family planning, conception, or simply gaining a better understanding of reproductive health [69, 116].
- **Genetic testing** for reproductive health: Genetic testing has evolved to provide insights into reproductive health. Women and couples can opt for genetic screening to assess the risk of certain genetic conditions in their offspring [73]. This information can inform family planning decisions and help manage potential genetic risks [18].
- **Machine learning and** artificial intelligence **(AI)** in diagnostics: Both machine learning and AI are being employed in diagnostics, particularly in the analysis of medical imaging. AI algorithms can assist in the early detection of conditions such as breast cancer through mammography or other imaging modalities [126].
- **Menstrual health wearables**: Wearable devices designed for menstrual health can track various aspects of the menstrual cycle, including flow, symptoms, and hormonal fluctuations. These wearable aims to provide a more comprehensive understanding of women's reproductive health beyond just fertility tracking [36].
- **Remote monitoring for pregnancy**: Wearable devices and remote monitoring tools are being developed to monitor pregnancies outside traditional clinical settings. These devices can track fetal heart rate, maternal health parameters, and provide real-time data to healthcare providers, enhancing prenatal care [59, 127].
- **Robotic surgery** for gynecological procedures: Robot-assisted surgery has become more common in gynecological procedures. Robotic systems provide surgeons with enhanced precision and control, leading to minimally invasive surgeries with reduced

recovery times for conditions such as endometriosis, fibroids, and hysterectomy [72, 78].

- **Smart breast pumps**: Technological advancements in breast pumps are designed to make breastfeeding more convenient for new mothers. Smart breast pumps can be connected to mobile apps, allowing women to track pumping sessions, milk production, and receive personalized breastfeeding tips [30, 61].
- **Telemedicine and virtual care**: Telemedicine has become a vital tool in providing healthcare services, allowing women to consult with healthcare professionals remotely. Virtual care platforms enable access to routine check-ups, consultations for family planning, and follow-ups on various health concerns from the convenience of home [96, 125].

The integration of new technologies like AI in female healthcare brings about various ethical considerations that need careful examination. While these technologies hold the potential to enhance diagnostics, treatment, and overall well-being, they also raise concerns related to privacy, informed consent, equity, and the appropriate use of sensitive health data [5, 51].

Many technologies involve the collection and storage of sensitive health data. Ensuring the privacy and security of women's health information is paramount. Ethical concerns arise regarding who has access to this data, how it is stored, and whether it is vulnerable to breaches or misuse [32]. As new technologies offer more sophisticated diagnostic and treatment options, ensuring informed consent becomes crucial. Women must be adequately informed about the purpose, risks, and potential benefits of using these technologies. Respecting women's autonomy involves providing them with the knowledge needed to make informed decisions about their healthcare. There is a risk of creating or exacerbating healthcare disparities if certain populations, especially those with limited access to technology or specific communities, are left behind in the adoption of these technologies [41].

Ethical considerations involve striving for equitable access to ensure that benefits are distributed across diverse socioeconomic and cultural groups. The accuracy and reliability of diagnostic technologies are critical ethical concerns. False positive or negative results may cause unwarranted concern or postpone medical intervention. Ensuring that these technologies are thoroughly tested, validated, and regularly updated is essential to maintain trust and ethical standards [54, 107].

The commercialization of healthcare technologies raises ethical questions about profit motives potentially influencing decisions related to research, development, and marketing. Ensuring that the primary focus remains on patient well-being rather than maximizing profits is crucial for ethical technology adoption. Advances in genetic testing technologies bring ethical considerations related to reproductive autonomy. Women should be empowered to make decisions based on genetic information, but there is a risk of creating pressure or stigma around certain genetic conditions [90]. Ensuring that genetic testing is accompanied by comprehensive counseling and support is essential. Algorithms and AI used in healthcare technologies may inherit biases present in the data used for their training. This raises ethical concerns related to the potential for biased outcomes, leading to disparities in care. Efforts to address and mitigate biases are crucial to ensure fair and equitable healthcare for all women.

In addressing these ethical implications, ongoing dialogue among healthcare professionals, technology developers, policymakers, and the public is essential. Establishing ethical guidelines, regulatory frameworks, and continuous monitoring of the impact of technologies on women's health can help ensure that technological advancements align with ethical principles and benefit all individuals equitably.

## 2.13 SUMMARY

Key ethical considerations in female health encompass a range of principles and concerns aimed at ensuring the well-being, autonomy, and dignity of women. These considerations span various aspects of healthcare, from reproductive rights to technological advancements.

Respecting women's autonomy involves providing comprehensive information and ensuring informed consent for medical interventions, treatments, and procedures. Women should have the right to make decisions about their own bodies and healthcare. Protecting the privacy and confidentiality of women's health information is crucial. Healthcare providers must implement measures to safeguard sensitive data and respect women's right to control the disclosure of their personal health details. Ethical considerations in female health include recognizing and upholding women's reproductive rights. This involves supporting access to family planning, contraception, safe abortion, and fertility services, allowing women to make choices aligned with their values and circumstances. Recognizing and respecting cultural diversity is essential in female healthcare. Cultural competence ensures that healthcare practices are sensitive to diverse backgrounds, beliefs, and practices, fostering an inclusive and respectful environment for all women. Ethical healthcare practices strive for equitable access to healthcare services for women, irrespective of socioeconomic status, race, ethnicity, or geographic location. Addressing disparities in healthcare access and outcomes is crucial for ethical care. Promoting gender equality involves addressing systemic biases and discriminatory practices in healthcare. Ethical considerations include working toward eliminating gender-based disparities in treatment, research, and access to medical resources. Ensuring the provision of high-quality and evidence-based care is an ethical imperative. Healthcare providers must stay informed about the latest advancements and guidelines to offer women the best possible medical care. Ethical considerations involve actively working against discrimination and stigma related to women's health issues. Creating an environment free from judgment and bias is essential to encourage open communication and ensure that women seek timely and appropriate care. The safety and well-being of women should be prioritized in healthcare practices. This includes measures to prevent medical errors, ensuring the efficacy of treatments, and providing a supportive environment for women to discuss and address their health concerns. With the integration of new technologies in healthcare, ethical considerations include ensuring the responsible and informed use of technologies, addressing issues such as data privacy, algorithmic biases, and the potential impact of technology on women's health outcomes. Special attention is given to ethical considerations in maternal and reproductive health, including comprehensive prenatal care, respectful maternity care, and addressing disparities in maternal mortality rates. Ethical care involves promoting the health and well-being of both mothers and infants.

In summary, ethical considerations in female health revolve around principles such as autonomy, privacy, equity, cultural sensitivity, and the promotion of gender equality. By upholding these principles, healthcare providers contribute to a healthcare system that respects and prioritizes the diverse needs and experiences of women.

## KEYWORDS

- **family planning services**
- **female**
- **informed consent**
- **pregnancy**
- **prenatal care**
- **reproductive rights**
- **violence**

## REFERENCES

1. (2000). A fifth amendment for the Declaration of Helsinki. *Lancet (London)*, *356*(9236), e1123.
2. Adinma, J. I., & Adinma, E. D. (2009). Ethical considerations in women's sexual and reproductive health care. *Nigerian Journal of Clinical Practice*, *12*(1), 92–98.
3. Akdeniz, M., Yardımcı, B., & Kavukcu, E. (2021). Ethical considerations at the end-of-life care. *SAGE Open Medicine*, *9*, article ID20503121211000918. doi: 10.1177/20503121211000918
4. Al Balushi, A. A. (2019). Female patients and informed consent: Oman's cultural background. *Sultan Qaboos University Medical Journal, 19*(1), e11–e14. doi: 10.18295/squmj.2019.19.01.003
5. Al-Hwsali, A., Alsaadi, B., Abdi, N., Khatab, S., Alzubaidi, M., Solaiman, B., & Househ, M. (2023). Scoping review: Legal and ethical principles of artificial intelligence in public health. *Studies in Health Technology and Informatics*, *305*, 640–643. doi: 10.3233/SHTI230579
6. Appleford, G., RamaRao, S., & Bellows, B. (2020). The inclusion of sexual and reproductive health services within universal health care through intentional design. *Sexual and Reproductive Health Matters, 28*(2), e1799589. doi: 10.1080/26410397.2020.1799589
7. Arousell, J., & Carlbom, A. (2016). Culture and religious beliefs in relation to reproductive health. Best practice & research. *Clinical Obstetrics & Gynecology*, *32*, 77–87. doi: 10.1016/j.bpobgyn.2015.08.011
8. Balarajan, Y., Selvaraj, S., & Subramanian, S. V. (2011). Health care and equity in India. *Lancet* (London), *377*(9764), 505–515. doi: 10.1016/S0140-6736(10)61894-6
9. Basheer, M. B., Bell, R., & Boyle, A. A. (2022). Systematic review of the effectiveness of advocacy interventions for adult victims of domestic violence within an emergency department setting. *Cureus, 14*(6), e25599. doi: 10.7759/cureus.25599

10. Bazzano, L. A., Durant, J., & Brantley, P. R. (2021). A modern history of informed consent and the role of key information. *Ochsner Journal, 21*(1), 81–85. doi: 10.31486/toj.19.0105
11. Bhattacharya, A., Yasmin, S., Bhattacharya, A., Baur, B., & Madhwani, K. P. (2020). Domestic violence against women: A hidden and deeply rooted health issue in India. *Journal of Family Medicine and Primary Care, 9*(10), 5229–5235. doi: 10.4103/jfmpc.jfmpc_506_20
12. Bohren, M. A., Vazquez Corona, M., Odiase, O. J., Wilson, A. N., Sudhinaraset, M., Diamond-Smith, N., Berryman, J., Tunçalp, Ö., & Afulani, P. A. (2022). Strategies to reduce stigma and discrimination in sexual and reproductive healthcare settings: A mixed-methods systematic review. *PLoS One, 2*(6), e0000582. doi: 10.1371/journal.pgph.0000582
13. Braveman, P., & Gruskin, S. (2003). Defining equity in health. *Journal of Epidemiology and Community Health, 57*(4), 254–258. doi: 10.1136/jech.57.4.254
14. Brito-Pons, G., & Librada-Flores, S. (2018). Compassion in palliative care: A review. *Current Opinion in Supportive and Palliative Care, 12*(4), 472–479. doi: 10.1097/SPC.0000000000000393
15. Bruno, B., Shalowitz, D. I., & Arora, K. S. (2021). Ethical challenges for women's healthcare highlighted by the COVID-19 pandemic. *Journal of Medical Ethics, 47*(2), 69–72. doi: 10.1136/medethics-2020-106646
16. Butcher, C. J., & Hussain, W. (2022). Digital healthcare: The future. *Future Healthcare Journal, 9*(2), 113–117. doi: 10.7861/fhj.2022-0046
17. Cain, J. M. (2000). A global overview of ethical issues in women's health. *International Journal of Gynaecology and Obstetrics: International Federation of Gynaecology and Obstetrics, 70*(1), 165–172. doi: 10.1016/s0020-7292(00)00229-0
18. Cariati, F., D'Argenio, V., & Tomaiuolo, R. (2019). The evolving role of genetic tests in reproductive medicine. *Journal of Translational Medicine, 17*(1), 267. doi: 10.1186/s12967-019-2019-8
19. Castillo, E. G., Ijadi-Maghsoodi, R., Shadravan, S., Moore, E., Mensah, M. O., 3rd, Docherty, M., Aguilera Nunez, M. G., Barcelo, N., Goodsmith, N., Halpin, L. E., Morton, I., Mango, J., Montero, A. E., Rahmanian Koushkaki, S., Bromley, E., Chung, B., Jones, F., Gabrielian, S., Gelberg, L., Greenberg, J. M., & Wells, K. B. (2019). Community interventions to promote mental health and social equity. *Current Psychiatry Reports, 21*(5), 35. doi: 10.1007/s11920-019-1017-0
20. Clark, P. A. (2000). The ethics of alternative medicine therapies. *Journal of Public Health Policy, 21*(4), 447–470.
21. Cocanour, C. S. (2017). Informed consent-It's more than a signature on a piece of paper. *American Journal of Surgery, 214*(6), 993–997. doi: 10.1016/j.amjsurg.2017.09.015
22. Colineaux, H., Neufcourt, L., Delpierre, C., Kelly-Irving, M., & Lepage, B. (2023). Explaining biological differences between men and women by gendered mechanisms. *Emerging Themes in Epidemiology, 20*(1), 2. doi: 10.1186/s12982-023-00121-6
23. Davidson, P. M., McGrath, S. J., Meleis, A. I., Stern, P., Digiacomo, M., Dharmendra, T., Correa-de-Araujo, R., Campbell, J. C., Hochleitner, M., Messias, D. K., Brown, H., Teitelman, A., Sindhu, S., Reesman, K., Richter, S., Sommers, M. S., Schaeffer, D., Stringer, M., Sampselle, C., Anderson, D., & Krassen Covan, E. (2011). The health of women and girls determines the health and well-being of our modern world:

A white paper from the International Council on Women's Health Issues. *Health Care for Women International, 32*(10), 870–886. doi: 10.1080/07399332.2011.603872

24. De La Rue, L., Ortega, L., & Rodriguez, G. C. (2023). System-based victim advocates identify resources and barriers to supporting crime victims. *International Review of Victimology, 29*(1), 16–26. doi: 10.1177/02697580221088340
25. Deb Roy, A., Das, D., & Mondal, H. (2023). The tribal health system in India: Challenges in healthcare delivery in comparison to the global healthcare systems. *Cureus, 15*(6), e39867. doi: 10.7759/cureus.39867
26. Dickens, B. M. (2001). Reproductive health services and the law and ethics of conscientious objection. *Medicine and Law, 20*(2), 283–293.
27. Donnelly, A., Haintz, G. L., McKenzie, H., & Graham, M. (2023). Influences on reproductive decision-making among forcibly displaced women resettling in high-income countries: A scoping review and thematic analysis. *International Journal for Equity in Health, 22*(1), 179. doi: 10.1186/s12939-023-01993-5
28. Dossett, E. C., Castañeda-Cudney, S. L., Nguyen, M. T., Olgun, M., Wang, J., Myrick, K. J., Hallmark, L., & Saks, E. R. (2023). Reproductive psychiatric advance directives: Promoting autonomy for perinatal people with serious mental illness diagnoses. *Archives of Women's Mental Health*, Advance online publication. doi: 10.1007/s00737-023-01382-5
29. D'Souza, P., Bailey, J. V., Stephenson, J., & Oliver, S. (2022). Factors influencing contraception choice and use globally: A synthesis of systematic reviews. *The European Journal of Contraception & Reproductive Health Care (European Society of Contraception), 27*(5), 364–372. doi: 10.1080/13625187.2022.2096215
30. Eglash, A., & Malloy, M. L. (2015). Breastmilk expression and breast pump technology. *Clinical Obstetrics and Gynecology, 58*(4), 855–867. doi: 10.1097/GRF.0000000000000141
31. Entwistle, V. A., Carter, S. M., Cribb, A., & McCaffery, K. (2010). Supporting patient autonomy: The importance of clinician-patient relationships. *Journal of General Internal Medicine, 25*(7), 741–745. doi: 10.1007/s11606-010-1292-2
32. Filkins, B. L., Kim, J. Y., Roberts, B., Armstrong, W., Miller, M. A., Hultner, M. L., Castillo, A. P., Ducom, J. C., Topol, E. J., & Steinhubl, S. R. (2016). Privacy and security in the era of digital health: What should translational researchers know and do about it? *American Journal of Translational Research, 8*(3), 1560–1580
33. Fitzpatrick, P. J. (2023). Improving health literacy using the power of digital communications to achieve better health outcomes for patients and practitioners. *Frontiers in Digital Health, 5*, e1264780. doi: 10.3389/fdgth.2023.1264780
34. Galletta, M., Piazza, M. F., Meloni, S. L., Chessa, E., Piras, I., Arnetz, J. E., & D'Aloja, E. (2022). Patient involvement in shared decision-making: Do patients rate physicians and nurses differently? *International Journal of Environmental Research and Public Health, 19*(21), 14229. doi: 10.3390/ijerph192114229
35. Garg, S., & Singh, R. (2014). Need for integration of gender equity in family planning services. *The Indian Journal of Medical Research, 140*(Suppl. 1), S147–S151.
36. Goodale, B. M., Shilaih, M., Falco, L., Dammeier, F., Hamvas, G., & Leeners, B. (2019). Wearable sensors reveal menses-driven changes in physiology and enable prediction of the fertile window: Observational study. *Journal of Medical Internet Research, 21*(4), e13404. doi: 10.2196/13404

37. Gronowski, A. M., & Schindler, E. I. (2014). Women's health. *Scandinavian Journal of Clinical and Laboratory Investigation, 244*, 2–7. doi: 10.3109/00365513.2014.936672
38. Gruskin, S., Zacharias, K., Jardell, W., Ferguson, L., & Khosla, R. (2021). Inclusion of human rights in sexual and reproductive health programming: Facilitators and barriers to implementation. *Global Public Health, 16*(10), 1559–1575. doi: 10.1080/17441692.2020.1828986
39. Gupte, S. (2021). Ethical challenges in the era of new realities in women's health. *International Journal of Gynaecology and Obstetrics (International Federation of Gynaecology and Obstetrics), 153*(1), 1–2. doi: 10.1002/ijgo.13336
40. Hackett, J. (2017). The Importance of holistic care at the end of life. *The Ulster Medical Journal, 86*(2), 143–144
41. Hadjiat, Y. (2023). Healthcare inequity and digital health-A bridge for the divide, or further erosion of the chasm? *PLoS Digital Health, 2*(6), e0000268. doi: 10.1371/journal.pdig.0000268
42. Hall, D. E., Prochazka, A. V., & Fink, A. S. (2012). Informed consent for clinical treatment. CMAJ *Canadian Medical Association Journal, 184*(5), 533–540. doi: 10.1503/cmaj.112120
43. Hall, K. S., Dalton, V., & Johnson, T. R. (2014). Social disparities in women's health service use in the United States: A population-based analysis. *Annals of Epidemiology, 24*(2), 135–143. doi: 10.1016/j.annepidem.2013.10.018
44. Heaman, M. (2001). Conducting health research with vulnerable women: Issues and strategies. *The Canadian Journal of Nursing Research, 33*(3), 81–86.
45. Hornbuckle, L. M., Amutah-Onukagha, N., Bryan, A., Skidmore Edwards, E., Madzima, T., Massey, K., May, L., & Robinson, L. E. (2017). Health disparities in women: Clinical medicine insights. *Women's Health, 10*, 1179562X17709546. doi: 10.1177/1179562X17709546
46. Idris, I. B., Hamis, A. A., Bukhori, A. B. M., Hoong, D. C. C., Yusop, H., Shaharuddin, M. A., Fauzi, N. A. F. A., & Kandayah, T. (2023). Women's autonomy in healthcare decision making: A systematic review. *BMC Women's Health, 23*(1), 643. doi: 10.1186/s12905-023-02792-4
47. Institute of Medicine (US) Committee on Women's Health Research. (2010). *Women's Health Research: Progress, Pitfalls, and Promise*. US National Academies Press.
48. International Conference on Population and Development. (1994). *Indian Medical Tribune, 2*(16), 3.
49. Jacobson, G. M., & Cain, J. M. (2009). Ethical issues related to patient use of complementary and alternative medicine. *Journal of Oncology Practice, 5*(3), 124–126. doi: 10.1200/JOP.0938501
50. Jansen, L. A. (2022). Medical beneficence, nonmaleficence, and patients' well-being. *The Journal of Clinical Ethics, 33*(1), 23–28.
51. Jobson, D., Mar, V., & Freckelton, I. (2022). Legal and ethical considerations of artificial intelligence in skin cancer diagnosis. *The Australasian Journal of Dermatology, 63*(1), e1–e5. doi: 10.1111/ajd.13690
52. Kassahun, A., & Zewdie, A. (2022). Decision-making autonomy in maternal health service use and associated factors among women in Mettu District, Southwest Ethiopia: A community-based cross-sectional study. *BMJ Open, 12*(5), e059307. doi: 10.1136/bmjopen-2021-059307

53. Kaur, R., & Garg, S. (2008). Addressing domestic violence against women: An unfinished agenda. *Indian Journal of Community Medicine (Indian Association of Preventive & Social Medicine), 33*(2), 73–76. doi: 10.4103/0970-0218.40871
54. Kerasidou, A. (2021). Ethics of artificial intelligence in global health: Explainability, algorithmic bias and trust. *Journal of Oral Biology and Craniofacial Research, 11*(4), 612–614. doi: 10.1016/j.jobcr.2021.09.004
55. Kingma, E. (2021). Harming one to benefit another: The paradox of autonomy and consent in maternity care. *Bioethics, 35*(5), 456–464. doi: 10.1111/bioe.12852
56. Konchak, P. S. (2023). Domestic violence: A primer for the primary care physician. *Journal of Osteopathic Medicine, 98*(s12), s11–s14. doi: 10.1515/jom-1998-0125
57. Krause, B., Lavretsky, H., & Dunn, L. B. (2018). Ethical challenges in complementary and alternative medicine. *Focus (American Psychiatric Publishing), 16*(1), 63–66. doi: 10.1176/appi.focus.20170054
58. Leenen, J. P., Scherrenberg, M., Bruins, W., Boyne, J., Vranken, J., Brunner la Rocca, H. P., Dendale, P., & van der Velde, A. E. (2023). Usability of a digital health platform to support home hospitalisation in heart failure patients: A multicenter feasibility study among healthcare professionals. *European Journal of Cardiovascular Nursing, zvad059*. doi: 10.1093/eurjcn/zvad059
59. Li, S., Yang, Q., Niu, S., & Liu, Y. (2023). Effectiveness of remote fetal monitoring on maternal-fetal outcomes: Systematic review and meta-analysis. *JMIR mHealth and uHealth, 11*, e41508. doi: 10.2196/41508
60. Li, T., Marinovich, M. L., & Houssami, N. (2018). Digital breast tomosynthesis (3D mammography) for breast cancer screening and for assessment of screen-recalled findings: Review of the evidence. *Expert Review of Anticancer Therapy, 18*(8), 785–791. doi: 10.1080/14737140.2018.1483243
61. Li, Y., Lozano, M. V., Peña, D., Gulati, I. K., & Jiang, L. (2023). SmartLact8: A bio-inspired robotic breast pump for customized and comfort milk expression. *Biomimetics (Basel, Switzerland), 8*(2), 190. doi: 10.3390/biomimetics8020190
62. Liberman, A. (2020). Ethical issues in women's healthcare: Practice and policy. *The Yale Journal of Biology and Medicine, 93*(4), 636–637.
63. Linton, P. B. (2007). The legal status of abortion in the states if Roe v. Wade is overruled. *Issues in Law & Medicine, 23*(1), 3–43.
64. Lippke, S., Derksen, C., Keller, F. M., Kötting, L., Schmiedhofer, M., & Welp, A. (2021). Effectiveness of communication interventions in obstetrics-a systematic review. *International Journal of Environmental Research and Public Health, 18*(5), 2616. doi: 10.3390/ijerph18052616
65. Liu, J. T., Kovar-Gough, I., Farabi, N., Animikwam, F., Weers, S. B., & Phillips, J. (2019). The role of primary care physicians in providing end-of-life care. *The American Journal of Hospice & Palliative Care, 36*(3), 249–254. doi: 10.1177/1049909118808232
66. Lloyd, K. B., & Hornsby, L. B. (2009). Complementary and alternative medications for women's health issues. *Nutrition in Clinical Practice (American Society for Parenteral and Enteral Nutrition), 24*(5), 589–608. doi: 10.1177/0884533609343001
67. López-Fernández, G., Barrios, M., Goberna-Tricas, J., & Gómez-Benito, J. (2017). Breastfeeding during pregnancy: A systematic review. *Women and birth:*

*Journal of the Australian College of Midwives, 30*(6), e292–e300. doi: 10.1016/j.wombi.2017.05.008
68. Lowe, N. K. (2018). Disparities in the health of women and children. *Journal of Obstetric, Gynecologic, and Neonatal Nursing (JOGNN), 47*(3), 273–274. doi: 10.1016/j.jogn.2018.04.001
69. Lyzwinski, L., Elgendi, M., & Menon, C. (2024). Innovative approaches to menstruation and fertility tracking using wearable reproductive health technology: Systematic review. *Journal of Medical Internet Research, 26*, e45139. doi: 10.2196/45139
70. Malicka, I., Kozłowska, A., Woźniewski, M., Rymaszewska, J., & Szczepańska-Gieracha, J. (2016). The role of social support in women's health and recovery processes. *Psychology, Health & Medicine, 21*(1), 81–91. doi: 10.1080/13548506.2015.1009378
71. Marmarosh, C. L., Sandage, S., Wade, N., Captari, L. E., & Crabtree, S. (2022). New horizons in group psychotherapy research and practice from third wave positive psychology: A practice-friendly review. *Research in Psychotherapy (Milano), 25*(3), 643. doi: 10.4081/ripppo.2022.643
72. Medical Advisory Secretariat. (2010). Robotic-assisted minimally invasive surgery for gynecologic and urologic oncology: An evidence-based analysis. *Ontario Health Technology Assessment Series, 10*(27), 1–118.
73. Mennuti, M. T. (2008). Genetic screening in reproductive health care. *Clinical Obstetrics and Gynecology, 51*(1), 3–23. doi: 10.1097/GRF.0b013e318160f241
74. Mercurio, M. R. (2016). Pediatric obstetrical ethics: Medical decision-making by, with, and for pregnant early adolescents. *Seminars in Perinatology, 40*(4), 237–246. doi: 10.1053/j.semperi.2015.12.013
75. Minh, L. H. N., Tawfik, G. M., Ghozy, S., Hashan, M. R., Nam, N. H., Linh, L. K., Abdelrahman, S. A. M., Quynh, T. T. H., Khoi Quan, N., Nhat Le, T., Ibrahim, H. Y., El-Nile, M. O., Kamel, A. M. A., Giang, H. T. N., & Huy, N. T. (2021). Feto-maternal outcomes of breastfeeding during pregnancy: A systematic review and meta-analysis. *Journal of Tropical Pediatrics, 67*(6), fmab097. doi: 10.1093/tropej/fmab097
76. Mondal, D., Karmakar, S., & Banerjee, A. (2020). Women's autonomy and utilization of maternal healthcare in India: Evidence from a recent national survey. *PLoS One, 15*(12), e0243553. doi: 10.1371/journal.pone.0243553
77. Mondal, H., Haldar, R., & Mondal, S. (2020). Informed consent for telemedicine. *Journal of Family Medicine and Primary Care, 9*(10), 5402–5403. doi: 10.4103/jfmpc.jfmpc_1752_20
78. Moon, A. S., Garofalo, J., Koirala, P., Vu, M. T., & Chuang, L. (2020). Robotic surgery in gynecology. *The Surgical Clinics of North America, 100*(2), 445–460. doi: 10.1016/j.suc.2019.12.007
79. Moylan, C. A., Herrenkohl, T. I., Sousa, C., Tajima, E. A., Herrenkohl, R. C., & Russo, M. J. (2010). The effects of child abuse and exposure to domestic violence on adolescent internalizing and externalizing behavior problems. *Journal of Family Violence, 25*(1), 53–63. doi: 10.1007/s10896-009-9269-9
80. Mullins, M. A., Ruterbusch, J. J., Clarke, P., Uppal, S., Wallner, L. P., & Cote, M. L. (2021). Trends and racial disparities in aggressive end-of-life care for a national sample of women with ovarian cancer. *Cancer, 127*(13), 2229–2237. doi: 10.1002/cncr.33488

81. Nair, A. R., Shivanna, Y. K. G., Illimoottil, J. P., Rachana, A., Mahasampath, G. S., Abraham, S., & Kurian, S. (2022). Common mental disorders among women and its social correlates in an urban marginalized populace in South India. *The International Journal of Social Psychiatry, 68*(7), 1394–1402. doi: 10.1177/00207640211025556
82. Nair, L., & Adetayo, O. A. (2019). Cultural competence and ethnic diversity in healthcare: Plastic and reconstructive surgery. *Global Open, 7*(5), e2219. doi: 10.1097/GOX.0000000000002219
83. Nigusie, A., Endehabtu, B. F., Angaw, D. A., Teklu, A., Mekonnen, Z. A., Feletto, M., Assan, A., Samuel, A., Sheikh, K., & Tilahun, B. (2022). Status of compassionate, respectful, and caring health service delivery: Scoping review. *JMIR Human Factors, 9*(1), e30804. doi: 10.2196/30804
84. Nimmon, L., & Stenfors-Hayes, T. (2016). The "Handling" of power in the physician-patient encounter: Perceptions from experienced physicians. *BMC Medical Education, 16*, 114. doi: 10.1186/s12909-016-0634-0
85. Nisha, Z. (2021). The medicalization of the female body and motherhood: Some biological and existential reflections. *Asian Bioethics Review, 14*(1), 25–40. doi: 10.1007/s41649-021-00185-z
86. Obaid, T. A. (2005). Religion and reproductive health and rights. *Journal of the American Academy of Religion, 73*(4), 1155–1173. doi: 10.1093/jaarel/lfi119
87. O'Neil, A., Sojo, V., Fileborn, B., Scovelle, A. J., & Milner, A. (2018). The #MeToo movement: An opportunity in public health? *Lancet (London), 391*(10140), 2587–2589. doi: 10.1016/S0140-6736(18)30991-7
88. Ormond, K. E., Borensztein, M. J., Hallquist, M. L. G., Buchanan, A. H., Faucett, W. A., Peay, H. L., Smith, M. E., Tricou, E. P., Uhlmann, W. R., Wain, K. E., Coughlin, & C. R. (2021). Defining the critical components of informed consent for genetic testing. *Journal of Personalized Medicine, 11*(12), 1304. doi: 10.3390/jpm11121304
89. Peters, S. A. E., Woodward, M., Jha, V., Kennedy, S., & Norton, R. (2016). Women's health: A new global agenda. *BMJ Global Health, 1*(3), e000080. doi: 10.1136/bmjgh-2016-000080
90. Pfledderer, C. D., Gren, L. H., Frost, C. J., Andrulis, I. L., Chung, W. K., Genkinger, J., Glendon, G., Hopper, J. L., John, E. M., Southey, M., Terry, M. B., & Daly, M. B. (2022). Women's thoughts on receiving and sharing genetic information: Considerations for genetic counseling. *Journal of Genetic Counseling, 31*(6), 1249–1260. doi: 10.1002/jgc4.1599
91. Pillai, V. K., & Gupta, R. (2011). Reproductive rights approach to reproductive health in developing countries. *Global Health Action, 4*. doi: 10.3402/gha.v4i0.8423
92. Pinter, B., Hakim, M., Seidman, D. S., Kubba, A., Kishen, M., & Di Carlo, C. (2016). Religion and family planning. *The European Journal of Contraception & Reproductive Health Care (European Society of Contraception), 21*(6), 486–495. doi: 10.1080/13625187.2016.1237631
93. Posadzki, P., Lee, M. S., Moon, T. W., Choi, T. Y., Park, T. Y., & Ernst, E. (2013). Prevalence of complementary and alternative medicine (CAM) use by menopausal women: A systematic review of surveys. *Maturitas, 75*(1), 34–43. doi: 10.1016/j.maturitas.2013.02.005

94. Prentice, R. L., & Anderson, G. L. (2008). The women's health initiative: Lessons learned. *Annual Review of Public Health, 29*, 131–150. doi: 10.1146/annurev.publhealth.29.020907.090947
95. Ranjit, A., Andriotti, T., Madsen, C., Koehlmoos, T., Staat, B., Witkop, C., Little, S. E., & Robinson, J. (2021). Does universal coverage mitigate racial disparities in potentially avoidable maternal complications? *American Journal of Perinatology, 38*(8), 848–856. doi: 10.1055/s-0040-1701195
96. Rayburn, W. F. (2020). The Role of telemedicine in improving women's health care. *Obstetrics and Gynecology Clinics of North America, 47*(2), xiii–xiv. doi: 10.1016/j.ogc.2020.03.002
97. Ren, Z., Bremer, A. A., & Pawlyk, A. C. (2021). Drug development research in pregnant and lactating women. *American Journal of Obstetrics and Gynecology, 225*(1), 33–42. doi: 10.1016/j.ajog.2021.04.227
98. Rosenbaum, S. (2011). The patient protection and affordable care act: Implications for public health policy and practice. *Public Health Reports (Washington, D.C., 1974), 126*(1), 130–135. doi: 10.1177/003335491112600118
99. Schenker, J. G. (2000). Women's reproductive health: Monotheistic religious perspectives. *International Journal of Gynaecology and Obstetrics, 70*(1), 77–86. doi: 10.1016/s0020-7292(00)00225-3
100. Schenker, J. G., & Eisenberg, V. H. (1997). Ethical issues relating to reproduction control and women's health. *International Journal of Gynaecology and Obstetrics, 58*(1), 167–176. doi: 10.1016/s0020-7292(97)02866-x
101. Schoen, C., Simantov, E., Gross, R., Brammli, S., & Leiman, J. (2003). Disparities in women's health and health care experiences in the United States and Israel: Findings from 1998 National Women's Health Surveys. *Women & Health, 37*(1), 49–70. doi: 10.1300/J013v37n01_04
102. Srikanthan, A., & Reid, R. L. (2008). Religious and cultural influences on contraception. *Journal of Obstetrics and Gynaecology Canada, 30*(2), 129–137. doi: 10.1016/S1701-2163(16)32736-0
103. Srivastava, K. (2012). Women and mental health: Psychosocial perspective. *Industrial Psychiatry Journal, 21*(1), 1–3. doi: 10.4103/0972-6748.110938
104. Stein, D. J., & Nair, M. G. (2000). Psychiatric aspects of women's health. *International Clinical Psychopharmacology, 15 Suppl 3*, S1–S4.
105. Stone, J. (2000). Ethical issues in complementary and alternative medicine. *Complementary Therapies in Medicine, 8*(3), 207–213. doi: 10.1054/ctim.2000.0385
106. Stotland, N. L. (2023). Reproductive rights and women's mental health. *The Psychiatric Clinics of North America, 46*(3), 607–619. doi: 10.1016/j.psc.2023.04.014
107. Tang, L., Li, J., & Fantus, S. (2023). Medical artificial intelligence ethics: A systematic review of empirical studies. *Digital Health, 9*, 20552076231186064. doi: 10.1177/20552076231186064
108. Taylor, R. M. (2013). Ethical principles and concepts in medicine. *Handbook of Clinical Neurology, 118*, 1–9. doi: 10.1016/B978-0-444-53501-6.00001-9
109. Teal, S., & Edelman, A. (2021). Contraception selection, effectiveness, and adverse effects: A review. *JAMA, 326*(24), 2507–2518. doi: 10.1001/jama.2021.21392
110. *The Fourth World Conference on Women*. (1995). *African Population Newsletter, 68*, 4–5.

111. Tjaden, K. (2015). Health disparities between rural and urban women in Minnesota. *Minnesota Medicine, 98*(10), 40–43.
112. Torralbas-Fernández, A., & Calcerrada-Gutiérrez, M. (2016). Using primary care to address violence against women in intimate partner relationships: Professional training needs. *MEDICC Review, 18*(4), 38–41. doi: 10.37757/MR2016.V18.N4.8
113. Tulchinsky, T. H. (2018). Ethical issues in public health. *Case Studies in Public Health,* 277–316. doi: 10.1016/B978-0-12-804571-8.00027-5
114. Tyrer, L. (1999). Introduction of the pill and its impact. *Contraception, 59*(1 Suppl), 11S–16S. doi: 10.1016/s0010-7824(98)00131-0
115. Vahdat, S., Hamzehgardeshi, L., Hessam, S., & Hamzehgardeshi, Z. (2014). Patient involvement in health care decision making: A review. *Iranian Red Crescent Medical Journal, 16*(1), e12454. doi: 10.5812/ircmj.12454
116. van de Roemer, N., Haile, L., & Koch, M. C. (2021). The performance of a fertility tracking device. *The European Journal of Contraception & Reproductive Health Care, 26*(2), 111–118. doi: 10.1080/13625187.2021.1871599
117. Varkey, B. (2021). Principles of clinical ethics and their application to practice. *Medical Principles and Practice, 30*(1), 17–28. doi: 10.1159/000509119
118. Vikas, H., Kini, A., Sharma, N., Gowda, N. R., & Gupta, A. (2021). How informed is the informed consent? *Journal of Family Medicine and Primary Care, 10*(6), 2299–2303. doi: 10.4103/jfmpc.jfmpc_2393_20
119. Webb Hooper, M., & Pérez-Stable, E. J. (2023). Health equity is not possible without addressing disparities. *Health Psychology, 42*(9), 625–627. doi: 10.1037/hea0001306
120. Weitzman, A. (2018). Does increasing women's education reduce their risk of intimate partner violence? Evidence from an education policy reform. *Criminology, 56*(3), 574–607. doi: 10.1111/1745-9125.12181
121. Wong, A. D., & Phillips, S. P. (2023). Gender disparities in end of life care: A scoping review. *Journal of Palliative Care, 38*(1), 78–96. doi: 10.1177/08258597221120707
122. Wright, P. M. (2017). Reducing health disparities for women through use of the medical home model. *Contemporary Nurse, 53*(1), 126–131. doi: 10.1080/10376178.2017.1281086
123. Wright, R. L., Fawson, P. R., Siegel, E., Jones, T., & Stone, K. (2018). Predictors of reproductive autonomy among a rural university population. *Health & Social Work, 43*(4), 235–242. doi: 10.1093/hsw/hly027
124. Wyn, R., & Solis, B. (2001). Women's health issues across the lifespan. *Women's Health Issues, 11*(3), 148–159. doi: 10.1016/s1049-3867(01)00081-0
125. Yoldemir, T. (2022). Telemedicine and women's health. *Climacteric, 25*(5), 425–426. doi: 10.1080/13697137.2022.2106725
126. Zheng, D., He, X., & Jing, J. (2023). Overview of artificial intelligence in breast cancer medical imaging. *Journal of Clinical Medicine, 12*(2), 419–422. doi: 10.3390/jcm12020419
127. Zielinska, A. P., Mullins, E., & Lees, C. (2022). The feasibility of multimodality remote monitoring of maternal physiology during pregnancy. *Medicine, 101*(26), e29566. doi: 10.1097/MD.0000000000029566

## CHAPTER 3

# Music and Aroma Therapy for Female Health: Principles, Methods, and Applications

ANUSHRI JADHAV and VIJAYAPANDI PANDY*

*Corresponding author

## ABSTRACT

This chapter examines the complementary therapeutic roles of essential oils and music therapy in enhancing psychological and physiological health. Essential oils, derived from various plant parts, modulate the hypothalamic–limbic axis, elevating relaxing hormones, while reducing stress-related neurotransmitters. These actions alleviate neuropsychological disturbances and sleep disorders, particularly in menopausal women. Through olfactory stimulation, aromatic compounds influence emotional regulation, while their antiseptic and permeation properties enhance circulation, relieve spasms, promote wound healing, and improve bone health due to their nutrient content. Music therapy, a practice rooted in antiquity, exerts significant psychophysiological benefits by modulating mood, cognition, and immune responses. It enhances neurotransmitter activity particularly, serotonin and dopamine thereby, alleviating anxiety, depression, and stress-related dysfunctions. Music-induced immunomodulation strengthens host defenses, while its regulatory effects on cardiovascular and endocrine systems mitigate the neurotoxic and immunosuppressive consequences of chronic stress. Together, essential oils and music therapy represent holistic, nonpharmacological approaches for restoring emotional balance and promoting overall well-being.

Holistic Approaches for Women's Sustainable Health, Volume 1: Foundations, Innovations, Challenges, and Management. Megh R. Goyal, Anamika Chauhan, and Junaid Ahmad Malik (Eds)


DOI: 10.1201/9781779641632-4

## 3.1 INTRODUCTION

### 3.1.1 AN OVERVIEW OF FEMALE HEALTH

Women's health refers to a wide range of conditions associated with women's mental, social, and physical well-being. Both biological and gender-related variations and sociocultural issues, such as discrimination, unequal power dynamics, and social norms, have an impact on women's health. If women's maternal health, reproductive health, and environmental health are affected, that can cause communicable diseases due to weakening of the immune system and noncommunicable diseases such as neuropsychiatric diseases, metabolic diseases, endocrine diseases, and even cancer [50, 51].

A crucial component of female health is mental wellness. Major depression and anxiety are the most common mental health issues prevalent in women. It is imperative to get guidance from neuropsychiatrist professionals to treat mental health issues. Nonpharmacological management, such as complementary and alternative therapy, is equally important as pharmacological management with available medications to treat depression and anxiety, targeting monoaminergic and GABAergic systems in the brain [50]. Stress can also affect women's reproductive health, such as irregularities in menstruation, earlier menopause, and polycystic ovary syndrome (PCOS), which can cause female infertility. Another crucial component of female health is sexual health. Chronic stress is found to affect sexual health through sympathetic overstimulation (e.g., hypertension) and decrease the blood supply to the genitals, thereby affecting genital arousal (lubrication and pain domains) [22].

### 3.1.2 AROMA AND MUSIC THERAPY IN WOMEN'S HEALTH: AN OVERVIEW

Research has demonstrated that music and aromatherapy can improve the overall health status of women. In comparison to separate interventions, combining aromatherapy and music therapy dramatically enhanced performance in research involving nursing students. Additionally, research has demonstrated that aromatherapy and music therapy together can enhance mental well-being and reduce anxiety, stress, and fear in a variety of contexts [44]. Essential oils obtained from aromatic plants are used in aromatherapy to enhance physical as well as mental wellness. These oils can enhance brain functions when inhaled, and when absorbed via the skin, they can support the healing process throughout the body by moving via the bloodstream. On the other side, music therapy employs music to help people with their social, emotional, cognitive, and physical requirements. It may enhance memory, improve communication, relieve pain, manage stress, and promote overall wellness [52]. There are exciting opportunities to improve female health and well-being owing to the synergistic benefits of aromatherapy and music therapy [44, 52].

This chapter comprehensively explores the potential of aroma and music therapy for the overall well-being of female health. This chapter recommends that music therapy can help to defend against certain bacterial and viral infections by elevating levels of certain defensive biomarkers.

## 3.2 AROMATHERAPY

### *3.2.1 HISTORY*

For millennia, essential oils served an integral part throughout numerous diverse civilizations across the world. Even the most ancient races acknowledged that fragrance essences had a particular influence.

The concept of aromatherapy was coined in 1937 by French scientist Rene-Maurice Gattefosse. Gattefosse discovered that lavender oil relieved his burn. Using essential oils to treat soldiers' wounds during World War II, French surgeon Jean Valnet demonstrated the medical benefits of aromatherapy.

Hippocrates made a substantial contribution to the knowledge of aromatherapy by recording the medicinal benefits of plant essential oils in classical Greek literature. He allegedly stated that having a scented massage and aromatic bath every day is the path to health, emphasizing the significance of aromatics in fostering well-being at the time. Aromatic flowers and incense have long been staples of our religious ceremonies and acts of worship. The natural fragrances were believed to be associated with soul-cleansing and spiritual development. The Buddha mentioned the use of aromatic plants in healing; Jivaka was the most well-known physician at that time.

The core scriptures of Ayurveda, Charaka Samhita, and Sushruta Samhita state that a significant portion of Ayurvedic remedies involves the use of aromatic plants and their parts for therapy and healing. Aromatic plants were used for therapy during the Buddha's time, despite mentioning the name of Jivaka, the most famous physician of that age.

The kings and queens often took baths in water enriched with extracts of aromatic plants, such as rose, jasmine, champaka, nag champa, and so on, for total body–mind relaxation. It is also claimed that the real key to the Mughal women's beauty was found in these luxurious baths [19].

### 3.2.2 PRINCIPLE

Aromatherapy is a subspecialty of complementary medicine that employs essential oils by massage, bathing, or direct inhalation. Unsaturated and saturated hydrocarbons, ketones, terpenes, phenols, oxides, esters, ethers, aldehydes, and alcohol are present in essential oils, which can give them a unique odor. Essential oils have gained recognition for their therapeutic properties on the body, mind, and soul. Numerous scientists have thoroughly documented their adaptable properties, which include being antibacterial, antiviral, and anti-inflammatory, as well as immune-boosting and having a relaxing effect, hormone, glandular, circulatory, emotional, and alertness- and memory-enhancing properties. The pharmacological effects of essential oil plants are given in Table 3.1.

**TABLE 3.1** Different Types of Essential Oil Plants and Their Pharmacological Effects

| Essential Oil Plant | Pharmacological Effects |
|---|---|
| **Bergamot** 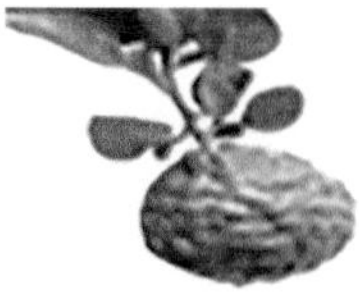 | Eases symptoms of menopause like hot flashes and mood swings |
| **Clary sage** 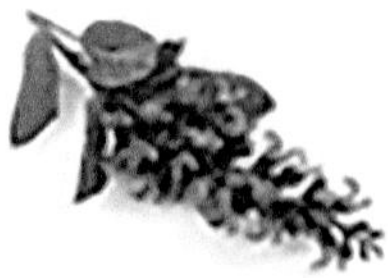 | Helps to maintain the hormonal balance and alleviates menstrual cramps and PMS (premenstrual syndrome) symptoms |

**TABLE 3.1** *(Continued)*

| Essential Oil Plant | Pharmacological Effects |
|---|---|
| **Frankincense** 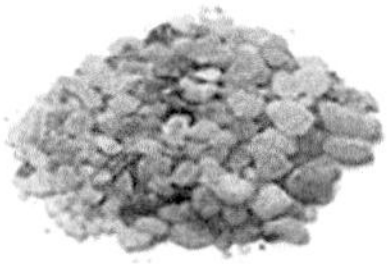 | Alleviates menstrual cramps and PMS symptoms |
| **Geranium** 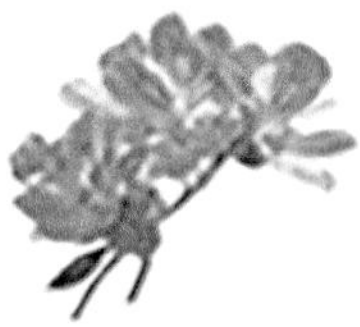 | Reduces physical and mental stress, promotes focus and calmness, and soothes symptoms of menstruation and menopause |
| **Lavender** 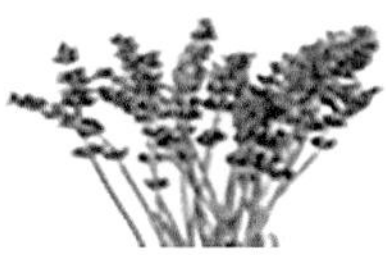 | Reduces stress and anxiety and promotes better sleep |
| **Lemon** 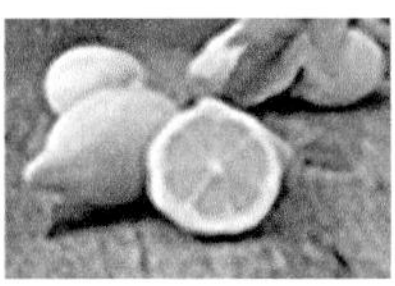 | Boosts energy and mood, and alleviates morning sickness during pregnancy |
| **Neroli** 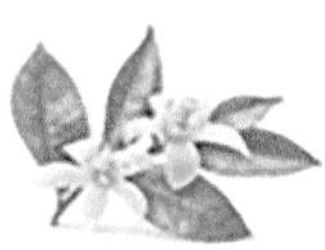 | Reverses depression and low libido during menopause |
| **Peppermint** 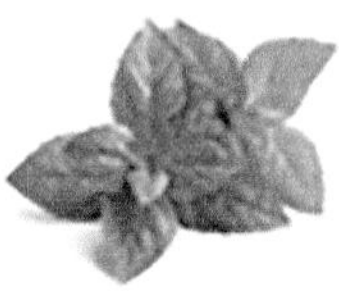 | Alleviates morning sickness during pregnancy |

The olfactory bulb relays the signal to the limbic and hypothalamic regions of the brain. These impulses trigger the brain to release neurotransmitters, such as endorphin and serotonin, which connect our nervous and other bodily systems, assuring the desired change and bringing about a feeling of relaxation. Calming oils release endorphins, noradrenaline, and serotonin, respectively, which have an intended impact on the body and mental health. The fundamental of aromatherapy is to inhale and externally apply the aromatic oil to balance the mental and physiological balance. These oils are known to reduce stress and provide people with a boost of energy, so they are ready to go back to work the next day [2, 27].

### *3.2.3 METHODS OF AROMATHERAPY*

#### *3.2.3.1 COSMETIC AROMATHERAPY*

Scientific research has demonstrated that essential oils show antioxidant, purifying, calming, whitening, and antiaging properties for the skin. Various benefits of essential oils are linked to their distinct chemical profile. Certain perfumes may be invigorating, boosting, or calming effect, which enhances the sensory experience with skincare regimens. Aromas have an important property in masking up odors of fatty acids, oils, and surfactants. Aromatherapy encourages the health of the hair and scalp by moisturizing it, enhancing blood circulation, and eliminating specific hair issues [2].

#### *3.2.3.2 MASSAGE AROMATHERAPY*

Massage is the artful stimulation of soft tissue with the hands, with the primary goal of promoting blood flow and releasing tension in the muscles. The body generates endorphins, which are painkillers when you massage your skin. A massage simply relieves muscle tension, which lowers stress hormones like cortisol that impair the immune system and induce feelings of comfort and well-being [2].

#### *3.2.3.3 OLFACTORY AROMATHERAPY*

Daily exposure to a variety of odorants showing olfactory enrichment is effective for improving memory and neurogenesis. To be effective pharmacologically, a volatile compound must enter the bloodstream *via* nasal or lung mucosa or diffuse directly into the olfactory neurons and limbic system of the brain. The relieving effect of aromatherapy against stress is accompanied by delightful scents that trigger olfactory memories [50].

### 3.2.4 SCIENTIFIC EVIDENCE RELATED TO AROMATHERAPY

The therapeutic potential of aromatherapy against various diseases and the probable mechanisms are shown in Figure 3.1.

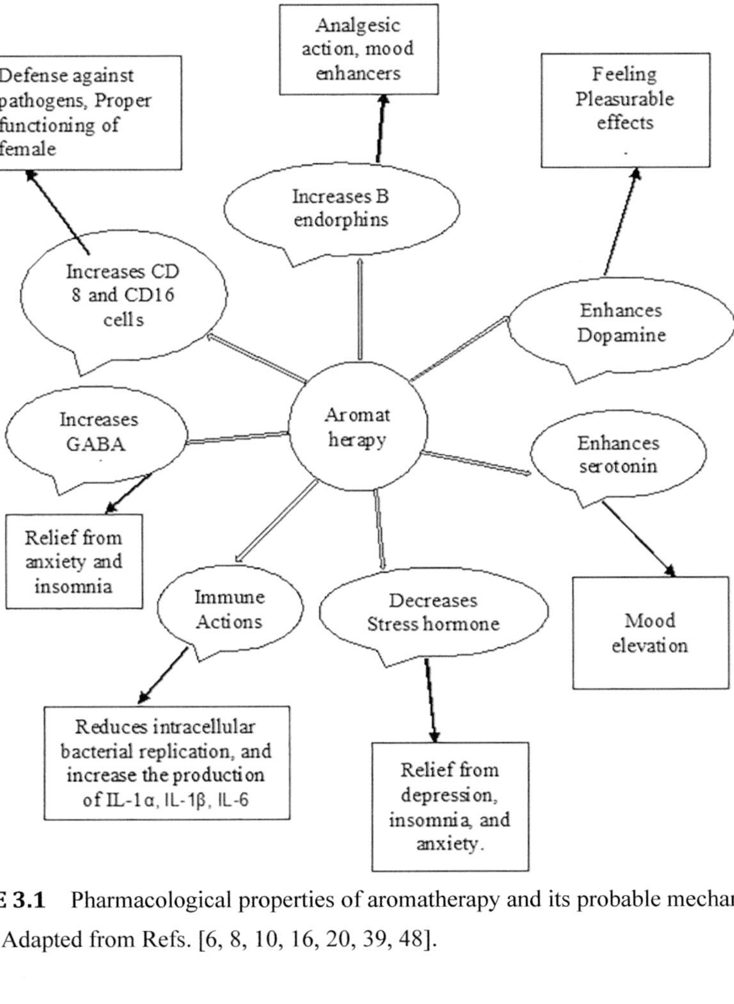


**FIGURE 3.1** Pharmacological properties of aromatherapy and its probable mechanisms.

*Source*: Adapted from Refs. [6, 8, 10, 16, 20, 39, 48].

### *3.2.5 IMPACT ON QUALITY OF LIFE OF FEMALE*

#### *3.2.5.1 DEPRESSION*

Depression is a severe mental illness that particularly impacts women. Clinical depression affects women approximately twice as frequently as males [29, 40]. It has been shown that aromatherapy (especially using essential oils such as bergamot, lavender, and chamomile) may help women cope with depression. Numerous research studies have demonstrated that massage and inhalation aromatherapies were found to minimize the various symptoms of major depression when compared to control groups. Interestingly, massage with aromatherapy seems to have more positive effects than aromatherapy inhalation [15, 23, 35, 42].

Aromatherapy may be therapeutically effective in treating symptoms of depression through multiple mechanisms, such as the augmentation of monoaminergic systems, importantly serotonergic-mediated mechanisms, stimulation of release of neurotrophic factor, the endocrine system's management, especially inhibition of stress hormone cortisol release, and overall, the encouragement of neurogenesis pathways [8]. In the case of depression, aromatherapy can facilitate the various responsible molecular mechanisms like cAMP element binding protein-signaling pathways, and neurotransmitter systems such as serotonin, dopamine, and GABA, and inhibit stress-mediated HPA axis [49]. Musk demonstrated to alleviate depressive-like symptoms by elevating brain-derived neurotrophic factor (BDNF) expression in the hippocampal regions [8]. Although essential oils are helpful as adjunctive therapies for depression, they should not be used without the supervision of a medical care expert.

#### *3.2.5.2 ANXIETY*

Women frequently have stresses and strains, such as managing jobs, family obligations, and cultural expectations, which can exacerbate anxiety. In addition, hormonal changes throughout adolescence, menstruation, pregnancy, childbirth, and menopause may contribute to the emergence of anxiety in women [3]. Aromatherapy has an impact on specific biomarkers for anxiety, such as the level of cortisol and salivary endocrinological stress markers. Studies have shown that controlling the activity of neurotransmitter systems, including the GABAergic, dopaminergic, and serotonergic systems, may be involved in the effectiveness of aromatherapy for anxiety [18].

Aromatherapy for anxiety is supported by various scientific evidence, and research has demonstrated that both massage and inhalation aromatherapies significantly reduced anxiety levels in a variety of circumstances [34]. Certain essential oils, such as orange, lavender, and rose, have been shown to have anxiolytic properties and to be beneficial in reducing anxiety symptoms [48]. Research has indicated that orange essence has anxiolytic properties, and that aromatherapy is a useful tool for easing anxiety symptoms in patients, especially in cases of postpartum women and those who are undergoing heart and stomach surgery [48].

#### *3 2.5.3 SCHIZOPHRENIA*

Women suffering from schizophrenia are more likely than men to be outwardly aggressive, physically active, domineering, have more sexual delusions, and are emotionally unstable [26]. Certain calming and soothing properties of certain essential oils are well known, and they may be able to alleviate some of the symptoms associated with schizophrenia [16]. Aromatherapy affects oxidative stress, neurotrophic factors, including BDNF, and inflammatory markers, are among the many biomarkers linked to schizophrenia itself.

#### *3.2.5.4 DEMENTIA*

Parkinson's disease (PD) and Alzheimer's disease (AD) have clinical and pathological similarities with dementia. Reports from the United States and much of Europe indicate that women account for up to two-thirds of clinically diagnosed cases of dementia and AD. Aromatherapy has demonstrated promising memory enhancement and protection against cognitive decline in AD and PD patients. The quality of life has been enhanced for dementia patients, especially when implemented in conjunction with specific essential oils like lavender and lemon balm [47].

#### *3.2.5.5 INSOMNIA*

The primary clinical features include challenges in both initiating and maintaining sleep, frequent awakenings throughout the night, struggles to return to sleep after waking up or waking up prematurely, with an inability to resume sleeping. These symptoms are often accompanied by fatigue, diminished energy levels, mood disruptions, and impaired cognitive functions, such as difficulties with attention, concentration, and memory. There is a substantial body of evidence indicating that women report experiencing insomnia more frequently compared to men. Aromatherapy, within the realm of complementary alternative medicine, has a significant effect on mood and sleep modulation. In case of insomnia, the inhalation of lavender oil for a short period is effective [39].

#### *3.2.5.6 REPRODUCTIVE HEALTH*

Aromatherapy has shown to reduce menopausal symptoms, especially anxiety, depression, and physical and vasomotor symptoms in a study using lavender inhalation. Serum levels of estrogens did not considerably decrease, but combined oil aromatherapy with fennel, lavender, rose, and geranium, dramatically enhanced sexual activity in the menopausal period. By improving blood circulation, diminishing stress hormone levels by increasing endorphin release, and raising serotonin release by encouraging parasympathetic activation, massage reduces the spasm that accompanies menstrual pain. Women benefit immensely from clary sage as its tonic, which is used to treat uterine and womb-related issues. It also regulates menstruation, relieves stress and cramps in the muscles, and has aphrodisiac and seductive properties [10].

#### *3.2.5.7 PREGNANCY AND POSTPARTUM*

The prevalence of nausea and vomiting was effectively reduced by using peppermint oil inhalation aromatherapy. It appears that the use of ginger, cardamom, lemon, and mint in aromatherapy was a useful way to manage symptoms of nausea and vomiting, with no adverse consequences [24]. Mothers who breastfeed their babies utilize herbs like ginger, fenugreek, garlic, chamomile, and thistle as complementary and alternative therapies in addition to massage, acupuncture, and chiropractic care to boost the production of milk [20].

#### *3.2.5.8 INFECTIONS*

In contrast to men, women are more susceptible to some infectious diseases, and their illnesses tend to be more severe for a variety of reasons, including biological variations, societal injustices, and societal norms [17]. Oils derived from the Eucalyptus plant have been utilized to treat respiratory disorders such as sinusitis, bronchitis, asthma, coughs, and throat infections. Several essential oils were evaluated for their antibacterial properties against both Gram-negative and Gram-positive bacteria and antifungal properties [6]. The tea tree itself possesses features that are immune-stimulating, antiviral, insecticidal, antibacterial, and anti-inflammatory. If carefully and thoroughly investigated, they can be excellent substitutes for antibiotics because tea tree oil has been shown to reduce reactivity to histamine of both flare and weal in humans. Tea tree oil is utilized in most head lice infestation preventative measures. Tea tree oil's anticholinesterase ability accounts for its insecticidal effects [2].

#### *3.2.5.9 GENERAL WELL-BEING*

Essential oils have the potential to mitigate a range of health issues that women encounter throughout their lives, including but not limited to menstruation, pregnancy, childbirth, the postpartum period, and menopause [6]. Excellent skin tonic qualities of essential oils used in aromatherapy can enhance the appearance and health of the skin. Certain essential oils, such as cedarwood, peppermint, and rosemary, are well known for their capacity to increase hair growth and decrease hair loss [37].

### ***3.2.6 CASE STUDIES***

#### *3.2.6.1 CHILDBIRTH AND PREGNANCY*

One study evaluated the impact of orange essential oil aromatherapy on labor anxiety. The results indicate that women's anxiety levels during labor were drastically lowered when they were exposed to orange essential oil [37].

#### *3.2.6.2 MENOPAUSE*

Another study examined the impact of aromatherapy using *Lavandula angustifolia* Mill-*Citrus bergamia* essential oil (lavender and bergamot) in conjunction with mindfulness-based intervention (MBI) on postmenopausal women's anxiety, depression, and sexual function [32]. The findings show that lavender–bergamot aromatherapy and MBI were equally successful in enhancing emotions, nervousness, and sexual function.

Furthermore, another study found that inhaling lavender oil considerably reduced menopausal hot flashes [16].

## 3.3 MUSIC THERAPY

Music possesses the remarkable ability to elevate the human spirit, provides solace to the heart, and ignites the soul with inspiration. Moreover, it can bolster immunity, rendering it a potent form of therapy [46]. Growing interest and studies have been carried out on the impacts of music therapy on the health of women, predominantly because of the desire to learn more about how music might improve the psychological, cognitive, and social elements of women's lives. Psychological stress cannot be eradicated, but it can be seen differently, and its capacity to cope with stressors is modified in certain ways. Studies have demonstrated that music has a calming effect on the cardiovascular and endocrine systems, which has led to its adaptation as a stress management tool. Music therapy has the power to elicit strong emotions and emotional catharsis [46]. This study explores the benefits of music therapy for women's health, looking at both the mechanisms that may underlie its therapeutic effects and the benefits supported by research. This study shed light on the various ways that music therapy can improve women's health and well-being, addressing both general health issues and particular requirements that are gender-specific, by evaluating new research and clinical applications [46].

### *3.3.1 HISTORY*

With incredible success, music therapy is being employed extensively in the hospital for patients in the gynecology and neurology departments. Like other artistic mediums, music has perpetually been regarded from an aesthetic point of view, and its restorative properties have been attested to in numerous global musical traditions. From fostering the development of strong emotional bonds between newborns and their parents to providing essential, compassionate, and sensitive palliative care toward the end of life, music may play a critical role in aiding individuals at all phases of life.

From ancient times, music was employed as a medium for social gatherings, entertainment, and religious prayer during religious events. Mantra chanting has been prevalent since the era of the Vedas. Vedic Richas or Mantras were chanted at different Yajnas utilizing various approaches and methodologies for satisfying worldly and spiritual objectives since they were seen to be energizing, powerful, and heavenly [43]. Considering this, spiritual leaders with skilled instrumentalists, good vocalists with a naturally melodic voice, knowledgeable about the Vedas and Vedic rites, and leaders experienced in these areas were deemed appropriate for this role. Music is represented by the Sama Veda among the four Vedas. Because of this, the Sama Veda is regarded as the most prominent of the four and is known as the source of Indian music [43].

Pythagoras, a Greek philosopher from the sixth century who is recognized as the father of both geometry and music therapy, felt that music had a profound effect on health and frequently recommended music and diet to maintain physical and mental balance [24].

### *3.3.2 PRINCIPLE*

Music possesses a greater ability to affect women since they are more sentimental and sensitive than men. According to a novel study, women are more prone than men to exhibit an increase in pain tolerance while listening to their favorite music. The application and effectiveness of music therapy in the context of female health are guided by several core principles. These guidelines highlight how evidence-based, modified, and holistic music therapy treatments are when they are designed to address the special requirements of women. The following are the key concepts of music therapy for women's health [33]:

- **Cultural sensitivity:** In the field of female health, music therapy promotes and integrates cultural diversity, realizing the impact of cultural backgrounds on health-related attitudes and behaviors.
- **Holistic approach:** Female health tends to comprise more than just physical issues throughout music therapy. To improve overall well-being, it addresses all aspects of a person by acknowledging the interconnection of physical, emotional, cognitive, and social components.
- **Individualized care:** To enhance therapeutic outcomes, music therapy adopts a tailored approach, adapting interventions to each woman's particular requirements, goals, and circumstances.
- **Strengths-based perspective:** The inherent qualities, resilient behavior, and coping strategies of women are emphasized and

strengthened through music therapy. Music therapy fosters women's empowerment, self-awareness, and positive self-esteem by promoting strengths rather than deficiencies. The development of empathy, compassion, and therapeutic interactions between therapists and women is essential to music therapy. Women can feel heard, acknowledged, and understood in a nonjudgmental and supportive environment provided by therapists, which builds emotional connection and trust.

Eliminating the avoidance strategy and facilitating the elaboration of feelings and distress can be achieved by bringing out emotions and thoughts through both verbal and nonverbal communication and exploration techniques, such as dance and body movement, artistic endeavors, and expressive writing [43]. Adrenaline, the adrenal medullary hormones, is released because of the sympathetic adrenal medullary system activating the autonomic nervous system. The anterior pituitary releases ACTH in response to the hypothalamus producing corticotropin-releasing factor, which is part of the hypothalamic-pituitary-adrenal system. Prolactin and glucocorticoids are subsequently released from the adrenal cortex in response to blood levels of ACTH. Moreover, glucocorticoids suppress the immune system's effectiveness by preventing the release and activity of cytokines and antibodies. It has been demonstrated that listening to music that soothes dramatically lowers cortisol and ACTH levels, increases salivary immunoglobulin A, and reduces subjective anxiety [43].

### 3.3.3 TYPES OF MUSIC NOTES

The 72 scales that together make up the Melakarta system is organized into two sections of six sectors each in the South Indian (Carnatic) musical system. Based on the mathematical formula used, certain emotional states are amplified through various tints in each sector. The various types of musical notes and their pharmacological effects are shown in Table 3.2 [4].

### 3.3.4 SCIENTIFIC EVIDENCE RELATED TO MUSIC THERAPY

The therapeutic benefits and probable mechanisms involved in music therapy are shown in Figure 3.2.

**TABLE 3.2** Types of Musical Notes and Their Pharmacological Effects [4]

| Types of Musical Notes | Pharmacological Effects |
|---|---|
| Dhirashankarabaranam | Evokes a cheerful, peaceful, and energetic vibe; express pleasant and uplifting feelings |
| Karaharapriya | Gradually eliminate sadness first, and subsequently promote peace and tranquility |
| Mayamalavagowla | Strengthens numerous intelligence-related skills, including focus, attention, memory, and the ability to build connections |
| Mlechakaliyani | Addresses sentimental and affective anxiety |

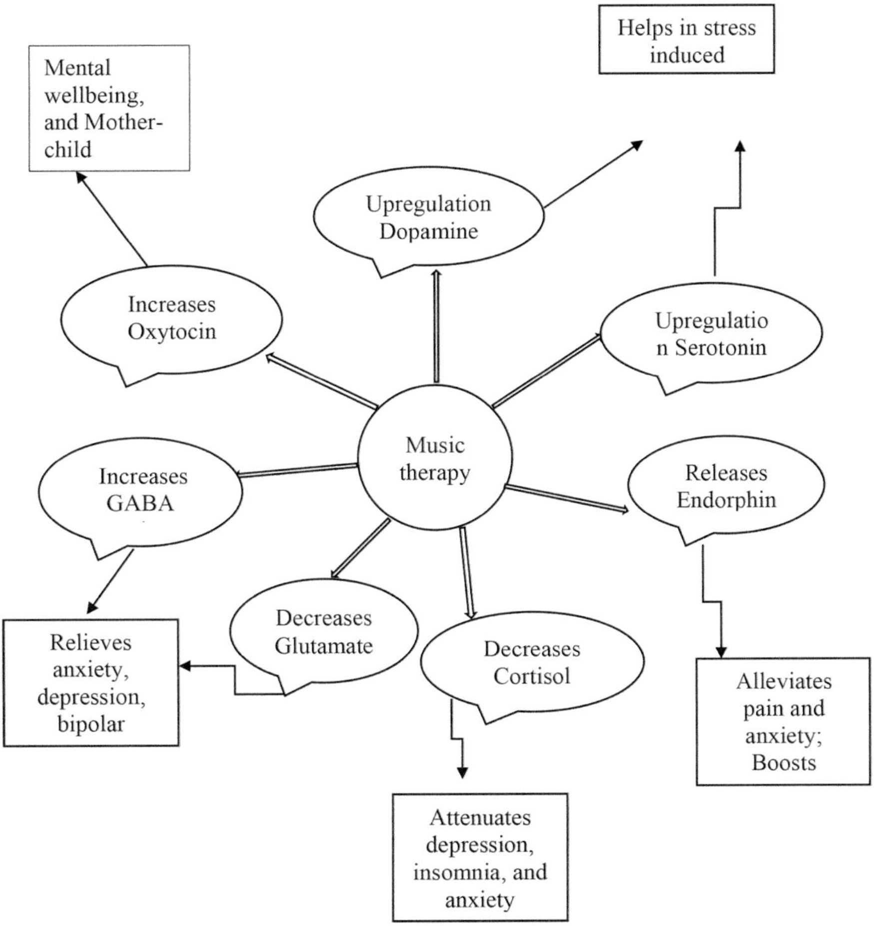


**FIGURE 3.2** Therapeutic benefits of music therapy and its probable mechanisms.

*Source*: Adapted from Refs. [11, 14, 25, 28, 30, 31, 33, 38, 41, 45].

### 3.3.5 IMPACT ON FEMALE'S QUALITY OF LIFE

#### 3.3.5.1 DEPRESSION

Music is a potent stimulant that generates and modifies feelings and emotions. In general, music therapy targets the emotional, cognitive, social, and neurobiological elements of depression, providing a comprehensive approach to treating the illness. It might not be an effective treatment on its own for severe depression, but it can be a useful adjuvant therapy to help with more conventional methods like medicine and psychotherapy [1]. According to studies, treatment as usual (TAU) combined with music therapy is more effective than TAU alone. Motivation, self-perception, and coping strategies with challenging emotional states might be influenced by music. The primary biological indicator of stress response is blood cortisol level. It has been demonstrated that listening to music that soothes dramatically lowers cortisol [45].

#### 3.3.5.2 ANXIETY

Women who have endured trauma can benefit from and integrate from music therapy. Singing and vocalizing, drumming, musical improvised music lyric assessment, composing music, and guided meditation with music comprise a few of the approaches. Research suggests that women's anxiety levels during pregnancy and caesarean delivery may be positively impacted by music therapy [7, 14]. In one study, researchers studied the way women's physiological parameters, anxiety levels, and satisfaction during gynecological exams were affected by music therapy. They discovered that music therapy can lower anxiety and raise contentment [14].

#### 3.3.5.3 SCHIZOPHRENIA

Music therapy can increase emotional expressiveness, improve general functioning and quality of life, and address the difficulties and symptoms of schizophrenia in women [21]. For patients who lack confidence and may find it difficult to talk openly about their challenges and trauma, music therapy, in which the patient and therapist come up with a song on the spot, improves their clinical outcome. In group treatment sessions, music therapy for schizophrenia usually entails a variety of activities such as composing songs, playing instruments, and listening to music. These activities are all intended to address the individual's particular challenges and symptoms [5].

### *3.3.5.4 DEMENTIA*

The syndrome of dementia is becoming more prevalent, and although medication is a choice, its potential benefits are restricted [28]. On the other hand, patients with dementia can retain music, particularly biographically relevant music, which can improve their quality of life by reducing symptoms associated with dementia and avoiding deficits. Benefits of music therapy for dementia patients include reduced depressive symptoms, greater joy, enhanced quality of life, and improved communication skills [9, 28].

### *3.3.5.5 INSOMNIA*

The insomnia is marked by symptoms that occur both during the day and at night. Music can quickly trigger emotions that generate interactions between cognitive and response systems. Patients suffering from insomnia may find that the music resonates with them, and listening to music has been suggested as a therapeutic technique for treating insomnia. Music therapy is a nonpharmacological way to improve sleep quality and may reduce the feeling of tiredness and frustration associated with insomnia [31, 33]. Women suffer from insomnia at a higher rate than men experience. One of the main signs of the menopause transition is changes in sleep patterns. The blood level of noradrenaline, which is linked to the onset of sleep, is lowered by music. Music can reduce the fatigue and frustration associated with insomnia and is a nonpharmacological intervention to enhance sleep [31, 33].

### *3.3.5.6 MUSIC AND EMOTIONAL HEALTH*

Many physiological parameters have been investigated in connection with music therapy for women's emotional health. The indicators include blood pressure, levels of cortisol, and the rhythm of the heart [41]. Additionally, it has been demonstrated that music therapy affects numerous brain regions related to emotion, mobility, cognition, and sensory processing, all of which can contribute to emotional well-being. All things considered, music therapy can benefit physiological indicators of women's mental well-being and emotional health [12].

### *3.3.5.7 NEURONAL HEALTH*

By modulating steroid hormone secretion, music listening promotes neurogenesis—the development, regeneration, and repair of cerebral nerves. In addition to influencing the levels of hormones like cortisol (C), testosterone (T), and estragon (E), scientists also think that music has an impact on the receptor genes and proteins that are linked to these hormones [11]. Hormone replacement therapy has been demonstrated to help preventing dementia and AD; nevertheless, side effects have also been reported, and the clinical implementation of this treatment faces significant obstacles [11]. It has been suggested that hormone replacement therapy, along with music therapy, improves the clinical outcome against memory impairment.

### *3.3.5.8 REPRODUCTIVE HEALTH*

Studies on the impact of music therapy on female reproductive health have looked specifically at assisted reproduction and stress management. Music therapy can also be used to better customize lifestyles and control stress in cases involving gynecological problems, such as PCOS, infertility, and so on [30]. Researchers included randomized controlled trials that examined music therapy with no music intervention in a study involving 793 IVF participants. This study discovered that music therapy significantly reduced pain and anxiety scores in the music therapy women group. Also, music therapy had a rise in the clinical pregnancy rate when compared to the nonmusical group; nevertheless, this difference was not statistically significant [36].

### *3.3.5.9 PREGNANCY*

When the thalamus is stimulated by music, it transfers impulses via the reticular activating system to the cerebrum, where it filters perceptual information that influences emotions, moods, and cognition [38]. In Ayurvedic prenatal care, Priya Shabda (pleasant voice/music) was highlighted to support both mother and fetal welfare and growth and development. Specific Mantras are also claimed to help with easy labor and to treat difficult or obstructed labor [43]. Research has demonstrated that a mother's contact and rhythmic motions, which she cocreates with her child when they engage in musical activities, are essential to the child's enjoyment and the well-being of the mother–child bond [38].

### *3.3.5.10 IMMUNOMODULATION*

Depressive state and psychological stress have an impact on the immune system and can lead to dysregulation, which alters humoral and cellular immunity and raises health risks. Psychoneuroimmunological impacts of music demonstrated that different neurotransmitters, cytokines, and hormones are being affected by music. The immune system is a sophisticated network of structures and functions that has developed over time to defend humans against illness. It is made up of both molecular and cellular components. After being exposed to a variety of musical genres, including both calming and stimulating music, salivary immunoglobulin A (s-IgA), a first-line defense against bacterial and viral infections and a trustworthy indicator of the functional state of the entire mucosal immune system, is particularly responsive to music. Researchers found that after singing, amateur choir members had a significant rise in s-IgA and that listening to choral music reduced their salivary cortisol levels [25].

### *3.3.5.11 GENERAL WELL-BEING*

The immune system's performance is improved by the social contact, emotional expression, and mutual support that music therapy group sessions offer. Social support stimulates neural pathways linked to resilience and stress interruptions, which lowers inflammation and boosts the immune system. Music therapy aids recovery from infections and enhances general immunological resilience by providing social connection and support [18]. Women's general well-being is boosted by engaging with music therapy groups, which can promote social connections and relationships. Women can benefit from music therapy in terms of strengthening their sense of identity, especially after significant life transitions or traumatic experiences [18].

### 3.3.6 CASE STUDIES

#### 3.3.6.1 MENTAL HEALTH

Research has shown that music therapy can assist in lowering depression and enhancing women's mental health. For instance, research comparing women receiving music therapy to those not receiving it revealed that the former had lower levels of sadness and less menopausal symptoms [13]. Another study that focuses on Taiwanese pregnant women demonstrated the beneficial effects of music therapy in lowering stress, anxiety, and depression during the gestational period [14].

#### 3.3.6.2 PREGNANCY

Pregnant women's mental health has also been reported to benefit from music therapy. According to studies, listening to music during pregnancy improves a woman's mood and reduces postpartum depression symptoms. To sum out, music therapy provides a safe and nonpharmacological way to enhance the mental health, menopausal symptoms, and pregnancy-related problems of women. For an exhaustive examination of the opportunities and mechanisms of music therapy in boosting women's health across various life phases, more research is required [14].

## 3.4 FUTURE PERSPECTIVES

The prospects of aromatherapy and music therapy suggest an upsurge in interest in combining these two complementary modalities for improved sensory experiences.

Future studies exploring the potential benefits of aromatherapy and music therapy in a variety of contexts, including managing stress and anxiety, relieving depression and psychotic symptoms, and improving the quality of sleep, learning, and overall well-being of female health, are likely to be carried out. It is feasible that these therapies will get greater acceptance and be incorporated into conventional medical procedures and wellness regimens as the understanding and importance of these complementary therapies increase.

Schematic description of the signaling cascade of opioidergic, serotoninergic, GABAergic, oxytocinergic, and dopaminergic systems and stress-associated HPA axis system involved in aromatherapy and music therapy.

| | |
|---|---|
| 5 HT—5-hydroxytryptamine | HPA—hypothalamic pituitary adrenal axis |
| cAMP—cyclic adenosine monophosphate | IP3—inositol triphosphate |
| CD38—cyclic ADP ribose hydrolase | MAPK—mitogen activated protein kinase |
| *CREB*—cAMP response element-binding protein | MEK2—mitogen-activated protein kinase 2 |
| CRH—corticotropin-releasing hormone | Myd88—myeloid differentiation primary response 88 |
| *DA—dopamine* | NF-κB—*nuclear factor kappa B* |
| DAG—diacylglycerol | OXTR—oxytocin receptor |
| EGFR—epidermal growth factor receptor | PKA—*protein kinase A* |
| ER β—estrogen receptor β | PLC—phospholipase C |
| ERK2—extracellular signal-regulated kinase 2 | SOD—superoxide dismutase |
| GABA—gamma-aminobutyric acid | TLR4—toll-like receptor |
| | TRPV4—transient receptor potential cation channel subfamily V member 4 |

## 3.5 SUMMARY

There are potential benefits of aroma and music therapy in lowering anxiety and stress levels and enhancing mood and efficiency. Aromatherapy utilizes essential oils to stimulate the olfactory system, which can influence emotions, memory, and even physiological responses.

Music therapy can engage various cognitive and emotional processes, offering therapeutic benefits for a wide range of conditions, from depression to neurological disorders. Figure 3.3 describes the effect of aroma and music therapy on the central nervous system for their neuropharmacological effects. Together alongside conventional medications to treat various CNS disorders, aromatherapy, and music therapy can provide complementary and synergistic therapeutic benefits to treat various neurological diseases such as depression, anxiety, and psychosis, and improve overall well-being in women's health.

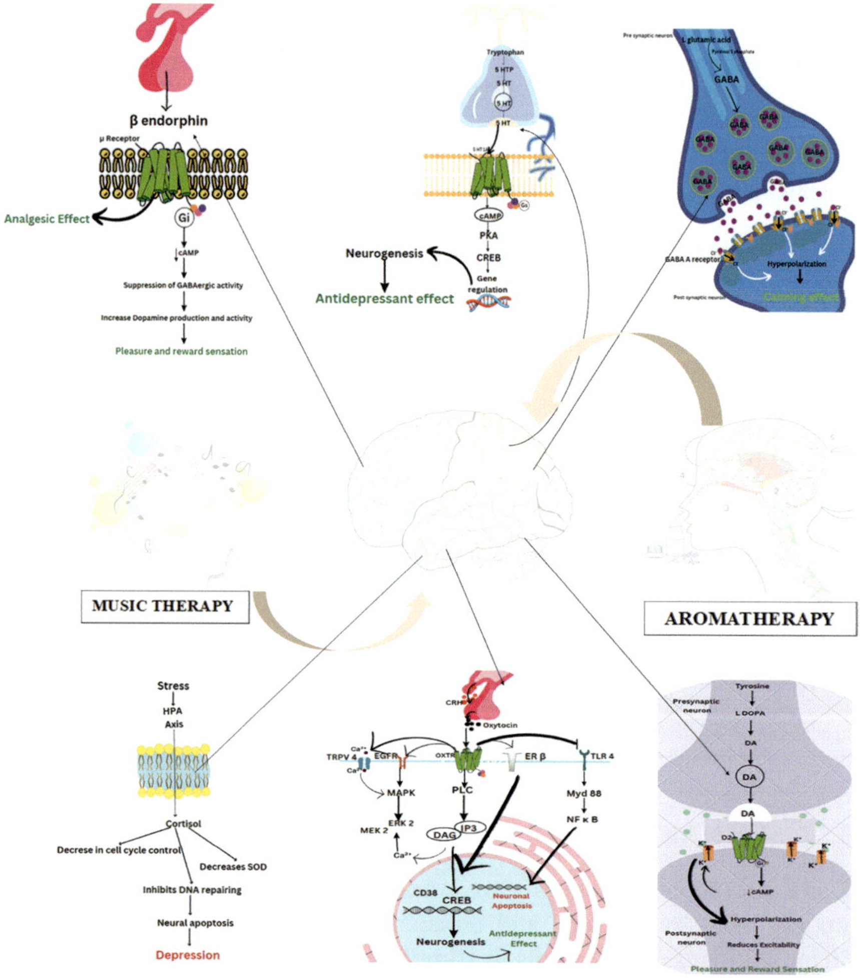


**FIGURE 3.3** Impact of aroma and music therapy on the central nervous system:


## ACKNOWLEDGMENTS

The authors thank Dr. Neeraj Mahindroo, the Dean of the School of Health Sciences and Technology, MIT WPU, Pune, for his constant encouragement and support for doing this research. The authors extend their sincere thanks to Canva software for the creation of the images presented in the manuscript.

## KEYWORDS


- **aroma therapy**
- **essential oils**
- **female health**
- **polycystic ovary syndrome**
- **pharmacological effects**


## REFERENCES


1. Aalbers, S., Fusar-Poli, L., Freeman, R. E., Spreen, M., Ket, J. C., Vink, A. C., Maratos, A., Crawford, M., Chen, X. J., & Gold, C. (2017). Music therapy for depression. *The Cochrane Database of Systematic Reviews*, *11*(11), CD004517. doi: 10.1002/14651858.CD004517.pub3
2. Babar, A., Naser, A., Saiba, S., Aftab, A., & Shah, A. (2015). Essential oils used in aromatherapy: A systemic review. *Asian Pacific Journal of Tropical Biomedicine*, *5*(8), 601–611. doi: 10.1016/j.apjtb.2015.05.007
3. Barati, F., Nasiri, A., Akbari, N., & Sharifzadeh, G. (2016). The effect of aromatherapy on anxiety in patients. *Nephro-urology Monthly*, *8*(5), e38347. doi: 10.5812/numonthly.38347
4. Barbara, L. W. (1983). A psychotherapeutic classification of music therapy practices: A continuum of procedures. *Music Therapy Perspectives*, *1*(2), 8–12. doi: 10.1093/mtp/1.2.8
5. Bleibel, M., El Cheikh, A., & Sadier, N. S. (2023). The effect of music therapy on cognitive functions in patients with Alzheimer's disease: A systematic review of randomized controlled trials. *Alzheimer's Research & Therapy*, *15*(1), 65. doi: 10.1186/s13195-023-01214-9
6. Burns, E., Zobbi, V., Panzeri, D., Oskrochi, R., & Regalia, A. (2007). Aromatherapy in childbirth: A pilot randomised controlled trial. *BJOG: International Journal of Obstetrics and Gynaecology*, *114*(7), 838–844. doi: 10.1111/j.1471-0528.2007.01381.x
7. Chang, S. C., & Chen, C. H. (2005). Effects of music therapy on women's physiologic measures, anxiety, and satisfaction during cesarean delivery. *Research in Nursing & Health*, *28*(6), 453–461. doi: 10.1002/nur.20102
8. Cui, J., Li, M., Wei, Y., Li, H., He, X., Yang, Q., Li, Z., Duan, J., Wu, Z., Chen, Q., Chen, B., Li, G., Ming, X., Xiong, L., & Qin, D. (2022). Inhalation aromatherapy via brain-targeted nasal delivery: Natural volatiles or essential oils on mood disorders. *Frontiers in Pharmacology*, *13*, 860043. doi: 10.3389/fphar.2022.860043
9. Ding, J., Huang, T., Hu, J., & Yuan, F. (2021). Effectiveness and safety of music therapy for insomnia disorder patients: A protocol for systematic review and meta-analysis. *Medicine*, *100*(26), e26399. doi: 10.1097/MD.0000000000026399

10. Domínguez-Solís, E., Lima-Serrano, M., & Lima-Rodríguez, J. S. (2021). Non-pharmacological interventions to reduce anxiety in pregnancy, labor and postpartum: A systematic review. *Midwifery*, *102*, 103126. doi: 10.1016/j.midw.2021.103126
11. Fleury, E. A. B., Approbato, M. S., Silva, T. M. D., & Maia, M. C. S. (2014). Music therapy in stress: Proposal of extension to assisted reproduction. *JBRA Assisted Reproduction*, *18*(2), 55–61. doi: 10.5935/1518-0557.20140006
12. Fukui, H., & Toyoshima, K. (2008). Music facilitates the neurogenesis, regeneration and repair of neurons. *Medical Hypotheses*, *71*(5), 765–769. doi: 10.1016/j.mehy.2008.06.019
13. Fung, T. K. H., Lau, B. W. M., Ngai, S. P. C., & Tsang, H. W. H. (2021). Therapeutic effect and mechanisms of essential oils in mood disorders: Interaction between the nervous and respiratory systems. *International Journal of Molecular Sciences*, *22*(9), 4844. doi: 10.3390/ijms22094844
14. Geretsegger, M., Mössler, K. A., Bieleninik, Ł., Chen, X. J., Heldal, T. O., & Gold, C. (2017). Music therapy for people with schizophrenia and schizophrenia-like disorders. *The Cochrane Database of Systematic Reviews*, *5*(5), CD004025. doi: 10.1002/14651858.CD004025.pub4
15. Gong, M., Dong, H., Tang, Y., Huang, W., & Lu, F. (2020). Effects of aromatherapy on anxiety: A meta-analysis of randomized controlled trials. *Journal of Affective Disorders*, *274*, 1028–1040. doi: 10.1016/j.ad.2020.05.118
16. Gürler, M., Kızılırmak, A., & Baser, M. (2020). The effect of aromatherapy on sleep and quality of life in menopausal women with sleeping problems: A non-randomized, placebo-controlled trial. *Complementary Medicine Research*, *27*(6), 421–430. doi: 10.1159/000507751
17. Hawkins, J., Hires, C., Keenan, L., & Dunne, E., (2022). Aromatherapy blend of thyme, orange, clove bud, and frankincense boosts energy levels in post-COVID-19 female patients: A randomized, double-blinded, placebo controlled clinical trial. *Complementary Therapies in Medicine*, *67*, e102823. doi: 10.1016/j.ctim.2022.102823
18. Healio. *Music Therapy Reduces Depression, Menopausal Symptoms*. https://www.healio.com/news/womens-health-ob-gyn/20220221/music-therapy-reduces-depression-menopausal-symptoms
19. Hedaoo, S. A., & Chandurkar, P. A. (2019). A review on aromatherapy. *World Journal of Pharmaceutical Research*, *8*(7), 635–651.
20. Hodgson, D. M., Nakamura, T., & Walker, A. K. (2007). Prophylactic role for complementary and alternative medicine in perinatal programming of adult health. *Forschende Komplementarmedizin*, *14*(2), 92–101. doi: 10.1159/000100958
21. Incadence (n.d.). Music therapy's benefits for patients with schizophrenia. *Incadence Music Therapy Blog*. https://www.incadence.org/post/music-therapys-benefits-for-patients-with-schizophrenia; (accessed on 25 April 2024).
22. Johns Hopkins Medicine. *Women's Health Conditions*. https://www.hopkinsmedicine.org/health/wellness-and-prevention/womens-health-conditions; (accessed on 25 April 2024).

23. Kim, M., Nam, E. S., Lee, Y., & Kang, H. J. (2021). Effects of lavender on anxiety, depression, and physiological parameters: Systematic review and meta-analysis. *Asian Nursing Research*, *15*(5), 279–290. doi: 10.1016/j.anr.2021.11.001
24. Koelsch, S. (2009). A neuroscientific perspective on music therapy. *Annals of the New York Academy of Sciences*, *1169*(1), 374–384. doi: 10.1111/j.1749-6632.2009.04592.x
25. Kok, B. E., Coffey, K. A., Cohn, M. A., Catalino, L. I., Vacharkulksemsuk, T., Algoe, S. B., Brantley, M., & Fredrickson, B. L. (2013). How positive emotions build physical health: Perceived positive social connections account for the upward spiral between positive emotions and vagal tone. *Psychological Science*, *24*(7), 1123–1132. doi: 10.1177/0956797612470827
26. Li, B. S. Y., Chan, C. W. H., Li, M., Wong, I. K. Y., & Yu, Y. H. U. (2021). Effectiveness and safety of aromatherapy in managing behavioral and psychological symptoms of dementia: A mixed-methods systematic review. *Dementia and Geriatric Cognitive Disorders Extra, 11*(3), 273–297. doi: 10.1159/000519915
27. Lv, X. N., Liu, Z. J., Zhang, H. J., & Tzeng, C. M., (2013). Aromatherapy and the central nerve system (CNS): Therapeutic mechanism and its associated genes. *Current Drug Targets*, *14*(8), 872–879. doi: 10.2174/1389450111314080007
28. Medical News Today. (n.d.). How music therapy benefits people with dementia and their caregivers. https://www.medicalnewstoday.com/articles/music-therapy-improves-well-being-in-people-with-dementia-and-caregivers; (accessed on 25 April 2024).
29. Medical News Today. (n.d.). Postpartum depression: Symptoms, causes, and diagnosis. https://www.medicalnewstoday.com/articles/237109; (accessed on 25 April 2024).
30. MediPass. (2023). Music and fertility. (2023). https://medipass.site/music-and-fertility/; (accessed on 25 April 2024).
31. Mejía-Rubalcava, C., Alanís-Tavira, J., Mendieta-Zerón, H., & Sánchez-Pérez, L. (2015). Changes induced by music therapy to physiologic parameters in patients with dental anxiety. *Complementary Therapies in Clinical Practice*, *21*(4), 282–286. doi: 10.1016/j.ctcp.2015.10.005
32. Mojtehedi, M., Salehi-Pourmehr, H., Ostadrahimi, A., Asnaashari, S., Esmaeilpour, K., & Farshbaf-Khalili, A. (2022). Effect of aromatherapy with essential oil of lavandula angustifolia mill- citrus bergamia and mindfulness-based intervention on sexual function, anxiety, and depression in postmenopausal women: A randomized controlled trial with factorial design. *Iranian Journal of Nursing and Midwifery Research*, *27*(5), 392–405. doi: 10.4103/ijnmr.ijnmr_129_21
33. Murrock, C. J., & Higgins, P. A. (2009). The theory of music, mood and movement to improve health outcomes. *Journal of Advanced Nursing*, *65*(10), 2249–2257. doi: 10.1111/j.1365-2648.2009.05108.x
34. Perry, N., & Perry, E., (2006). Aromatherapy in the management of psychiatric disorders: Clinical and neuropharmacological perspectives. *CNS Drugs*, *20*(4), 257–280. doi: 10.2165/00023210-200620040-00001
35. Priority Group. (2022). *Anxiety in Women: Anxiety Symptoms in Women.* https://www.priorygroup.com/mental-health/anxiety-treatment/anxiety-in-women; (accessed on 25 April 2024).

36. Raglio, A., Attardo, L., Gontero, G., Rollino, S., Groppo, E., & Granieri, E. (2015). Effects of music and music therapy on mood in neurological patients. *World Journal of Psychiatry*, *5*(1), 68–78. doi: 10.5498/wjp.v5.i1.68
37. Rashidi-Fakari, F., Tabatabaeichehr, M., & Mortazavi, H. (2015). The effect of aromatherapy by essential oil of orange on anxiety during labor: A randomized clinical trial. *Iranian Journal of Nursing and Midwifery Research*, *20*(6), 661–664. doi: 10.4103/1735-9066.170001
38. Rebecchini, L. (2021). Music, mental health, and immunity. *Brain, Behavior, & Immunity —Health*, *18*, e100374. doi: 10.1016/j.bbih.2021.100374
39. Safajou, F., Soltani, N., Taghizadeh, M., Amouzeshi, Z., & Sandrous, M. (2020). The effect of combined inhalation aromatherapy with lemon and peppermint on nausea and vomiting of pregnancy: A double-blind, randomized clinical trial. *Iranian Journal of Nursing and Midwifery Research*, *25*(5), 401–406. doi: 10.4103/ijnmr.IJNMR_11_19
40. Sánchez-Vidaña, D. I., Ngai, S. P., He, W., Chow, J. K., Lau, B. W., & Tsang, H. W. (2017). The effectiveness of aromatherapy for depressive symptoms: A systematic review. *Evidence-based Complementary and Alternative Medicine: eCAM*, *2017*, 5869315. doi: 10.1155/2017/5869315
41. Save The Music Foundation. (2024). *Understanding the Psychology and Benefits of Music Therapy*. https://www.savethemusic.org/blog/music-therapy-and-mental-health/
42. Shamsunisha, Y., Arunesh, A., Pandiaraja, M., Venugopal, V., Poonguzhali, S., & Kuppusamy, M. (2023). Aromatherapy for postpartum depression: A systematic review and meta-analysis. *Journal of Family & Reproductive Health*, *17*(1), 1–7. doi: 10.18502/jfrh.v17i1.11970
43. Sivanandan, A. (2022). Role of music as a therapeutic measure in women's health. *International Research Journal of Ayurveda & Yoga*, *5*(10), 124–129.
44. Son, H. K., So, W. Y., & Kim, M. (2019). Effects of aromatherapy combined with music therapy on anxiety, stress, and fundamental nursing skills in nursing students: A randomized controlled trial. *International Journal of Environmental Research and Public Health*, *16*(21), 4185. doi: 10.3390/ijerph16214185
45. Tang, Q., Huang, Z., Zhou, H., & Ye, P. (2020). Effects of music therapy on depression: A meta-analysis of randomized controlled trials. *PLoS One*, *15*(11), e0240862. doi: 10.1371/journal.pone.0240862
46. Thaut, M. H. (2015). Music as therapy in early history. *Progress in Brain Research*, *217*, 143–158. doi: 10.1016/bs.pbr.2014.11.025
47. Tillett, J., & Ames, D. (2010). The uses of aromatherapy in women's health. *The Journal of Perinatal & Neonatal Nursing*, *24*(3), 238–245. doi: 10.1097/JPN.0b013e3181ece75d
48. VineVida. (n.d.). *Essential Oils and Schizophrenia*. https://www.vinevida.com/blogs/adhoc-aromatics/essential-oils-and-schizophrenia; (accessed on 25 April 2024).
49. Więdłocha, M., Zborowska, N., Marcinowicz, P., Dębowska, W., Dębowska, M., Zalewska, A., Maciejczyk, M., Waszkiewicz, N., & Szulc, A. (2023). Oxidative stress biomarkers among schizophrenia inpatients. *Brain Sciences*, *13*(3), 490. doi: 10.3390/brainsci13030490

50. World Health Organization. (9 March 2020). *Ten Top Issues for Women's Health.* https://www.who.int/news-room/commentaries/detail/ten-top-issues-for-women's-health; (accessed on 25 April 2024).
51. World Health Organization. *Women's Health.* https://www.who.int/health-topics/women-s-health; (accessed on 25 April 2024).
52. Zamanifar, S., Bagheri-Saveh, M. I., Nezakati, A., Mohammadi, R., & Seidi, J. (2020). The effect of music therapy and aromatherapy with chamomile-lavender essential oil on the anxiety of clinical nurses: A randomized and double-blind clinical trial. *Journal of Medicine and Life*, *13*(1), 87–93. doi: 10.25122/jml-2019-0105

CHAPTER 4

# Nurturing Women's Health Through Yoga and Meditation in the Post-COVID-19 Era

RAHUL SAXENA,* SUYASH SAXENA, and AJIT PAL SINGH

*Corresponding author

## ABSTRACT

Millions of people have died because of pandemics caused by variety of deadly diseases during the past few centuries. In this regard, the COVID-19 pandemic's tremendous loss of global health has been a tragic event. During the COVID-19 epidemic, women of all ages had greater rates of sadness, worry, terror, insomnia, and severe uncontrollable mental disturbances, according to several studies. Furthermore, the regulatory bodies and government agencies suggested social distancing, quarantine, and lockdown steps to stop the virus's spread that accelerated the pandemic's disruptive and detrimental effects on women's social environments as well as business, education, and employment. Through the application of various traditional and spiritual ways (such as yoga and meditation), a great deal of emphasis has been focused on helping the women population to overcome the disruption brought on by the uncertainty of the pandemic in the post-COVID-19 age, which is characterized by obsessive fear, anxiety, and stress. It is noteworthy that yoga and meditation have been extensively studied as alternative treatment strategies for various pandemic diseases impacting women's health, such as diabetes, cardiovascular problems, chronic pulmonary obstruction, and mental stress. As a result, yoga and meditation are useful and proactive strategies for managing women's stress and the subsequent issues that

Holistic Approaches for Women's Sustainable Health, Volume 1: Foundations, Innovations, Challenges, and Management. Megh R. Goyal, Anamika Chauhan, and Junaid Ahmad Malik (Eds)


DOI: 10.1201/9781779641632-5

are linked to it. There is, however, a dearth of research on the impact of yoga and meditation on health and wellness in the post-COVID-19 age, particularly among women.

## 4.1 INTRODUCTION

Yoga is a Sanskrit term meaning association, originating from the word YUJ. One distinctive way to live a healthy life is through yoga. It is an age-old method of figuring out maximum potential of a person. To maintain congruency between the body, mind, and spirit, it is anything but a strict regimen. When one is in this state of congruity, one feels united with the cosmos and connected to within.

Yoga is mentioned in the old literature dating back to more than 5000 years. Even while yoga has its roots in Hinduism, its knowledge transcends all religions [4]. Regardless of where it originated from, knowledge—whether it be logical, scientific, or extraterrestrial—it has universal applications. For example, many logical advancements are applied globally, even though they were developed in Western countries. People in the Eastern countries would be innocent to claim that just because refrigerators and cell phones were invented in the West, therefore, they will not use these. Similarly, it would be somewhat disapproved for non-Hindus to claim that they will not practice yoga since it is a part of Hinduism, even though there are legitimate benefits of yoga and meditation.

This chapter offers a thorough analysis of the impact of yoga and meditation on women's population in the post-COVID-19 era, and it can be regarded as a useful strategy for preserving their normal homeostasis as well as better and enhanced health.

## 4.2 TYPES OF YOGA

The numerous ancient literatures contain information and ideas of yoga. Yoga and meditation have been mentioned in several religious books, such as *Bhagavad Gita, Patanjali Yoga Sutras, Gheranda Samhita, Hatha Yoga*, and *Hatha Yoga Pradipika*. In the ancient literature, a wide sort of yoga has been endorsed, such as [3]:

- **Ashtanga Yoga:** The mind is regularly busy in a variety of mental activities, most of which lack attention. The mind gets increasingly confused with the complex daily activities without awareness. A higher level of awareness leads to a calmer mind [1]. A tranquil mind sees more clearly and remains free of tensions and anxieties. According to the ancient *Yogi Patanjali*, the purpose of yoga is to restrain waves of concerns. He collected concise teachings of yoga known as "*Patanjali's Yoga Sutras*," where he outlines a method of using eight appendages of our body for prosperity and self-sanitization. The term "*Ashtanga Yoga*" refers to this eight-limb system, and it does not imply a methodical approach. This approach is far from employing multidimensional asanas, which make use of all eight appendages simultaneously. The eight limbs of yoga are as follows:

1. ***Yamas*** (the five social ethics or the universal vows):
   - ***Asteya:*** Physically and psychologically nonstealing (not wanting things that belong to others).
   - ***Brahmacharya*** includes celibacy (moderation in all joys) and perpetually being in the consciousness of the divine consciousness.
   - ***Ahimsa*****:** Nonviolence in words, deeds, and ideas.
   - ***Aparigraha*****:** Not needlessly gathering possessions.
   - ***Satyam*****:** Being sincere in the intentions and staying rooted in the greater reality.
2. ***Niyamas*** includes five personal ethics: *Tapas*—austerity and self-discipline; *Santosha*—contentment and happiness; ***Shaucha***—cleanliness of the body and mind; *Svadhyaya*—investigating and dwelling in the self; and *Ishvarapranidhana*—submitting to and respecting the divine.
3. ***Pranayamas*** involve using certain breathing techniques to properly regulate *prana* or life force.
4. ***Asanas*** includes yoga poses.
5. ***Dharana*** is a one-pointed focus.
6. ***Pratyahara*** consists of taking the awareness inward.
7. ***Dhyana*** includes meditation.
8. ***Samadhi*** involves becoming one with the self that implies an unfathomably superconscious condition.

- ***Bhakti Yoga* (path of devotion)**: Knowing, respecting, and being devoted to God.
- ***Gyana Yoga* (path of knowledge)**: Studying sacred writings, receiving guidance directly from your spiritual teacher, and applying this knowledge in daily life.
- ***Hatha Yoga* (Hatha implies solid assurance)**: Making a conscious effort to achieve mental and physical well-being, with a focus on practicing the asanas and pranayamas.
- ***Karma Yoga* (path of action):** Helping humanity with altruism and allocating all of one's efforts in a competent and sincere manner.
- ***Raja Yoga* (royal path: the effortless path):** Subsequent to the expending energy, one ought to have ease. The emphasis is on calm contemplation and continuing with life without struggle.

## 4.3 ROLE OF YOGA IN WOMEN HEALTH

Normal rehearsing of yoga has extraordinary influence on the body, mind, and soul (spirit). Many of these benefits cannot be expressed in words. Certain advantages are beyond description and must be experienced directly [3]. The body, mind, and soul is related to yoga as follows:

- **Yoga and body:** The numerous advantages of yoga at actual level include [1, 2] (1) improved adaptability of muscles; (2) improved posture and body arrangement; (3) greater range of motion in the joints; (4) better bone and muscle health and strength; (5) enhanced neurological and endocrine organ function; (6) better resistance, dispersal, and processing; (7) prevention and relief from various physical illnesses and chronic pain; and (8) overall, the body feels rejuvenated, energized, and full of vitality.
- **Yoga and mind:** Everything feels fantastic if the brain is functioning properly. For this reason, the mental health of a yoga practitioner is highly valued. With consistently rehearsing yoga, one can encounter

many of the several advantages, such as (1) improved sharpness and clearness, (2) increased significant serenity, (3) decreased dependence on drugs, (4) expanded centralization of brain, (5) increased capacity to manage short- and long-haul stresses, (6) developed confidence, (7) greater energy, and (8) eagerness forever.

- **Yoga and spirit:** Yoga helps us to understand the spirit within us in a proper way. As we feel oneness with everyone, it enables us to recognize the divine presence in one another and ourselves. This gives our lives a meaningful purpose and provides us with unqualified personal contentment. It is from this sense of fulfillment that we can share others' experience our joy.

## 4.4 COORDINATION OF YOGA WITH FOUR PILLARS OF SPIRITUALITY

Yoga integrates four pillars of spirituality that encompass every essential aspects of life, enabling the full realization of women's potential [3]. Yoga takes us back to our regular self, thus upholding all the ethical principles that we are brought into the world these pillars of spirituality, such as:

1. **Knowledge** refers to pearls of intelligence that one can apply in day-to-day life whether with the end goal of thought or capably managing everyday life circumstances.
2. **Meditation** is the process of redirecting your thoughts to calm the body, mind, and soul.
3. **Satsang (being with the truth):** An opportunity to be in the company of like-minded individuals who seek spiritual growth.
4. **Seva (service)** is a chance to engage in different service projects for others.

## 4.5 IMPACT OF COVID-19 PANDEMIC ON WOMEN HEALTH

Infectious disease pandemics have substantial impact on both the physical and mental health of the populace, which has increased the death rate [5–7]. This terrible trend has persisted into the present millennium as well, manifesting itself as COVID-19, which is most likely the result of the novel zoonotic severe acute respiratory syndrome coronavirus 2 (SARS-CoV-2) virus that was first discovered in bat species. There have been 180 million confirmed COVID-19 cases to date, and 3.91 million deaths have been reported globally [4, 9]. Both symptomatic and asymptomatic patients' droplets are the primary means of airborne SARS-CoV-2 transmission. There is, however, a dearth of information regarding asymptomatic patients' mediated transmission. Furthermore, studies on asymptomatic viral contamination are currently being conducted throughout the world to help understand why COVID-19 is so common and deadly. Furthermore, it is still unclear what caused COVID-19 and what cellular mechanism underlies the devastating symptoms that relate to the virus [2]. There is a need to investigate more innovative therapy targets, as the current attempts to delay or prevent this debilitating disease have not been very successful.

## 4.6 TRIUMPH OF YOGA IN OVERALL WELLNESS: HOPE TO COPE IN POST-COVID-19 ERA

Yoga is a useful and proactive method for managing stress and the secondary problems that come with it. In the psychosocial assessment and rehabilitation of COVID-19 patients under isolation and quarantine, this could play a crucial role. Yoga is very beneficial for overcoming the tension and emotions of anxiety. Yoga assumes a fundamental role in the administration and treatment of COVID-19, complementing all other interventions. The following goals are offered for yoga-based lifestyle modules that can be employed by different segments of society in the current post-COVID-19 age:

- Prerehabilitation for patients in isolation or disconnection with mild side effects, as well as for children, the elderly, and those with comorbid diseases, including diabetes and hypertension.
- To boost population immunity or universal susceptibility.
- To incorporate more yoga-based meditations and meditation practices into COVID-19 clients that are hospitalized for psychosocial care and are being disconnected.

Adopting a Common Yoga Protocol, along with practices such as *Jala Neti, Sutra Neti, Bhastrika Kriyas,* and *Yoga Nidra* on an empty stomach, has been shown to enhance immunity and promote overall health [3]. Dr Taneja [7] recently published on the function of *Bhramari Pranayama* in investigating the role of yoga against the harmful effects of COVID-19, based on the physiological principles of nitric oxide, carbon dioxide, and pH of the body. He claims that *Bhramari Pranayama* not only increases nitric oxide expression because of serendipity humming but also increases $CO_2$ and alkaline pH by prolonged expiration, preventing COVID-19-driven coagulopathies and morbidity. Furthermore, by directing the release of feel-good hormones during a relaxed phase and visualizing it, the cortisol level is lowered, thus improving general well-being, immunological response, and physiological recovery.

## 4.7 YOGIC DIET AND ITS SIGNIFICANCE

The ideas from yoga should be incorporated to enhance women mental health while adhering to the dietary guidelines prescribed by the doctor if one has diabetes, heart disease, or another medical condition. This includes a variety of freshly prepared, nutritious, and home-cooked meals that are burnt through at regular intervals [5–7]. It also includes a lot of fresh vegetables and natural goods, with the addition of conventional flavors in moderation depending on your illness status. It includes abstaining from substance abuse (such as alcohol, tobacco, and other habit-forming drugs) to reduce the risk of sickness in populations at high risk. This guideline [3] recommends safe, fundamental, and evidence-based yoga poses as discussed above that improve respiratory, cardiovascular, and safety framework health.

## 4.8 YOGA-BASED LIFESTYLE IN HOSPITALIZED CASES WITHOUT ACUTE RESPIRATORY DISTRESS

The COVID-19 patients who are hospitalized and remain in bed without respiratory complications [7] are advised to engage in repeated practice of reflective practices without breath mindfulness. It is recommended to exercise deep relaxation of the body, slowing down of the respiration rate, and mental calm using any yoga practice for 20 minutes, repeated once every 3–4 hours during the day with clear instructions. Some examples of these types of meditation are progressive relaxation, deep relaxation, yoga nidra, transcendental meditation, and so on. Aside from this, morning prayers, neck, shoulder, and trunk development, breathing exercises, and introspection can all be the start of yoga practices for anticipation, recovery, and immune enhancement [7, 8].

## 4.9 SUMMARY

It has been observed that the health of women has been significantly affected by the COVID-19 pandemic, with potential long-lasting effects persisting for years. This global crisis has exacerbated physical, mental, and economic health deterioration worldwide. Data suggests an increased prevalence of common psychiatric disorders and suicide in the post-COVID-19 era. Interestingly, yoga has garnered considerable research attention in recent decades as an alternative therapeutic approach for epidemic diseases such as mental stress, chronic obstructive pulmonary disease, diabetes, and cardiovascular complications. Therefore, yoga serves as an effective preventive measure for managing stress and its associated complications. However, literature on the impact of yoga on health and wellness in the post-COVID-19 era remains limited, indicating the need for more comprehensive research in this area. Overall, the importance of yoga practices for women's health in the post-COVID-19 era cannot be overlooked, as it is considered a valuable approach to restore normal homeostasis and enhance immune resilience.

## KEYWORDS

- **depression**
- **homeostasis**
- **mental stress**
- **obsessive anxiety**
- **obsessive fear**

## REFERENCES

1. Chong, C. S., Tsunaka, M., & Chan, E. P. (2021). Effects of yoga on stress management in healthy adults: A systematic review. *Alternative Therapies in Health and Medicine*, *17*(1), 32–36.
2. Contini, C., Caselli, E., Martini, F., Maritati, M., Torreggiani, E., Seraceni, S., Vesce, F., Perri, P., Rizzo, L., & Tognon, M. (2020). COVID-19 is a multifaceted challenging

pandemic, which needs urgent public health interventions. *Microorganisms, 8*(8), 1228–1234.
3. *Guidelines for Yoga practitioners for COVID-19*. Ministry of Ayush, Government of India: New Delhi. [Ayush.gov.in]
4. https://www.worldometers.info/coronavirus/; (accessed on May 31, 2024).
5. Lederberg, J. (1988). Medical science, infectious disease, and the unity of humankind. *JAMA, 260*, 684–685.
6. Posadzki, P., Cramer, H., Kuzdzal, A., Lee, M. S., & Ernst, E. (2014). Yoga for hypertension: A systematic review of randomized clinical trials. *Complementary Therapies in Medicine*, *22*(3), 511–522.
7. Ranjita, R., Hankey, A., Nagendra, H. R., & Mohanty, S. (2016). Yoga-based pulmonary rehabilitation for the management of dyspnea in coal miners with chronic obstructive pulmonary disease: A randomized controlled trial. *Journal of Ayurveda and Integrative Medicine*, *7*(3), 158–166.
8. Tandeja, M. K. (2020). Modified Bhramari Pranayama in Covid-19 infection. *Indian Journal of Otolaryngology and Head & Neck Surgery*, *72*(3), 395–397.
9. World Health Organization (WHO). (2021). *Novel Coronavirus (2019-nCoV) Situation Report-1*.

# CHAPTER 5

# Holistic Approach to Depression and Migrant Headache in Females

N. L. SWATHI,* MUHAMMAD MUZZAMIL, SURJABHA PAL, ISHWAR BASAVAN, AKHIL ARUN, MARYAM NISA, and TAHMINA BEGUM

*Corresponding author

## ABSTRACT

The chapter emphasizes the importance of cultural sensitivity for diagnosing, treating, and communicating with individuals in this demographic by highlighting the prevalence and risk factors associated with both conditions. Providing culturally competent care requires overcoming language barriers, addressing stigma, and tailoring therapeutic approaches to meet individual needs and sociocultural backgrounds. The chapter explores a range of treatment modalities, acknowledging both the strengths and limitations of pharmacological and psychotherapeutic interventions. It further examines the therapeutic value of lifestyle modifications, mind–body practices, and evidence-based integrative medicine approaches in enhancing overall well-being and supporting symptom management. In addition, the role of community support systems, including peer support networks and improved access to healthcare through telemedicine services, is emphasized. Effective collaboration among healthcare professionals, policymakers, and community organizations is identified as vital to addressing persistent challenges and reducing disparities in research and care delivery. In summary, navigating the complex challenges faced by female migrants

Holistic Approaches for Women's Sustainable Health, Volume 1: Foundations, Innovations, Challenges, and Management. Megh R. Goyal, Anamika Chauhan, and Junaid Ahmad Malik (Eds)


DOI: 10.1201/9781779641632-6

experiencing depression and migraine necessitates an interdisciplinary strategy focused on education, stigma reduction, and ensuring equitable and culturally appropriate healthcare. Through evidence-based interventions, supportive policies, and coordinated efforts, it is possible to empower female migrants to better manage their health and thrive in their new environments.

## 5.1 INTRODUCTION

Depression and migraine are common disorders that have a substantial negative influence on quality of life, especially in the case of female migrants who may also be dealing with additional stressors such as social isolation, difficulty in adjusting to a new culture, and financial issues [93, 119]. Given the complexity of depression and migraines in this population, a comprehensive approach to treatment is necessary.

Complex neurological pathways, including vascular dysfunction, proinflammatory states, oxidative stress, activation of the trigeminovascular system, and cortical spreading depression, are involved in the pathogenesis of migraines [119]. Potential modulators of these processes have been investigated through dietary treatments. For example, low-glycemic diets may reduce inflammation, while ketogenic diets may enhance mitochondrial function [119].

Through inflammatory processes, obesity has also been connected to headaches. General medical conditions, such as disorders of the immune or neurological systems, musculoskeletal disorders, cardiovascular diseases, endocrine abnormalities, migraine, anxiety, posttraumatic stress disorder (PTSD), attention-deficit/hyperactivity disorder, chronic primary pain, chronic overlapping pain conditions, and functional somatic disorders, are linked to treatment-resistant depression. This implies a reciprocal relationship in which one state makes the other worse. By impairing gap junction activities, which are essential for cellular communication within neural tissues, environmental variables such as exposure to chemical pollutants can exacerbate brain diseases. Neurobehavioral problems such as major depressive disorders or neurodevelopmental disorders such as autism spectrum disorders may be linked to this disturbance [62, 93, 100].

Preventive care for migraines frequently entails taking drugs that can have serious side effects that restrict their use. As an illustration, β-adrenergic blockers have the potential to cause cardiovascular problems, while antiepileptic medications such as valproate should not be used when pregnant due to teratogenic hazards [156]. The chronic pain-causing disease endometriosis has been linked to genes implicated in estrogen pathways through genomic studies, indicating that hormonal regulation may be a factor in the etiology of the disorder. The co-occurring conditions of endometriosis and migraines highlight the necessity for all-encompassing treatment plans that take hormones and pain management into account [132]. Children with headaches and migraines frequently use complementary medicines, suggesting a preference for nonpharmacological methods, perhaps because of the negative effects or limited effectiveness of traditional treatments [32].

Although recovery times following sports-related concussions vary, it is nevertheless evident that the initial severity of symptoms is a reliable indicator of lengthier recovery times. Premorbid conditions, including a history of migraines or depression/anxiety, might alter the course of recovery, highlighting the significance of individualized treatment regimens created based on each patient's risk profile [8]. A genetic study on cluster headaches has found many loci that are shared by migraine and cluster headaches, suggesting that these two headache syndromes share similar pathophysiology foundations. It has been suggested that smoking is a causative risk factor, highlighting the importance of environmental factors in addition to genetics in the presentation of disease [165]. Incorporating targeted dietary modifications, environmental risk assessment, pharmacological preventive strategies, genomic-driven insights, and appropriate adjunctive therapies, along with structured psychological support, enables a comprehensive approach for preventing and managing complex headache disorders, especially in individuals with coexisting psychiatric vulnerabilities [34, 116].

This chapter focuses on a holistic approach to treating depression and migraine headaches in females.

## 5.2 UNDERSTANDING DEPRESSION AND MIGRAINES IN MIGRANT FEMALES

Migraine is a prevalent headache-related illness and one of the most debilitating conditions worldwide. It is a common and ongoing medical condition characterized by recurring headaches accompanied by other symptoms [46]. Migraine affects about one billion persons annually worldwide. On a global scale, migraine ranked as the second most significant factor in terms of disability-adjusted life years [6]. Headache disorders are 52.0% worldwide, with "migraine" contributing to 14.0% [11]. Its global prevalence in females is 18.9% [57].

There are several potential occurrences of psychological issues with migraine. Depression and migraine are very common illnesses [37]. Depressive disorders affect almost 80% of those with migraines at one time or another [65, 67]. Depression is the main cause of disability globally and contributes significantly to disease burden, according to the World Health Organization (WHO) [88]. Depression affects 3.8% of the population, with 5% of adults being affected (6% of whom are women). Depression affects approximately 50% more women than males [33]. An estimated 280 million individuals worldwide suffer from depression [169].

Adolescent depression symptoms are 12% and 24.6% in the United States and China, respectively, making the situation worse. Migraine has a substantial influence on interpersonal, physical, and occupational functioning [57]. There is a correlation between migraine and several mental health diseases, including anxiety and depression, as well as stress-related diseases, such as PTSD. Epidemiological studies have shown that the incidence of migraines is two to three times higher in females than in males [4, 66].

Migraines may be caused by several factors, such as genes, hormones, the environment, the dietary choices the individual makes, the quality of sleep, and the psychological component. Several hypothesized migraine mechanisms have led to the identification of certain risk factors, such as age, brain injury, poor socioeconomic status, excessive use of caffeine or medicines, anxiety, difficulty in sleeping (such as snoring), being overweight, and a pain condition (either proinflammatory or prothrombotic) [125]. Lifestyle variables may dramatically impact migraine risk and quality of life. Overuse of acute migraine medication, depression, obesity, and stress are the main modifiable risk factors for migraine. Identifying and managing environmental, dietary, and behavioral causes might prevent it [11]. If not managed consistently over an extended period, it gives rise to comorbidities with numerous conditions, including cardiovascular disease, sleep disorders, mental health illness (such as anxiety), and neurological disorders (for instance, Alzheimer's disease) [14].

Depression is a common psychiatric disorder often seen in those who suffer from migraine headaches. Depression in those who experience migraines is believed to heighten the probability of developing chronic migraines, diminish the effectiveness of migraine treatments, contribute to the misuse of medications, trigger suicidal thoughts associated with psychiatric problems, and negatively impact the overall quality of life for those who experience migraines. Depression is caused by several factors, such as social, family-related, educational, residential, psychological, and hereditary characteristics [133]. Females have a greater incidence of depression compared to males, and this gender discrepancy may be linked to their hormonal profiles, including estrogen and progesterone [169]. Migrant females had a threefold higher likelihood of developing depression compared to nonmigrants [39]. Another research found that "cultural differences" affect the mental well-being of migrant females [88].

There is a significantly increased likelihood of mental health issues developing among female migrants [108]. Traumatic events before, during, and after migration make women migrants more susceptible to migration-related stresses and mental health suffering. Immigrant depression is increased by extreme poverty and violence preceding migration [148]. It is possible that those who suffer from PTSD also have a higher chance of getting migraines. "Some genes and pathways are shared by both PTSD and migraine," so that they share certain risk factors. If this is the case, then the comorbidity of the two disorders may be partially explained [9]. Female migrants, especially refugees, are more likely to develop perinatal depression and PTSD [45].

Migraine is associated with depression, anxiety, cardiovascular illness, sleep difficulties, and neurological diseases, including Alzheimer's disease and PTSD. Women regularly have more cases of migraine, depression, anxiety, and PTSD than males [15]. A study of over 6000 persons found that migraineurs are twice as likely to report mental illness [151]. In general, depressed patients are twice as likely to experience the onset of migraines [65]. This may be due to "hypothalamic–pituitary–adrenal axis" activity lowering serotonin during migraines [139]. Migraine is prevalent in individuals diagnosed with bipolar illness. The prevalence of migraines in individuals diagnosed with "bipolar disorder" may reach up to 39%. These two disorders have some common risk factors, such as genetic and environmental variables, oxidative stress, and disruptions in inflammatory cytokines [155].

## 5.3 CULTURAL CONSIDERATIONS

Culture refers to the unique spiritual, material, cognitive, and emotional characteristics of a community or group of individuals. It incorporates many aspects such as art, literature, lifestyles, social interactions, value systems, traditions, and beliefs [124]. Culture may contain predisposing variables, but it cannot reflect a patient's complexity and actual views. Additionally, culture comprises race, ethnicity, religion, and socioeconomic status [109]. The occurrence of migraines is influenced by biological factors such as sex, age, and sex hormones, which play a significant part in defining the condition. However, migraines are also influenced by "culture," since women are more susceptible to social pressure and relationship issues, while sexual minorities experience stigma and different forms of discrimination [26].

About 16% of global migrants reside in high-income nations with extremely diverse cultures. If cultural context is not considered, medical care may provide improper assessments, diagnoses, and treatments. Cultural identities may affect these women's mental health and sickness reactions. First, culture might affect immigrant women's healthcare access by affecting their symptoms, help-seeking, decision-making, illness role expectations, coping style, and health provider communication. Second, culture affects immigrant women's mental illness stigma [64]. Scientific study relating spirituality and religion to health has increased in recent decades. Spirituality and religion affect mental health, survival, hospitalization, and suffering. About 50% of pain sufferers find relief via prayer, religion, and spirituality [90].

Religion has been linked to active and passive coping mechanisms among Arab Muslim patients, with the former improving well-being [118]. Cultural ideas and practices influence how rural Africans perceive, diagnose, and treat migraines. Rural Africans' health is harmed by cultural customs and poor healthcare availability. Without proper treatment, migraines may become persistent, causing pain and lowering the quality of life [106]. Rural Africans' headache understanding and management are heavily influenced by cultural beliefs and behaviors. Traditional healers may cure headaches caused by bad spirits or curses. In certain societies, obtaining medical attention, especially for minor diseases, is stigmatized [77].

## 5.4 MEDICAL PERSPECTIVES AND INTERVENTIONS

### *5.4.1 PHARMACOLOGICAL INTERVENTIONS*

Pharmacological interventions are crucial in treating migraine and depression symptoms, especially in women, who experience these conditions more frequently than men [167]. Gender-specific factors, such as hormonal fluctuations, reproductive health, and potential drug interactions, require careful consideration [91]. Estrogen fluctuations during menstruation and pregnancy can affect migraine patterns and treatment response, necessitating individualized treatment strategies. Women are more susceptible to adverse drug reactions, impacting 20–25% of migraine patients. Effective management strategies are insufficient [158]. Migraine treatment aims to reduce intensity, duration, functional capacity, dependence on acute relief medications, and minimize adverse effects using conventional pharmacotherapeutic modalities [22, 87, 96, 149, 163]. Over-the-counter medications such as naproxen, ibuprofen, acetaminophen, and aspirin are recommended for acute migraine management due to their advantages such as ease of administration, affordability, and effectiveness [25, 104]. Triptans, such as sumatriptan, are first-line treatments for migraines due to their selective serotonin agonism. Introduced in 1991, it works on serotonin receptors, causing vasoconstriction and inhibiting neurogenic inflammation. Available in tablets, nasal spray, and subcutaneous injections, it is preferred for severe headaches and patients with excessive nausea or vomiting [48, 120, 163, 164].

Alternative triptans such as zolmitriptan, almotriptan, frovatriptan, naratriptan, eletriptan, and rizatriptan offer different pharmacokinetic profiles and suitability for specific patient cohorts. Opioids should be avoided for addiction and medication sensitization [34, 99, 119, 135, 150]. Menstrual migraines are severe and recurrent, with oral contraceptives, naproxen, and acute therapies aiding in mitigation, but caution is advised for aura migraines due to stroke risk [8, 92]. Prophylactic pharmacological strategies for migraine prophylaxis include beta-blockers such as propranolol and metoprolol and antiepileptic drugs such as topiramate and valproate. Propranolol is effective for first-line migraine prophylaxis, while other beta-blockers are recommended for underlying cardiovascular conditions [78]. While antiepileptic drugs may confer benefits, concerns regarding teratogenicity and adverse effects necessitate cautious evaluation, particularly in women of childbearing potential [127]. Calcium channel blockers (e.g., verapamil, flunarizine) have also exhibited efficacy in mitigating migraine frequency and severity, albeit with potential side effects such as hypotension and constipation [114]. Antidepressants (Figure 5.1) regulate mood and behavior by targeting specific neurotransmitters, enhancing serotonin and norepinephrine within the synaptic cleft, and inhibiting nerve terminal reuptake [60].

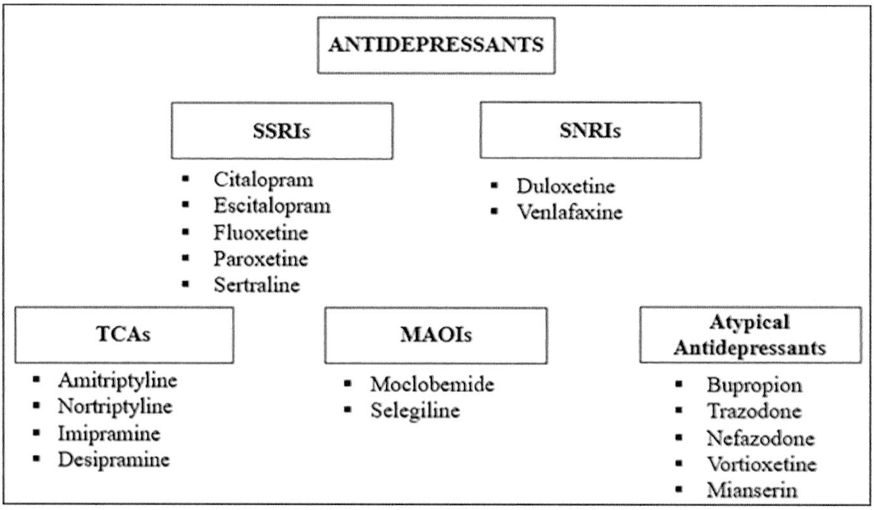


**FIGURE 5.1** Classification of antidepressants. SSRIs: selective serotonin reuptake inhibitors, SNRIs: serotonin–norepinephrine reuptake inhibitors, TCAs: tricyclic antidepressants, MAOIs: monoamine oxidase inhibitors

*Source*: Adapted from Ref. [79].

SSRIs are the first-line treatment for depression, blocking serotonin reuptake and prolonging neurotransmission. They increase cyclic adenosine monophosphate signaling, phosphorylation of transcription factors, and brain-derived neurotrophic factor expression while causing side effects such as sexual dysfunction and headache [16, 129, 130].

SNRIs inhibit serotonin and norepinephrine reuptake in synaptic cleft, increasing postsynaptic receptor stimulation. Milnacipran and levomilnacipran exhibit greater selectivity for norepinephrine reuptake [82]. Some side effects of this medication include hypertension, headache, diaphoresis, and bone resorption [140].

Tricyclic antidepressants such as amitriptyline block norepinephrine and serotonin reuptake, causing sedation and side effects. MAOIs inhibit this enzyme, preventing side effects. MAOIs, first antidepressants, are not first-line treatment for depression due to adverse effects. Migraine-preventive medication selection depends on psychiatric condition severity, patient preferences, risk of adverse events, and treatment history [101].

### *5.4.2 LIMITATIONS IN MIGRANT POPULATIONS*

Migration exposes individuals to circumstances that can affect their physical, social, and mental well-being. The migration journey itself can induce stress, evoke feelings of loss, and lead to social marginalization, rendering migrants more susceptible to health issues, including anxiety and depression [40]. These populations often face challenges in accessing mental health care, including language barriers and cultural stigmas [74]. Women face an elevated risk of perinatal depression stemming from the stressors encountered before, during, and after migration. Therefore, healthcare providers must be aware of these factors and provide culturally sensitive and comprehensive support to mitigate the risk and address the mental health needs of this population during the perinatal period [44]. Migrant populations may also exhibit distinct genetic variations impacting drug metabolism and efficacy. Pharmacogenetic testing could offer personalized insights to enhance treatment efficacy (US Department of Health and Human Services, 2018). Addressing these disparities through targeted interventions and social support structures is essential for optimizing treatment outcomes.

### *5.4.3 NONPHARMACOLOGICAL INTERVENTIONS*

Biopsychological intervention effectively manages migraines through accurate diagnosis; patient education; multidimensional assessment; and strategic interventions such as nutraceuticals, neuromodulation techniques, and psychotherapeutics. These have been recommended for pregnant women, adolescents, and those with drug restrictions [7, 69, 81, 163]. Transcranial magnetic stimulation induces electrical currents in the brain, affecting cortical excitability, which is used to treat chronic migraines and migraines with and without aura [12, 28]. Supraorbital nerve stimulation, a treatment option for migraines, operates through single-pulse and repetitive stimulation, potentially inhibiting nociceptive transmission in pain-transmitting fibers [136].

Transcranial direct current stimulation (tDCS) is a cost-effective, portable, and noninvasive neurostimulation technique that alters the resting membrane potential of cortical neurons, modulating their excitability [134]. tDCS is currently used in two modalities: (1) cathodal and (2) anodal, with the former reportedly decreasing cortical excitability and the latter reportedly increasing it [141]. Electroconvulsive therapy is a treatment option for patients with treatment-resistant depression or severe major depression that significantly affects their ability to perform daily tasks [128].

Biofeedback is a therapeutic technique that helps individuals' control and regulate their physiological responses, enhancing physical and mental well-being by improving self-regulation, coping mechanisms, and modifying maladaptive responses [54]. Cognitive–behavioral therapy (CBT) is a psychotherapeutic method that focuses on identifying and modifying dysfunctional thoughts, behaviors, and stress responses that can worsen or perpetuate headaches [117]. Hypnosis is characterized by a state marked by heightened focus and decreased peripheral awareness [83].

Dating back to the 18th century, hypnosis has been utilized in pain management as hypnotherapy. It has shown promising results in reducing headache activity, decreasing medication usage, and enhancing quality of life in adults, with no reported adverse effects [47]. Psychoeducation is a treatment approach that enhances patients' emotional resilience and understanding of their illness. It involves thorough diagnosis, education, and follow-up appointments. It focuses on symptom management and motivation for active participation. Active psychoeducation involves direct interaction with patients, while passive psychoeducation involves providing materials for independent reading and assimilation [38, 115, 131].

Migraine sufferers are often stigmatized due to cultural associations and belief systems. These myths, rooted in early 18th-century Britain, often lead to delayed diagnoses and skepticism toward modern medicine. Factors such as vulnerability, social connection, language, culture, insurance, stigma, disengagement, information, and family dynamics should be considered when providing treatment for migraine and depression [49, 103, 154].

## 5.5 HOLISTIC FRAMEWORK: INTEGRATING PHYSICAL AND MENTAL WELL-BEING

### *5.5.1 LIFESTYLE MODIFICATIONS*

Migraine is a recurrent, debilitating headache lasting 4–72 h, which is more prevalent in females, especially in the reproductive age group [58, 80, 157]. A holistic approach to managing migraine includes engaging in physical activity, effectively addressing obesity, adopting a nutritious diet, and embracing a healthier lifestyle that includes sufficient sleep and the avoidance of substance abuse (Figure 5.2). This approach helps to reduce the impact of this migraine on an individual's family, social, professional, and economic aspects of life [2].

| | |
|---|---|
| **S – Sleep** | • Dark and cool room<br>• Quiet<br>• No screen<br>• Fixed time to go to bed and wake-up<br>• Bedtime relaxation techniques |
| **E – Exercise** | • Start exercising with a goal of 30–60 minutes, alternate days a week<br>• Start small and slowly increase exercise duration and frequency to make it a habit<br>• Choose an activity you enjoy |
| **E – Eat** | • Avoid skipping meals<br>• Balanced meals at least 3 times a day<br>• Elimination diets depending on individual's triggers and comorbidities<br>• Aim for optimal weight (body mass index 18.5 to 25 kg/m2)<br>• Stay hydrated<br>• Stop caffeine or consistently use less than 200 mg/day |
| **D – Diary** | • Track your headaches in a migraine diary<br>• Rescue medications should be used fewer than 2 days per week to avoid a rebound headache called "medication-overuse headache" |

**FIGURE 5.2** SEED (representing Sleep, Exercise, Eat, and Diary) captures the necessary lifestyle changes to enhance migraine management.

#### *5.5.1.1 NUTRITION AND DIETARY CONSIDERATIONS*

Diet plays a crucial role in overall health (Table 5.1). Migraineurs who are overweight are advised to reduce their carbohydrate and fat intake and increase the amount of protein in their diet to keep their weight in check, as well as for pristine cardiovascular health. Elimination diets, nutrient-rich diets, and epigenetic diets are a few dietary approaches that have shown promise in alleviating migraine symptoms.

**TABLE 5.1** Examples of Elimination Diets, which Involve Identifying and Removing Specific Dietary Triggers Known to Provoke Migraines

| Elimination Diets | Restricted Food Items |
|---|---|
| Gluten-free diets | Wheat, rye, and barley |
| IgG[a] elimination diets | Foods that serve as antigens for IgG |
| Antihistamine diets | Fermented diary, vegetables, soy products, wine, beer, and alcohol |
| Tyramine-free diets | Aged cheese, cured or smoked meats and fish, and beer |
| Low-fat diets | |
| Low-glycemic index diets | |

[a]IgG: immunoglobulin G.

An individual's mood and general disposition can differ based on the food they intake. Depression, stress, and anxiety can cause marked loss in appetite or a sudden urge to binge eat. Hence, alteration in food habits can prove to be a window to the psychological status of an individual [2].

Diets, including whole grains, nonstarchy vegetables, fruits, and lean proteins, have a low glycemic index and have been shown to improve the migraine frequency [41]. Eating an excess of omega-6 fatty acid-rich diet, especially when not balanced with omega-3 fatty acids, can contribute to inflammation and may increase the risk of certain chronic diseases such as migraine [145].

Diets tailored for migraine patients work by improving the function of mitochondria, correcting abnormal serotonin levels, lowering levels of calcitonin gene-related peptide, protecting the neurons, and reducing inflammation in the nervous system, thus protecting the brain from inflammation [144].

Patients experiencing migraines have elevated sodium levels in their cerebrospinal fluid, especially during migraine attacks. Recommendations regarding sodium intake should be customized based on the specific characteristics of patient populations, such as age, sex, and comorbidities [123].

Research indicates low levels of these micronutrients in the plasma and brain of migraineurs (Figure 5.3). Supplementing these micronutrients may potentially alleviate the intensity of the headaches.

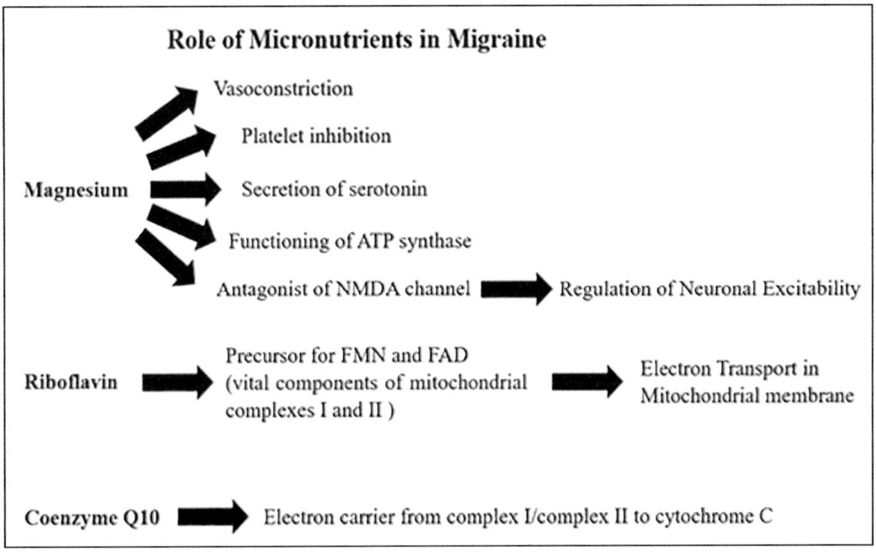


**FIGURE 5.3** The mitochondria require riboflavin, magnesium, and coenzyme Q10 to function.

Migraine attacks are more susceptible during fasting [123]. Certain religious practices among specific groups require individuals, especially women, to fast, thus worsening migraine symptoms [1]. Skipping meals, especially breakfast, reduces energy level, causes low-grade inflammation, and may alter glucose metabolism, thereby triggering migraine attacks. Individuals with migraines are, therefore, advised to consume regular meals [2]. Fluid restriction and dehydration can lead to headaches, primarily because of inadequate oxygenation of the brain resulting from decreased blood volume [50]. Improving hydration status can lead to a balance of plasma osmolality and ion concentrations, which may decrease the severity of migraine headaches [20]. The suggested quantity of daily water consumption ranges between 1.8 and 4 L [123].

Caffeine intake is a significant factor to consider in managing migraines. Caffeine is a nonspecific adenosine receptor antagonist, which affects the

2A receptor, which is linked to the neuropathophysiology of migraine. The risk of headaches is dependent on the dose of caffeine, and most studies advise consuming less than 200 mg/day or discontinue it entirely [143]. It must be kept in mind that due to the heightened sensitivity to caffeine cessation, alteration in the daily amount of caffeine intake may also lead to migraine attacks [123].

For most migraineurs, alcohol serves as a potent trigger. The effects of alcohol involve vasodilation, dehydration, and release of inflammatory modulators (such as histamine, tyramine, sulfites), all of which lead to inflammation. Red wine is considered the most common form of alcohol to cause migraine attacks. Smoking, especially exceeding five cigarettes per day, may precipitate a migraine attack due to the direct action of nicotine on the central nervous system [110, 123].

#### *5.5.1.2 EXERCISE AND PHYSICAL ACTIVITY*

A sedentary lifestyle is a probable cause of migraine. There are reduced levels of beta-endorphins in the cerebrospinal fluid of migraineurs. Physical activity may increase these levels and, in effect, reduce headache frequency [1, 123]. Migraineurs are encouraged to participate in gradually intensified moderate cardiorespiratory exercise, spanning 30–60 minutes, on three to five occasions per week (equivalent to 150 minutes weekly). For those who are inactive or have limited exercise endurance, beginning with shorter sessions once a week may be a more feasible starting point [80, 123].

Obese people are prone to more frequent and severe migraine attacks [2, 19]. This connection exhibits a sexual dimorphism, with a more pronounced impact on women than men, often correlated with estrogen levels and hormonal changes throughout the life cycle [152]. In obese individuals with migraines, disruptions in the hypothalamus result in changes to peptides, neurotransmitters, and adipocytokines that regulate energy balance and feeding, notably through the orexinergic system [56]. Obesity's reward circuitry overactivation may lead to food addiction [121]. Chronic migraine is linked to insulin resistance [43]. Additionally, some migraine medications may cause weight gain. Therefore, weight loss is a primary intervention in the case of migraine management. The prescription of exercise should be guided by patients' clinical presentation and the expertise of clinicians, following the best recommendations from the current evidence [80].

#### *5.5.1.3 SLEEP HYGIENE*

Inadequate sleep is recognized as both a potential trigger and an effect of migraine headaches. Sleep apnea and insomnia lead to a diminished quality of life, increased chances of mood disorders, increased stress levels, and a greater likelihood of engaging in unhealthy lifestyle habits [123].

Stimulus control therapy utilizes different prompts and signals to initiate sleep. Patients are encouraged to create a calm, peaceful, dimly lit, comfortable setting in their bedroom, and maintain a regular sleep schedule. If they struggle to fall asleep within half an hour, leaving the room is recommended to avoid associating the bed with frustration and anxiety. Digital audio–visual gadgets cause sleep disruption and are discouraged before bedtime as they cause difficulty in falling asleep [27, 159].

### ***5.5.2 MIND–BODY PRACTICES***

#### *5.5.2.1 MEDITATION AND MINDFULNESS*

Migraine patients exhibit cognitive and emotional reactions to the repetitive sensory aspects of migraine attacks. This includes anticipatory anxiety due to uncertainty about attack onset and pain catastrophizing triggered by fear of recurring incapacitating episodes, often resulting in avoidance behaviors driven by hypervigilance, all of which can be addressed through mindfulness interventions.

Mindfulness-based interventions contribute to stress reduction and have a positive influence on overall well-being. Mindfulness meditation is an intervention, which teaches the patient to refocus their attention toward any simple physical function such as their breath. With practice, patients are trained to refocus their awareness of their pain, thus helping the experience of a migraine attack be less traumatizing. By honing the skill of meditation, one is more aware and accepting of one's emotions, thoughts, and bodily sensations [71].

Mindfulness-based stress reduction (MBSR) is a technique targeted to acquire, assimilate, and implement mindfulness in one's daily life. MBSR is a conglomeration of mindfulness meditation, Hatha Yoga (physical postures of yoga), and active, nonjudgmental conversation, which allows migraineurs to talk about their experiences, identify their stereotypes and stigmas, and be more accepting of themselves [68, 162].

Mindfulness-based cognitive therapy blends elements of both MBSR and CBT. The approach is to change thoughts and behaviors by practicing mindfulness, problem-solving, and psychoeducation [137].

#### *5.5.2.2 YOGA AND ITS CULTURAL VARIATIONS*

Yoga is a holistic practice involving three elements: (1) breathing exercises, (2) physical alignment poses (asanas), and (3) mindfulness practices (meditations). Its level of difficulty ranges from gentle to intense, encompassing aspects such as strength, balance, coordination, and flexibility. Studies indicate that yoga-based approaches contribute to chronic pain management by restoring autonomic balance and reducing associated disabilities [75, 105, 166]. It helps in restoring a peaceful mind and body, thus reducing stress and anxiety levels. Yoga is also used to augment the treatment of depression. A few yoga postures recommended for migraine patients are *Trikonasana*, *Bhujangasana*, and *Shavasana* with breath awareness.

### ***5.5.3 INTEGRATIVE MEDICINE APPROACHES***

#### *5.5.3.1 HERBAL AND NATURAL REMEDIES*

Certain herbal remedies show promise in improving migraine treatment due to their various physiological effects. Early research suggests that curcumin, citron, and coriander may be beneficial for preventing migraines, while menthol and chamomile could be helpful for immediate relief [18, 21, 89].

Feverfew (*Tanacetum parthenium*) has been used since ancient Greece. It was commonly used for headaches, insect bites, and pain relief. It has mild side effects such as bloating, canker sores, and nausea. Pregnant women and those on blood thinners should avoid using feverfew [36, 113]. Numerous herbal remedies utilize a refined extract derived from the root of butterbur (*Petasites hybridus*), known as *Petasites*, in tablet form to alleviate headaches and migraines [17, 63].

Ginger powder demonstrates a statistically comparable effectiveness to sumatriptan in treating common migraine attacks and with lesser adverse effects [94]. In traditional Ayurvedic medicine, coriander seed (*Coriandrum sativum*) was employed to ease sinus pressure and headaches through the inhalation of steam produced by pouring hot water over fresh seeds [146].

Caution should always be exercised when contemplating herbal treatments for migraines. Before initiating or discontinuing any medical or herbal treatment, the decision should be discussed with a healthcare professional, as many herbs can interfere with other medications.

#### *5.5.3.2 ACUPUNCTURE AND ACUPRESSURE*

Acupuncture has gained attention as a potential treatment for migraines. In this traditional Chinese method, needles are inserted into precise points on the body to balance the flow of energy [85, 160]. Activating different sensory nerves with acupuncture leads to blocking pain signals and releasing endorphins, dopamine, serotonin, and nitric oxide, which in turn relieves pain. Additionally, it lowers levels of serum matrix metalloproteinase, offering alleviation from migraine headaches [42]. Studies demonstrate that acupuncture significantly decreases the frequency of migraines and shows prophylactic effects [86, 160]. While more research is needed, these conclusions imply that acupuncture could be a valuable complementary therapy for migraine management.

## 5.6 CULTURAL SENSITIVITY IN MENTAL HEALTH CARE

Over 200 million foreign migrants face challenges in identifying and addressing psychological issues due to language, cultural differences, and migration-related stressors [117]. The "healthy immigrant effect" initially shows lower rates of mental health issues [84], but over time, depression and other conditions increase. Cultural nuances and understanding of evolving mental health patterns among immigrants are crucial [61]. Cultural factors can impact the causes, progression, and outcomes of major mental illnesses [72, 76]. Researchers, policymakers, analysts [73], and service providers face additional challenges due to the lack of culturally competent methods for diagnosing inadequacies in long-term information for refugees and immigrants.

Cultural competency is crucial for organizations and professionals to function effectively in cross-cultural environments, especially in medical care. It helps understand patients and their families better, and culturally sensitive treatment methods can improve patient outcomes and engagement. Miscommunication can negatively impact patient satisfaction, staff retention, and care quality. Overcoming language barriers, cognitive, behavioral, and emotional barriers is essential for effective cross-cultural understanding [93, 95]. An all-encompassing approach, including culturally competent care, multilingual materials, ongoing training, and professional interpretation services, is required. Health providers must practice ongoing adaptation and active awareness to manage these issues effectively [107].

The stigma surrounding mental illness hinders mental wellness services and the overall well-being of individuals, families, communities, and medical professionals. Research by the Canadian Mental Health Association revealed widespread misunderstandings about mental disorders, including the idea that people with mental health disorders are violent, dangerous, or have low intelligence. Strategies to combat stigma include stigma-busting, education, contact, and political activism. Stigma-busting involves criticizing inaccurate media representations of mental health patients, while education programs such as the UK's Royal College of Psychiatrists' "Changing Minds" initiative aim to eliminate stigmas and raise awareness. Contact aims to make mental patients more visible, while political activism advocates for improved access to care and changes to discriminatory policies [5]. The WHO's "Stop exclusion. Dare to care" initiative uses legal advocacy and education to promote equitable mental health care and combat stigma [112].

## 5.7 COMMUNITY SUPPORT AND RESOURCES

Approximately 26.6 million individuals were anticipated to be seeking protection in mid-2021, according to the United Nations Refugee Agency [5]. Unfortunately, health exams of refugees frequently fail to mention headaches, probably due to the misconception that headaches are not serious or life-threatening. Consequently, research on the frequency of headaches among immigrant groups is severely lacking. Inequalities are both violent and structural since they harm individuals and are rooted in the social, political, and economic systems in which we exist. As an example, structural injustices and structural violence lead to discrimination, racism (both institutional and individual), poverty, and social exclusion, all of which influence people's health and their ability to get the medical treatment they need [24]. Both public health and human rights considerations highlight the critical requirement of attending to migrant communities' healthcare demands. Problems with funding, administration, culture, and law are also impeding this endeavor. While it is widely recognized that including the people who will be receiving health care is essential for resolving these issues, very little has been done to include migrating populations in setting priorities [126].

Worldwide, primary headache disorders are a major concern for public health due to their high incidence and impact. Despite this, many individuals with primary headache disorders still do not have enough medical care. It is possible to address and overcome the main issues that are contributing to this scenario, which include a lack of public information, societal stigma, inadequately trained personnel, and inadequate healthcare systems and legislation. Even while headache advocacy has come a long way, support for research, provision of specialized medical care, and standards of care have all remained stagnant. Due to the substantial obstacles that people in low- and middle-income countries face when attempting to obtain medical treatment, the situation is very complex and urgently needs advocacy for headaches [53].

### *5.7.1 CHALLENGES*

Worldwide, migraines and other main headache diseases are the second leading cause of disability-adjusted life years, according to the WHO [161]. While there has been some progress in understanding migraines, the amount of government support for migraine research remains tragic, and access to therapy and medical care is still limited [31, 70].

According to recent studies, the stigma associated with migraine and other headache diseases is a major factor in the gap between their treatment and knowledge. A study that aimed to shed light on the stigmatization of migraines found that it is independently linked to impairment due to migraines and emotional well-being, and it has medium to large connections with symptoms of mental illness and migraine outcomes. The stigma associated with migraines strongly influences the correlation between migraine frequency and migraine outcomes. Migrants or refugees, those seeking medical treatment frequently, faced discrimination and uneven access to services. Research shows that healthcare practitioners are more prone to discrimination against patients [138] because of their nationality and proficiency in the language of the nation where they are receiving treatment. Cultural mediation and linguistic support are two ways that healthcare services can be enhanced to make them more accessible. Minority patients, women migrants, and those with a history of frequent relocations were more likely to experience discrimination when seeking medical care [52].

### 5.7.2 MITIGATION STRATEGIES

The use of telemedicine and online consultations has recently grown commonplace. Migraine treatment and diagnosis should be core competencies for all physicians. Additionally, medical professionals should stay up to date on the latest recommendations and guidelines because they might change quickly. To provide successful treatment for migraine patients, doctors must rapidly adjust to this new reality [29].

A community neurology practice has implemented an Electronic Health Record-integrated mobile app for migraine management. This study's findings support the notion that the Migraine Interactive Care Plan can enhance patient engagement and access to treatment without burdening care teams with additional tasks or necessitating participation from a broader spectrum of patients. Additional research is necessary to ascertain its impact on primary care [168].

A comprehensive and ever-changing community experience can be provided for individuals with long-term health issues by analyzing the application of this adaptive engagement model in Online Health Communities. This model's three basic components are (1) social support, (2) engagement, and (3) moderation. Mutual aid can take many forms, including the sharing and affirmation of information, the demonstration of empathy, and the provision of encouraging words to those around us [55].

Findings from a study showed that taking zinc supplements helped reduce the frequency of migraine attacks in people who suffer from them. Yet, other features of migraine episodes, such as headache severity, attack duration, and impairment rating due to headaches, were unaffected by zinc supplementation. Additional research in this area is needed to determine the efficacy of long-term interventions in helping migraine patients [3]. The outcomes from research in Jeddah, Saudi Arabia, highlighted the importance of primary care doctors continuing their education. Unfortunately, primary care physicians' lack of training in chronic migraine diagnosis and treatment may influence their decision to refer patients to hospitals or other specialized clinics. Based on these findings, it seems that primary healthcare providers and medical students would benefit from enhanced medical education programs that provide ongoing training to boost their expertise [3].

Having few options for treatment and social stigma to overcome, migraine is a major problem in global health, especially for women migrants. We need a holistic strategy that incorporates community involvement, cultural awareness, and medical progress to solve this problem. To close the information gap and enhance early diagnosis and treatment, telemedicine and educational programs for patients and healthcare professionals are crucial. Building trust and removing barriers to getting treatment requires culturally competent care, which includes language support and attention to any prejudice [62].

Community-based therapies, such as online support groups, can provide women with helpful peer support and the tools they need to manage their disease on their own. Research into nonpharmacological therapies, such as zinc supplementation, shows potential for alleviating symptoms. When it comes down to it, the complicated issues that female migrants with migraine face need an intersectional approach that includes healthcare providers, legislatures, and community leaders. Reclaiming women's health and wellness can be achieved through prioritizing education, decreasing stigma, and encouraging accessible, culturally appropriate care [5, 62].

## 5.8 CHALLENGES AND FUTURE DIRECTIONS

Migraine and depression are comorbid conditions, with 80% of migraine patients suffering from depression. Treatment for depression presents clinical challenges, healthcare system, and societal and cultural barriers. Clinicians face persistent challenges in treating female migraine patients, with low success rates due to societal stigma and inefficiency. This module focuses on future research and policy implications [65].

Studies have shown that the prevalence of depression and anxiety in female migraine patients is significantly higher due to societal stigma associated with mood changes, behavioral alterations, aggression, and low self-respect [102, 111]. Migraine is also associated with various schizoaffective and anxiety disorders, making it difficult and embarrassing to seek timely care. The prevalence of depression with migraine is higher in women compared to men and is often underdiagnosed, leading to gender-based disparity in reporting rates [10, 59, 97]. The progression of depression in migraine patients increases exponentially in middle-aged and older women, highlighting the impact of age on the disease [13, 23, 59]. Women with migraine and significant depression are more likely to have experienced childhood maltreatment, especially if the abuse occurs before and after the age of 12 years [98, 122].

The healthcare system is essential for female migraine sufferers' mental health, but barriers such as access barriers, fragmented care, and lack of cultural competency can hinder efficient delivery [153].

To improve understanding and outcomes, it is crucial to address research gaps and prioritize key areas. This includes conducting comprehensive epidemiological investigations to understand the frequency, variables, and progression patterns of depression and migraines in female migrants [30]. Interventional research should focus on assessing integrative techniques and culturally appropriate therapies to reduce the burden of these conditions [147]. Health services research should focus on healthcare consumption, access, and delivery patterns to shape legislative initiatives to address care gaps. The management of depression in female migraine patients requires a comprehensive approach, including optimal treatment, patient education, and consideration of the overall functional impairment associated with migraines. However, there is a lack of research on specific priorities and gaps in managing depression in this population, indicating a need for further investigation [51].

To effectively treat female migrant headache and depression, a comprehensive approach is needed. This includes culturally competent care training for healthcare professionals, integrating care approaches, and multisector collaboration [13]. A mixture of behavioral therapies, supportive psychotherapy, and antidepressant therapy should be used holistically [30]. The healthcare system's inadequacies, cultural hurdles, and societal stigma must be addressed. Research on interventions, health services, and epidemiology is crucial to close gaps [35]. Evidence-based initiatives and policies can guarantee equal access to appropriate treatment for female migrant headache and depression patients, improving their overall well-being [142].

## 5.9 SUMMARY

By examining the experience of migraines and depression through the lens of female migration, this chapter explores the unique interplay of factors that exacerbate these conditions. It sheds light on the specific challenges they face and their impact on mental and physical health. We support a comprehensive approach that incorporates physical, psychological, and social variables, acknowledging the constraints of relying simply on medical interventions. The text emphasizes the importance of cultural sensitivity in diagnosing, treating, and communicating with individuals in this demographic by highlighting the prevalence and risk factors linked with both illnesses. Providing culturally competent care involves overcoming language hurdles, confronting stigmas, and customizing treatment approaches to suit individual needs and backgrounds. The chapter explores different treatment possibilities, recognizing the effectiveness and constraints of pharmacological and psychotherapy therapies. The significance of community support through networks, peer support programs, and enhanced access to healthcare services, such as telemedicine possibilities, is highlighted. Collaboration among healthcare professionals, governments, and communities is essential to tackle ongoing challenges and close gaps in research and healthcare services. In summary, successfully coping with the intricate challenges encountered by female migrants with depression and migraine requires an interdisciplinary strategy. Emphasizing education, decreasing stigma, and guaranteeing accessible, culturally suitable care are essential actions to improve the health and well-being of this vulnerable group. By utilizing evidence-based interventions, legislation, and joint efforts, we may work toward a future where female migrants are empowered to handle their situations and flourish in their new communities.

## KEYWORDS


- **community**
- **depression**
- **holistic approach**
- **migraine**
- **policy**


## REFERENCES


1. Abu-Salameh, I., Plakht, Y., & Ifergane, G. (2010). Migraine exacerbation during Ramadan fasting. *The Journal of Headache and Pain*, *11*(6), 6. doi: 10.1007/s10194-010-0242-z
2. Agbetou, M., & Adoukonou, T. (2022). Lifestyle modifications for migraine management. *Frontiers in Neurology*, *13*, e719467. doi: 10.3389/fneur.2022.719467
3. Ahmadi, H., Mazloumi-Kiapey, S. S., Sadeghi, O., Nasiri, M., Khorvash, F., Mottaghi, T., & Askari, G. (2020). Zinc supplementation affects favorably the frequency of migraine attacks: A double-blind randomized placebo-controlled clinical trial. *Nutrition Journal*, *19*(1), 101. doi: 10.1186/s12937-020-00618-9
4. Al-Hassany, L., Haas, J., Piccininni, M., Kurth, T., Maassen Van Den Brink, A., & Rohmann, J. L. (2020). Giving researchers a headache – Sex and gender differences in migraine. *Frontiers in Neurology*, *11*, online. https://www.frontiersin.org/articles/10.3389/fneur.2020.549038
5. Al-Nuaimi, S. K., & Qoronfleh, M. W. (2020). Mental health and psycho-social-spiritual support for muslim populations in emergency settings. *Journal of Muslim Mental Health*, *14*(1), doi: 10.3998/jmmh.10381607.0014.105
6. Amiri, P., Kazeminasab, S., Nejadghaderi, S. A., Mohammadinasab, R., Pourfathi, H., Araj-Khodaei, M., Sullman, M. J. M., Kolahi, A. A., & Safiri, S. (2022). Migraine: A review on its history, global epidemiology, risk factors, and comorbidities. *Frontiers in Neurology*, *12*, e800605. doi: 10.3389/fneur.2021.800605
7. Andrasik, F., Flor, H., & Turk, D. C. (2005). An expanded view of psychological aspects in head pain: The biopsychosocial model. *Neurological Sciences*, *26*(S2), s87–s91. doi: 10.1007/s10072-005-0416-7
8. Antonaci, F., Ghiotto, N., Wu, S., Pucci, E., & Costa, A. (2016). Recent advances in migraine therapy. *SpringerPlus*, *5*(1), 637. doi: 10.1186/s40064-016-2211-8
9. *Are Migraines and PTSD Linked?* (2021, June 22). https://www.psychiatrictimes.com/view/are-migraines-and-ptsd-linked
10. Ayata, C., Jin, H., Kudo, C., Dalkara, T., & Moskowitz, M. A. (2006). Suppression of cortical spreading depression in migraine prophylaxis. *Annals of Neurology*, *59*(4), 652–661. doi: 10.1002/ana.20778

11. Babateen, O., Althobaiti, F. S., Alhazmi, M. A., Al-Ghamdi, E., Alharbi, F., Moffareh, A. K., Matar, F. M., Tawakul, A., Samkari, J. A., Babateen, O., Althobaiti, F. S., Alhazmi, M. A., Al-Ghamdi, E., Alharbi, F., Moffareh, A. K., Matar, F. M., Tawakul, A., & Samkari, J. A. (2023). Association of migraine headache with depression, anxiety, and stress in the population of Makkah City, Saudi Arabia: A cross-sectional study. *Cureus*, *15*(5), e39788. doi: 10.7759/cureus.39788
12. Barker, A. T., & Shields, K. (2017). Transcranial magnetic stimulation: Basic principles and clinical applications in migraine. *Headache*, *57*(3), 517–524. doi: 10.1111/head.13002
13. Baskin, S. M., & Smitherman, T. A. (2009). Migraine and psychiatric disorders: Comorbidities, mechanisms, and clinical applications. *Neurological Sciences*, *30*(1), 61–65. doi: 10.1007/s10072-009-0071-5
14. Bazargan, M., Comini, J., Kibe, L. W., Assari, S., & Cobb, S. (2023a). Association between migraine and quality of life, mental health, sleeping disorders, and health care utilization among older African American adults. *Journal of Racial and Ethnic Health Disparities*. *11*(3), 1530–1540 doi: 10.1007/s40615-023-01629-y
15. Bagley, C. L., Rendas-Baum, R., Maglinte, G. A., Yang, M., Varon, S. F., Lee, J., & Kosinski, M. (2012). Validating migraine-specific quality of life questionnaire v2. 1 in episodic and chronic migraine. *Headache*, *52*(3), 409–421.
16. Beach, S. R., Kostis, W. J., Celano, C. M., Januzzi, J. L., Ruskin, J. N., Noseworthy, P. A., & Huffman, J. C. (2014). Meta-analysis of selective serotonin reuptake inhibitor-associated QTc prolongation. *The Journal of Clinical Psychiatry*, *75*(5), e441–e449. doi: 10.4088/JCP.13r08672
17. Benemei, S., De Logu, F., Li Puma, S., Marone, I. M., Coppi, E., Ugolini, F., Liedtke, W., Pollastro, F., Appendino, G., Geppetti, P., Materazzi, S., & Nassini, R. (2017). The anti-migraine component of butterbur extracts, isopetasin, desensitizes peptidergic nociceptors by acting on TRPA1 cation channel. *British Journal of Pharmacology*, *174*(17), 2897–2911. doi: 10.1111/bph.13917
18. Bhaskaran, N., Shukla, S., Srivastava, J. K., & Gupta, S. (2010). Chamomile: An anti-inflammatory agent inhibits inducible nitric oxide synthase expression by blocking RelA/p65 activity. *International Journal of Molecular Medicine*, *26*(6), 935–940. doi: 10.3892/ijmm_00000545
19. Bigal, M. E., & Lipton, R. B. (2006). Obesity is a risk factor for transformed migraine but not chronic tension-type headache. *Neurology*, *67*(2), 252–257. doi: 10.1212/01.wnl.0000225052.35019.f9
20. Blau, J. N. (2005). Water deprivation: A new migraine precipitant. *Headache*, *45*(6), 757–759. doi: 10.1111/j.1526-4610.2005.05143_3.x
21. Borhani Haghighi, A., Motazedian, S., & Rezaii, R. (2007). Therapeutic potentials of menthol in migraine headache: Possible mechanisms of action. *Medical Hypotheses*, *69*(2), 455. doi: 10.1016/j.mehy.2006.12.024
22. Brandes, J. L., Kudrow, D., Stark, S. R., O'Carroll, C. P., Adelman, J. U., O'Donnell, F. J., Alexander, W. J., Spruill, S. E., Barrett, P. S., & Lener, S. E. (2007). Sumatriptan-naproxen for acute treatment of migraine: A randomized trial. *JAMA*, *297*(13), 1443–1454. doi: 10.1001/jama.297.13.1443

23. Breslau, N., Davis, G. C., & Andreski, P. (1991). Migraine, psychiatric disorders, and suicide attempts: An epidemiologic study of young adults. *Psychiatry Research, 37*(1), 11–23. doi: 10.1016/0165-1781(91)90102-U
24. Browne, A. J., Varcoe, C. M., Wong, S. T., Smye, V. L., Lavoie, J., Littlejohn, D., Tu, D., Godwin, O., Krause, M., Khan, K. B., Fridkin, A., Rodney, P., O'Neil, J., & Lennox, S. (2012). Closing the health equity gap: Evidence-based strategies for primary health care organizations. *International Journal for Equity in Health, 11*(1), 59. doi: 10.1186/1475-9276-11-59
25. Bushra, R., & Aslam, N. (2010). An overview of clinical pharmacology of ibuprofen. *Oman Medical Journal, 25*(3), 1655–1661. doi: 10.5001/omj.2010.49
26. Calabrò, R. S. (2022). Gender effect on migraine: Nature or culture? *Journal of Integrative Neuroscience, 21*(1), 1. doi: 10.31083/j.jin2101018
27. Calhoun, A. H., & Ford, S. (2007). Behavioral sleep modification may revert transformed migraine to episodic migraine. *Headache, 47*(8), 1178–1183. doi: 10.1111/j.1526-4610.2007.00780.x
28. Chervyakov, A. V., Chernyavsky, A. Yu., Sinitsyn, D. O., & Piradov, M. A. (2015). Possible mechanisms underlying the therapeutic effects of transcranial magnetic stimulation. *Frontiers in Human Neuroscience, 9*. doi: 10.3389/fnhum.2015.00303
29. Chowdhury, D., & Datta, D. (2020). Managing migraine in the times of COVID-19 pandemic. *Annals of Indian Academy of Neurology, 23*(7), 33. doi: 10.4103/aian.AIAN_296_20
30. Cook, C. L., & Shedd, G. C. (2018). Diagnosis and treatment of migraine in the patient with depression. *Journal of the American Association of Nurse Practitioners, 30*(11), 630–637. doi: 10.1097/JXX.0000000000000075
31. D'Amico, D., Grazzi, L., Curone, M., Di Fiore, P., Proietti Cecchini, A., Leonardi, M., Scaratti, C., & Raggi, A. (2015). Difficulties in work activities and the pervasive effect over disability in patients with episodic and chronic migraine. *Neurological Sciences, 36*(S1), 9–11. doi: 10.1007/s10072-015-2130-4
32. Dennis, A., Matthew, L. J., Yan, Z., & Holger, C. (2022). Predictors of headache/migraine and the use of complementary medicine in U.S. Children: A population-based analysis of 2017 national health interview survey data. *Journal of Integrative and Complementary Medicine, 28*(1), 60–66. doi: 10.1089/jicm.2021.0117
33. *Depressive disorder (depression)*. (n.d.). accessed January 24, 2024 from https://www.who.int/news-room/fact-sheets/detail/depression
34. Di Stefano, V., Iacono, S., Gagliardo, A., Maggio, B., Guggino, G., Gangitano, M., Monastero, R., Maggio, V. R., Bolognini, N., & Brighina, F. (2022). Sound-induced flash illusions support cortex hyperexcitability in fibromyalgia. *Pain Research & Management, 2022*, 7355102. doi: 10.1155/2022/7355102
35. Diamond, M. (2007). The impact of migraine on the health and well-being of women. *Journal of Women's Health, 16*(9), 1269–1280. doi: 10.1089/jwh.2007.0388
36. Diener, H., Pfaffenrath, V., Schnitker, J., Friede, M., & Zepelin, H. H. H.(2005). Efficacy and safety of 6.25 mg t.i.d. feverfew $CO_2$-extract (MIG-99) in migraine prevention: A randomized, double-blind, multicentre, placebo-controlled study. *Cephalalgia, 25*(11), 1031–1041. doi: 10.1111/j.1468-2982.2005.00950.x
37. Dresler, T., Caratozzolo, S., Guldolf, K., Huhn, J.-I., Loiacono, C., Niiberg-Pikksööt, T., Puma, M., Sforza, G., Tobia, A., Ornello, R., & Serafini, G. (2019). Understanding

the nature of psychiatric comorbidity in migraine: A systematic review focused on interactions and treatment implications. *The Journal of Headache and Pain*, *20*(1), 51. doi: 10.1186/s10194-019-0988-x

38. Elisa, A., & Federica, G. (2016). Psychological treatment for headache: A pilot study on the efficacy of joint psychoeducational group and relaxation training. *Journal of Neurology & Neurophysiology*, *7*(3). doi: 10.4172/2155-9562.1000379
39. Erulkar, A., & Medhin, G. (2022). Factors associated with depression among young female migrants in Ethiopia. *BMC Women's Health*, *22*(1), 432. doi: 10.1186/s12905-022-02017-0
40. Essayagh, F., Essayagh, M., Essayagh, S., Marc, I., Bukassa, G., El otmani, I., Kouyate, M. F., & Essayagh, T. (2023). The prevalence and risk factors for anxiety and depression symptoms among migrants in Morocco. *Scientific Reports*, *13*(1), 1. doi: 10.1038/s41598-023-30715-8
41. Evcili, G. (2018). Early and long period follow-up results of low-glycemic index diet for migraine prophylaxis. *Ağrı*. doi: 10.5505/agri.2017.62443
42. Farahmand, S., Shafazand, S., Alinia, E., Bagheri-Hariri, S., & Baratloo, A. (2018). Pain management using acupuncture method in migraine headache patients: A single blinded randomized clinical trial. *Anesthesiology and Pain Medicine*, *8*(6), e81688. doi: 10.5812/aapm.81688
43. Fava, A., Pirritano, D., Consoli, D., Plastino, M., Casalinuovo, F., Cristofaro, S., Colica, C., Ermio, C., De Bartolo, M., Opipari, C., Lanzo, R., Consoli, A., & Bosco, D. (2014). Chronic migraine in women is associated with insulin resistance: A cross-sectional study. *European Journal of Neurology*, *21*(2), 267–272. doi: 10.1111/ene.12289
44. Fellmeth, G., Plugge, E., Fazel, M., Nosten, S., Oo, M. M., Pimanpanarak, M., Phichitpadungtham, Y., Fitzpatrick, R., & McGready, R. (n.d.). Perinatal depression in migrant and refugee women on the Thai–Myanmar border: Does social support matter? *Philosophical Transactions of the Royal Society B: Biological Sciences*, *376*(1827), 20200030. doi: 10.1098/rstb.2020.0030
45. Fellmeth, G., Plugge, E., Fazel, M., Oo, M. M., Pimanpanarak, M., Phichitpadungtham, Y., Wai, K., Charunwatthana, P., Simpson, J. A., Nosten, F., Fitzpatrick, R., & McGready, R. (2020). Prevalence and determinants of perinatal depression among labor migrant and refugee women on the Thai–Myanmar border: A cohort study. *BMC Psychiatry*, *20*(1), 168. doi: 10.1186/s12888-020-02572-6
46. Ferrari, M. D., Goadsby, P. J., Burstein, R., Kurth, T., Ayata, C., Charles, A., Ashina, M., van den Maagdenberg, A. M. J. M., & Dodick, D. W. (2022). Migraine. *Nature Reviews. Disease Primers*, *8*(1), 2. doi: 10.1038/s41572-021-00328-4
47. Flynn, N. (2018). Systematic review of the effectiveness of hypnosis for the management of headache. *The International Journal of Clinical and Experimental Hypnosis*, *66*(4), 343–352. doi: 10.1080/00207144.2018.1494432
48. Fowler, P. A., Lacey, L. F., Thomas, M., Keene, O. N., Tanner, R. J. N., & Baber, N. S. (2008). The clinical pharmacology, pharmacokinetics and metabolism of sumatriptan. *European Neurology*, *31*(5), 291–294. doi: 10.1159/000116756
49. Foxhall, K. (2019). *Migraine: A History*. Johns Hopkins University Press. http://www.ncbi.nlm.nih.gov/books/NBK544082/

50. Gaul, C., Diener, H.-C., & Danesch, U. (2015). Improvement of migraine symptoms with a proprietary supplement containing riboflavin, magnesium and Q10: A randomized, placebo-controlled, double-blind, multicenter trial. *The Journal of Headache and Pain*, *16*, 516. doi: 10.1186/s10194-015-0516-6
51. Ghajarzadeh, M., Jalilian, R., Togha, M., Azimi, A., Hosseini, P., & Babaei, N. (2014). Depression, poor sleep, and sexual dysfunction in migraineurs women. *International Journal of Preventive Medicine*, *5*(9), 1113–1118.
52. Gil-Salmerón, A., Katsas, K., Riza, E., Karnaki, P., & Linos, A. (2021). Access to healthcare for migrant patients in Europe: Healthcare discrimination and translation services. *International Journal of Environmental Research and Public Health*, *18*(15), e7901. doi: 10.3390/ijerph18157901
53. Gouider, R., Lorenz, D. H., Craven, A., Grisold, W., & Dodick, D. W. (2023). Advocacy for patients with headache disorders. *eNeurologicalSci*, *31*, e100466. doi: 10.1016/j.ensci.2023.100466
54. Grazzi, L., Toppo, C., D'Amico, D., Leonardi, M., Martelletti, P., Raggi, A., & Guastafierro, E. (2021). Non-pharmacological approaches to headaches: Non-invasive neuromodulation, nutraceuticals, and behavioral approaches. *International Journal of Environmental Research and Public Health*, *18*(4), 1503. doi: 10.3390/ijerph18041503
55. Green, B. M., Van Horn, K. T., Gupte, K., Evans, M., Hayes, S., & Bhowmick, A. (2020). Assessment of adaptive engagement and support model for people with chronic health conditions in online health communities: Combined content analysis. *Journal of Medical Internet Research*, *22*(7), e17338. doi: 10.2196/17338
56. Guldiken, B., Guldiken, S., Demir, M., Turgut, N., & Tugrul, A. (2008). Low leptin levels in migraine: A case control study. *Headache*, *48*(7), 1103–1107. doi: 10.1111/j.1526-4610.2008.01152.x
57. Haghdoost, F., & Togha, M. (2022a). Migraine management: Non-pharmacological points for patients and health care professionals. *Open Medicine*, *17*(1), 1869–1882. doi: 10.1515/med-2022-0598
58. Haghdoost, F., & Togha, M. (2022b). Migraine management: Non-pharmacological points for patients and health care professionals. *Open Medicine (Warsaw, Poland)*, *17*(1), 1869–1882. doi: 10.1515/med-2022-0598
59. Hamelsky, S. W., & Lipton, R. B. (2006). Psychiatric Comorbidity of Migraine. *Headache*, *46*(9), 1327–1333. doi: 10.1111/j.1526-4610.2006.00576.x
60. Harmer, C. J., Duman, R. S., & Cowen, P. J. (2017). How do antidepressants work? New perspectives for refining future treatment approaches. *The Lancet—Psychiatry*, *4*(5), 409–418. doi: 10.1016/S2215-0366(17)30015-9
61. Harmer, C. J., Goodwin, G. M., & Cowen, P. J. (2009). Why do antidepressants take so long to work? A cognitive neuropsychological model of antidepressant drug action. *The British Journal of Psychiatry*, *195*(2), 102–108.
62. Henningsen, P., Hausteiner-Wiehle, C., & Häuser, W. (2022). Migraine in the context of chronic primary pain, chronic overlapping pain disorders, and functional somatic disorders: A narrative review. *Headache*, *62*(10), 1272–1280. doi: 10.1111/head.14419
63. Holland, S., Silberstein, S. D., Freitag, F., Dodick, D. W., Argoff, C., & Ashman, E. (2012). Evidence-based guideline update: NSAIDs and other complementary

treatments for episodic migraine prevention in adults. *Neurology*, *78*(17), 1346–1353. doi: 10.1212/WNL.0b013e3182535d0c

64. Iba, C., Ohtani, S., Lee, M. J., Huh, S., Watanabe, N., Nakahara, J., Peng, K. P., & Takizawa, T. (2023). Migraine triggers in Asian countries: A narrative review. *Frontiers in Neurology*, *14*, online. https://www.frontiersin.org/articles/10.3389/fneur.2023.1169795
65. Jahangir, S., Adjepong, D., Al-Shami, H. A., & Malik, B. H. (n.d.). Is there an association between migraine and major depressive disorder? A narrative review. *Cureus*, *12*(6), e8551. doi: 10.7759/cureus.8551
66. J. Katon, W. (2011). Epidemiology and treatment of depression in patients with chronic medical illness. *Dialogues in Clinical Neuroscience*, *13*(1), 7–23.
67. Kabat-Zinn, J. (1982). An outpatient program in behavioral medicine for chronic pain patients based on the practice of mindfulness meditation: Theoretical considerations and preliminary results. *General Hospital Psychiatry*, *4*(1), 33–47. doi: 10.1016/0163-8343(82)90026-3
68. Kabat-Zinn, J., Lipworth, L., & Burney, R. (1985). The clinical use of mindfulness meditation for the self-regulation of chronic pain. *Journal of Behavioral Medicine*, *8*(2), 163–190. doi: 10.1007/BF00845519
69. Kabbouche, M. A., Powers, S. W., Vockell, A. B., LeCates, S. L., Ellinor, P. L., Segers, A., Manning, P., Burdine, D., & Hershey, A. D. (2005). Outcome of a multidisciplinary approach to pediatric migraine at 1, 2, and 5 years. *Headache*, *45*(10), 1298–1303. doi: 10.1111/j.1526-4610.2005.00261.x
70. Katsarava, Z., Mania, M., Lampl, C., Herberhold, J., & Steiner, T. J. (2018). Poor medical care for people with migraine in Europe—Evidence from the Eurolight study. *The Journal of Headache and Pain*, *19*(1), 10. doi: 10.1186/s10194-018-0839-1
71. Kerr, C. E., Sacchet, M. D., Lazar, S. W., Moore, C. I., & Jones, S. R. (2013). Mindfulness starts with the body: Somatosensory attention and top-down modulation of cortical alpha rhythms in mindfulness meditation. *Frontiers in Human Neuroscience*, *7*, 12. doi: 10.3389/fnhum.2013.00012
72. Kirland, J. L., Mukku, V. R., Hardy, M., & Stancel, G. M. (1984). Hormonal control of uterine growth: Alterations in luminal epithelial deoxyribonucleic acid synthesis after intraluminal application of estrogen. *Endocrinology*, *114*(3), 969–973.
73. Kirmayer, L. J. (2001). Cultural variations in the clinical presentation of depression and anxiety: Implications for diagnosis and treatment. *The Journal of Clinical Psychiatry*, *62*(13), 22–28, discussion 29–30.
74. Kirmayer, L. J., Narasiah, L., Munoz, M., Rashid, M., Ryder, A. G., Guzder, J., Hassan, G., Rousseau, C., & Pottie, K. (2011a). Common mental health problems in immigrants and refugees: General approach in primary care. *Canadian Medical Association Journal*, *183*(12), E959–E967. doi: 10.1503/cmaj.090292
75. Kisan, R., Sujan, M., Adoor, M., Rao, R., Nalini, A., Kutty, B. M., Chindanda Murthy, B., Raju, T., & Sathyaprabha, T. (2014). Effect of Yoga on migraine: A comprehensive study using clinical profile and cardiac autonomic functions. *International Journal of Yoga*, *7*(2), 126–132. doi: 10.4103/0973-6131.133891
76. Kleinman, A., Eisenberg, L., & Good, B. (1978). Culture, illness, and care: Clinical lessons from anthropologic and cross-cultural research. *Annals of Internal Medicine*, *88*(2), 251–258. doi: 10.7326/0003-4819-88-2-251

77. Krah, E., de Kruijf, J., & Ragno, L. (2018). Integrating traditional healers into the health care system: Challenges and opportunities in Rural Northern Ghana. *Journal of Community Health*, *43*(1), 157–163. doi: 10.1007/s10900-017-0398-4
78. Kumar, A., & Kadian, R. (2024). Migraine prophylaxis. In: *StatPearls*. StatPearls Publishing. http://www.ncbi.nlm.nih.gov/books/NBK507873/
79. Kumral, E. (2020). The role of neurologist in the assessment and treatment of depression. *Turkish Journal of Neurology*, *26*(1), 1–9. doi: 10.4274/tnd.2019.44341
80. La Touche, R., Fierro-Marrero, J., Sánchez-Ruíz, I., Rodríguez de Rivera-Romero, B., Cabrera-López, C. D., Lerma-Lara, S., Requejo-Salinas, N., de Asís-Fernández, F., Elizagaray-García, I., Fernández-Carnero, J., Matesanz-García, L., Pardo-Montero, J., Paris-Alemany, A., & Reina-Varona, Á. (2023). Prescription of therapeutic exercise in migraine, an evidence-based clinical practice guideline. *The Journal of Headache and Pain*, *24*(1), 68. doi: 10.1186/s10194-023-01571-8
81. Lake, A. E., Saper, J. R., & Hamel, R. L. (2009). Comprehensive inpatient treatment of refractory chronic daily headache. *Headache*, *49*(4), 555–562. doi: 10.1111/j.1526-4610.2009.01364.x
82. Lambert, O., & Bourin, M. (2002). SNRIs: Mechanism of action and clinical features. *Expert Review of Neurotherapeutics*, *2*(6), 849–858. doi: 10.1586/14737175.2.6.849
83. Lanfranco, R. C., Canales-Johnson, A., & Huepe, D. (2014). Hypnoanalgesia and the study of pain experience: From Cajal to modern neuroscience. *Frontiers in Psychology*, *5*, online. https://www.frontiersin.org/articles/10.3389/fpsyg.2014.01126
84. Lewis-Fernández, R., & Díaz, N. (2002). (No title found). *Psychiatric Quarterly*, *73*(4), 271–295. doi: 10.1023/A:1020412000183
85. Li, Z., Zeng, F., Yin, T., Lan, L., Makris, N., Jorgenson, K., Guo, T., Wu, F., Gao, Y., Dong, M., Liu, M., Yang, J., Li, Y., Gong, Q., Liang, F., & Kong, J. (2017). Acupuncture modulates the abnormal brainstem activity in migraine without aura patients. *NeuroImage: Clinical*, *15*, 367–375. doi: 10.1016/j.nicl.2017.05.013
86. Linde, K., Allais, G., Brinkhaus, B., Fei, Y., Mehring, M., Vertosick, E. A., Vickers, A., & White, A. R. (2016). Acupuncture for the prevention of episodic migraine. *The Cochrane Database of Systematic Reviews*, *2016*(6), CD001218. doi: 10.1002/14651858.CD001218.pub3
87. Lipton, R. B., Baggish, J. S., Stewart, W. F., Codispoti, J. R., & Fu, M. (2000). Efficacy and safety of acetaminophen in the treatment of migraine: Results of a randomized, double-blind, placebo-controlled, population-based study. *Archives of Internal Medicine*, *160*(22), 3486–3492. doi: 10.1001/archinte.160.22.3486
88. Lommel, L., Hu, X., Sun, M., & Chen, J. L. (2020). Frequency of depressive symptoms among female migrant workers in China: Associations with acculturation, discrimination, and reproductive health. *Public Health*, *181*, 151–157. doi: 10.1016/j.puhe.2019.12.006
89. Lopresti, A. L., Smith, S. J., & Drummond, P. D. (2020). Herbal treatments for migraine: A systematic review of randomized-controlled studies. *Phytotherapy Research: PTR*, *34*(10), 2493–2517. doi: 10.1002/ptr.6701
90. Lucchetti, G., Koenig, H. G., & Lucchetti, A. L. G. (2021). Spirituality, religiousness, and mental health: A review of the current scientific evidence. *World Journal of Clinical Cases*, *9*(26), 7620–7631. doi: 10.12998/wjcc.v9.i26.7620

91. MacGregor, E. A. (2006). Migraine and the menopause. *The Journal of the British Menopause Society*, *12*(3), 104–108. doi: 10.1258/136218006778234048
92. MacGregor, E. A. (2015). Migraine management during menstruation and menopause. *CONTINUUM: Lifelong Learning in Neurology*, *21*(4), 990. doi: 10.1212/CON.0000000000000196
93. Madsen, K. B., Momen, N. C., Petersen, L. V., Plana-Ripoll, O., Haarman, B. C. M., Drexhage, H., Mortensen, P. B., McGrath, J. J., & Munk-Olsen, T. (2021). Bidirectional associations between treatment-resistant depression and general medical conditions. *European Neuropsychopharmacology: The Journal of the European College of Neuropsychopharmacology*, *51*, 7–19. doi: 10.1016/j.euroneuro.2021.04.021
94. Maghbooli, M., Golipour, F., Moghimi Esfandabadi, A., & Yousefi, M. (2014). Comparison between the efficacy of ginger and sumatriptan in the ablative treatment of the common migraine. *Phytotherapy Research: PTR*, *28*(3), 412–415. doi: 10.1002/ptr.4996
95. Magis, D., & Schoenen, J. (2012). Advances and challenges in neurostimulation for headaches. *The Lancet Neurology*, *11*(8), 708–719. doi: 10.1016/S1474-4422(12)70139-4
96. Marmura, M. J., Silberstein, S. D., & Schwedt, T. J. (2015). The acute treatment of migraine in adults: The American Headache Society Evidence Assessment of Migraine Pharmacotherapies. *Headache*, *55*(1), 3–20. doi: 10.1111/head.12499
97. Martin, P. R., Aiello, R., Gilson, K., Meadows, G., Milgrom, J., & Reece, J. (2015). Cognitive behavior therapy for comorbid migraine and/or tension-type headache and major depressive disorder: An exploratory randomized controlled trial. *Behavior Research and Therapy*, *73*, 8–18. doi: 10.1016/j.brat.2015.07.005
98. Mattsson, P., & Ekselius, L. (2002). Migraine, major depression, panic disorder, and personality traits in women aged 40–74 years: A population-based study. *Cephalalgia*, *22*(7), 543–551. doi: 10.1046/j.1468-2982.2002.00407.x
99. McKeage, K. (2016). Zolmitriptan nasal spray: A review in acute migraine in pediatric patients 12 years of age or older. *Pediatric Drugs*, *18*(1), 75–81. doi: 10.1007/s40272-015-0160-2
100. Mesnil, M., Defamie, N., Naus, C., & Sarrouilhe, D. (2020). Brain disorders and chemical pollutants: A gap junction link? *Biomolecules*, *11*(1), 51. doi: 10.3390/biom11010051
101. Minen, M. T., Dhaem, O. B. D., Diest, A. K. V., Powers, S., Schwedt, T. J., Lipton, R., & Silbersweig, D. (2016). Migraine and its psychiatric comorbidities. *Journal of Neurology, Neurosurgery & Psychiatry*, *87*(7), 741–749. doi: 10.1136/jnnp-2015-312233
102. Mongini, F., Keller, R., Deregibus, A., Raviola, F., Mongini, T., & Sancarlo, M. (2003). Personality traits, depression and migraine in women: A longitudinal study. *Cephalalgia*, *23*(3), 186–192. doi: 10.1046/j.1468-2982.2003.00519.x
103. Mortel, D., Kawatu, N., Steiner, T. J., & Saylor, D. (2022). Barriers to headache care in low- and middle-income countries. *eNeurologicalSci*, *29*, e100427. doi: 10.1016/j.ensci.2022.100427
104. Moyer, S. (1986). Pharmacokinetics of naproxen sodium. *Cephalalgia*, *6*(4_suppl), 77–80. doi: 10.1177/03331024860060S409

105. Nayar, D., Mahapatro, M., & Nayar, P. (2022). Role of yoga as an adjunct in the management of migraine headache-current status and future indications. *International Journal of Yoga*, *15*(1), 12–18. doi: 10.4103/ijoy.ijoy_173_21
106. Nicholas, A. (2023). The Impact of cultural beliefs and practices on the diagnosis and management of headaches in rural African communities. *Advances in Medical, Dental and Health Sciences*, *6*(1), 18–20. doi: 10.5530/amdhs.2023.1.3
107. Novins, D. K., Bechtold, D. W., Sack, W. H., Thompson, J., Carter, D. R., & Manson, S. M. (1997). The DSM-IV outlines for cultural formulation: A critical demonstration with American Indian children. *Journal of the American Academy of Child & Adolescent Psychiatry*, *36*(9), 1244–1251. doi: 10.1097/00004583-199709000-00017
108. Nyikavaranda, P., Pantelic, M., Jones, C. J., Paudyal, P., Tunks, A., & Llewellyn, C. D. (2023). Barriers and facilitators to seeking and accessing mental health support in primary care and the community among female migrants in Europe: A "feminisms" systematic review. *International Journal for Equity in Health*, *22*(1), 196. doi: 10.1186/s12939-023-01990-8
109. Palermo, T. M., Davis, K. D., Bouhassira, D., Hurley, R. W., Katz, J. D., Keefe, F. J., Schatman, M., Turk, D. C., & Yarnitsky, D. (2023). Promoting inclusion, diversity, and equity in pain science. *The Journal of Pain*, *24*(2), 187–191. doi: 10.1016/j.jpain.2022.11.005
110. Panconesi, A. (2008). Alcohol and migraine: Trigger factor, consumption, mechanisms: A review. *The Journal of Headache and Pain*, *9*(1), 1. doi: 10.1007/s10194-008-0006-1
111. Pareja-Angel, J., & Campo-Arias, A. (2004). The prevalence of symptoms of anxiety and depression in female migraine sufferers. *Revista de Neurologia*, *39*(8), 711–714.
112. Parker, M. (2007). Ethnography/ethics. *Social Science & Medicine, 65*(11), 2248–2259. doi: 10.1016/j.socscimed.2007.08.003
113. Pittler, M. H., & Ernst, E. (2004). Feverfew for preventing migraine. In *Cochrane Database of systematic reviews* (e-document CD002286.pub2). John Wiley & Sons, Ltd. doi: 10.1002/14651858.CD002286.pub2
114. Pringsheim, T., Davenport, W. J., Mackie, G., Worthington, I., Aubé, M., Christie, S. N., Gladstone, J., & Becker, W. J. (2012). Canadian Headache Society guideline for migraine prophylaxis. *The Canadian Journal of Neurological Sciences*, *39*(Suppl 2), S1–S59.
115. Pryse-Phillips, W. E. M., Dodick, D. W., Edmeads, J. G., Gawel, M. J., Nelson, R. F., Purdy, R. A., Robinson, G., Stirling, D., & Worthington, I. (n.d.). Guidelines for the nonpharmacologic management of migraine in clinical practice. *Canadian Headache Society (CMAJ)*, *159*(1), 47–54.
116. Putukian, M., Purcell, L., Schneider, K. J., Black, A. M., Burma, J. S., Chandran, A., Boltz, A., Master, C. L., Register-Mihalik, J. K., Anderson, V., Davis, G. A., Fremont, P., Leddy, J. J., Maddocks, D., Premji, Z., Ronksley, P. E., Herring, S., & Broglio, S. (2023). Clinical recovery from concussion-return to school and sport: A systematic review and meta-analysis. *British Journal of Sports Medicine*, *57*(12), 798–809. doi: 10.1136/bjsports-2022-106682
117. Raggi, A., Grignani, E., Leonardi, M., Andrasik, F., Sansone, E., Grazzi, L., & D'Amico, D. (2018). Behavioral approaches for primary headaches: Recent advances. *Headache*, *58*(6), 913–925. doi: 10.1111/head.13337

118. Rajkumar, R. P. (2023). The influence of cultural and religious factors on cross-national variations in the prevalence of chronic back and neck pain: An analysis of data from the global burden of disease 2019 study. *Frontiers in Pain Research*, *4*, e1189432. https://www.frontiersin.org/articles/10.3389/fpain.2023.1189432
119. Razeghi Jahromi, S., Ghorbani, Z., Martelletti, P., Lampl, C., & Togha, M. (2019). Association of diet and headache. *The Journal of Headache and Pain*, *20*(1), 106. doi: 10.1186/s10194-019-1057-1
120. Razzaque, Z., Pickard, J. D., Ma, Q. -P., Shaw, D., Morrison, K., Wang, T., & Longmore, J. (2002). 5-$HT_{1B}$-receptors and vascular reactivity in human isolated blood vessels: Assessment of the potential craniovascular selectivity of sumatriptan. *British Journal of Clinical Pharmacology*, *53*(3), 266–274. doi: 10.1046/j.0306-5251.2001.01536.x
121. Recober, A., & Goadsby, P. J. (2010). Calcitonin gene-related peptide: A molecular link between obesity and migraine? *Drug News & Perspectives*, *23*(2), 112. doi: 10.1358/dnp.2010.23.2.1475909
122. Rist, P. M., Schürks, M., Buring, J. E., & Kurth, T. (2013). Migraine, headache, and the risk of depression: Prospective cohort study. *Cephalalgia*, *33*(12), 1017–1025. doi: 10.1177/0333102413483930
123. Robblee, J., & Starling, A. J. (2019). SEEDS for success: Lifestyle management in migraine. *Cleveland Clinic Journal of Medicine*, *86*(11), 741–749. doi: 10.3949/ccjm.86a.19009
124. Rogger, R., Bello, C., Romero, C. S., Urman, R. D., Luedi, M. M., & Filipovic, M. G. (2023). Cultural framing and the impact on acute pain and pain services. *Current Pain and Headache Reports*, *27*(9), 429–436. doi: 10.1007/s11916-023-01125-2
125. Rosignoli, C., Ornello, R., Onofri, A., Caponnetto, V., Grazzi, L., Raggi, A., Leonardi, M., & Sacco, S. (2022). Applying a biopsychosocial model to migraine: Rationale and clinical implications. *The Journal of Headache and Pain*, *23*(1), 100. doi: 10.1186/s10194-022-01471-3
126. Roura, M., Bisoffi, F., Navaza, B., & Pool, R. (2015). "Carrying ibuprofen in the bag": Priority health concerns of Latin American migrants in Spain: A participatory qualitative study. *PLoS One*, *10*(8), e0136315. doi: 10.1371/journal.pone.0136315
127. Sacco, S., Bendtsen, L., Ashina, M., Reuter, U., Terwindt, G., Mitsikostas, D.-D., & Martelletti, P. (2019). European headache federation guideline on the use of monoclonal antibodies acting on the calcitonin gene related peptide or its receptor for migraine prevention. *The Journal of Headache and Pain*, *20*(1), 6. doi: 10.1186/s10194-018-0955-y
128. Salik, I., & Marwaha, R. (2024). Electroconvulsive Therapy. In *StatPearls*. StatPearls Publishing. http://www.ncbi.nlm.nih.gov/books/NBK538266/
129. Sangkuhl, K., Klein, T. E., & Altman, R. B. (2009). Selective serotonin reuptake inhibitors pathway. *Pharmacogenetics and Genomics*, *19*(11), 907–909. doi: 10.1097/FPC.0b013e32833132cb
130. Santarelli, L., Saxe, M., Gross, C., Surget, A., Battaglia, F., Dulawa, S., Weisstaub, N., Lee, J., Duman, R., Arancio, O., Belzung, C., & Hen, R. (2003). Requirement of hippocampal neurogenesis for the behavioral effects of antidepressants. *Science (New York, N.Y.)*, *301*(5634), 805–809. doi: 10.1126/science.1083328
131. Sarkhel, S., Singh, O. P., & Arora, M. (2020). Clinical practice guidelines for psychoeducation in psychiatric disorders general principles of psychoeducation.

*Indian Journal of Psychiatry*, *62*(Suppl 2), S319–S323. doi: 10.4103/psychiatry.IndianJPsychiatry_780_19

132. Saunders, P. T. K. (2022). Insights from genomic studies on the role of sex steroids in the etiology of endometriosis. *Reproduction & Fertility*, *3*(2), R51–R65. doi: 10.1530/RAF-21-0078
133. Schmidt, M., Wilhelmy, S., & Gross, D. (2020). Retrospective diagnosis of mental illness: Past and present. *The Lancet Psychiatry*, *7*(1), 14–16. doi: 10.1016/S2215-0366(19)30287-1
134. Schoenen, J., Roberta, B., Magis, D., & Coppola, G. (2016). Noninvasive neurostimulation methods for migraine therapy: The available evidence. *Cephalalgia*, *36*(12), 1170–1180. doi: 10.1177/0333102416636022
135. Schwedt, T. J., & Shapiro, R. E. (2009). Funding of research on headache disorders by the National Institutes of Health. *Headache*, *49*(2), 162–169. doi: 10.1111/j.1526-4610.2008.01323.x
136. Schwedt, T. J., & Vargas, B. (2015). Neurostimulation for treatment of migraine and cluster headache. *Pain Medicine*, *16*(9), 1827–1834. doi: 10.1111/pme.12792
137. Segal, Z. V., Williams, J. M. G., & Teasdale, J. D. (2002). *Mindfulness-based Cognitive Therapy for Depression: A New Approach to Preventing Relapse* (pp. 351). Guilford Press.
138. Seng, E. K., Shapiro, R. E., Buse, D. C., Robbins, M. S., Lipton, R. B., & Parker, A. (2022). The unique role of stigma in migraine-related disability and quality of life. *Headache*, *62*(10), 1354–1364. doi: 10.1111/head.14401
139. Sharpe, L., McDonald, S., Correia, H., Raue, P. J., Meade, T., Nicholas, M., & Arean, P. (2017). Pain severity predicts depressive symptoms over and above individual illnesses and multimorbidity in older adults. *BMC Psychiatry*, *17*(1), 166. doi: 10.1186/s12888-017-1334-y
140. Shea, M. L. O., Garfield, L. D., Teitelbaum, S., Civitelli, R., Mulsant, B. H., Reynolds, C. F., Dixon, D., Doré, P., & Lenze, E. J. (2013). Serotonin-norepinephrine reuptake inhibitor therapy in late-life depression is associated with increased marker of bone resorption. *Osteoporosis International*, *24*(5), 1741–1749. doi: 10.1007/s00198-012-2170-z
141. Shirahige, L., Melo, L., Nogueira, F., Rocha, S., & Monte-Silva, K. (2016). Efficacy of noninvasive brain stimulation on pain control in migraine patients: A systematic review and meta-analysis. *Headache*, *56*(10), 1565–1596. doi: 10.1111/head.12981
142. Silberstein, S. D. (1998). Comprehensive management of headache and depression. *Cephalalgia*, *18*(Suppl 21), 50–55. doi: 10.1177/0333102498018s2113
143. Silverman, K., Evans, S. M., Strain, E. C., & Griffiths, R. R. (1992). Withdrawal syndrome after the double-blind cessation of caffeine consumption. *The New England Journal of Medicine*, *327*(16), 1109–1114. doi: 10.1056/NEJM199210153271601
144. Slavin, M., & Ailani, J. (2017). A clinical approach to addressing diet with migraine patients. *Current Neurology and Neuroscience Reports*, *17*(2), 17. doi: 10.1007/s11910-017-0721-6
145. Soares, A. de A., Louçana, P. M. C., Nasi, E. P., Sousa, K. M. de H., Sá, O. M. de S., & Silva-Néto, R. P. (2018). A double-blind, randomized, and placebo-controlled clinical trial with omega-3 polyunsaturated fatty acids (OPFA ω-3) for the prevention of

migraine in chronic migraine patients using amitriptyline. *Nutritional Neuroscience, 21*(3), 219–223. doi: 10.1080/1028415X.2016.1266133

146. Soman, A., Venkatram, S., Chikkanna, U., Ramakrishna, K. K., Bhargav, H., Mailankody, P., & Varambally, S. (2022). Ayurveda for management of migraine: A narrative review of clinical evidence. *Journal of Family Medicine and Primary Care, 11*(8), 4228. doi: 10.4103/jfmpc.jfmpc_2109_21
147. Stuginski-Barbosa, J., Dach, F., Bigal, M., & Speciali, J. G. (2012). Chronic pain and depression in the quality of life of women with migraine: A controlled study. *Headache, 52*(3), 400–408. doi: 10.1111/j.1526-4610.2012.02095.x
148. *Supporting Mental Health of Immigrant Women.* (2023, March 27). https://www.samhsa.gov/blog/supporting-mental-health-immigrant-women
149. Suthisisang, C. C., Poolsup, N., Suksomboon, N., Lertpipopmetha, V., & Tepwitukgid, B. (2010). Meta-analysis of the efficacy and safety of naproxen sodium in the acute treatment of migraine. *Headache, 50*(5), 808–818. doi: 10.1111/j.1526-4610.2010.01635.x
150. Tfelt-Hansen, P., De Vries, P., & Saxena, P. R. (2000). Triptans in migraine. *Drugs, 60*(6), 1259–1287. doi: 10.2165/00003495-200060060-00003
151. The link between migraine and mental health. (2021, February 25). https://www.medicalnewstoday.com/articles/evidence-connecting-migraine-and-mental-health
152. Thierry, A., Mendinatou, A., Aude, G., Bohr, S. C., & Dismand, H. (2018). Migraine and obesity in Parakou in 2017: Case-control study. *Pain Studies and Treatment, 6*(3), 3. doi: 10.4236/pst.2018.63003
153. Tietjen, G. E., Brandes, J. L., Digre, K. B., Baggaley, S., Martin, V. T., Recober, A., Geweke, L. O., Hafeez, F., Aurora, S. K., Herial, N. A., Utley, C., & Khuder, S. A. (2007). History of childhood maltreatment is associated with comorbid depression in women with migraine. *Neurology, 69*(10), 959–968. doi: 10.1212/01.wnl.0000271383.60376.67
154. Uebelacker, L. A., Marootian, B. A., Pirraglia, P. A., Primack, J., Tigue, P. M., Haggarty, R., Velazquez, L., Bowdoin, J. J., Kalibatseva, Z., & Miller, I. W. (2012). Barriers and facilitators of treatment for depression in a Latino community: A focus group study. *Community Mental Health Journal, 48*(1), 114–126. doi: 10.1007/s10597-011-9388-7
155. *Understanding the Link between Bipolar Disorder, Migraine.* (2021, February 10). AJMC. https://www.ajmc.com/view/understanding-the-link-between-bipolar-disorder-migraine
156. Vécsei, L., Majláth, Z., Szok, D., Csáti, A., & Tajti, J. (2015). Drug safety and tolerability in prophylactic migraine treatment. *Expert Opinion on Drug Safety, 14*(5), 667–681. doi: 10.1517/14740338.2015.1014797
157. Verrotti, A., Di Fonzo, A., Penta, L., Agostinelli, S., & Parisi, P. (2014). Obesity and headache/migraine: The importance of weight reduction through lifestyle modifications. *BioMed Research International, 2014*, e420858. doi: 10.1155/2014/420858
158. Vetvik, K. G., & MacGregor, E. A. (2021). Menstrual migraine: A distinct disorder needing greater recognition. *The Lancet. Neurology, 20*(4), 304–315. doi: 10.1016/S1474-4422(20)30482-8

159. Vgontzas, A., & Pavlović, J. M. (2018). Sleep disorders and migraine: Review of literature and potential pathophysiology mechanisms. *Headache*, *58*(7), 1030–1039. doi: 10.1111/head.13358
160. Vickers, A. J., Vertosick, E. A., Lewith, G., MacPherson, H., Foster, N. E., Sherman, K. J., Irnich, D., Witt, C. M., & Linde, K. (2018). Acupuncture for chronic pain: Update of an individual patient data meta-analysis. *The Journal of Pain*, *19*(5), 455–474. doi: 10.1016/j.jpain.2017.11.005
161. Vos, T., Allen, C., Arora, M., Barber, R. M., Bhutta, Z. A., Brown, A., Carter, A., Casey, D. C., Charlson, F. J., Chen, A. Z., Coggeshall, M., Cornaby, L., Dandona, L., Dicker, D. J., Dilegge, T., Erskine, H. E., Ferrari, A. J., Fitzmaurice, C., Fleming, T., & Murray, C. J. L. (2016). Global, regional, and national incidence, prevalence, and years lived with disability for 310 diseases and injuries, 1990–2015: A systematic analysis for the Global Burden of Disease Study 2015. *The Lancet*, *388*(10053), 1545–1602. doi: 10.1016/S0140-6736(16)31678-6
162. Wells, R. E., O'Connell, N., Pierce, C. R., Estave, P., Penzien, D. B., Loder, E., Zeidan, F., & Houle, T. T. (2021). Effectiveness of mindfulness meditation vs headache education for adults with migraine: A randomized clinical trial. *JAMA Internal Medicine*, *181*(3), 317–328. doi: 10.1001/jamainternmed.2020.7090
163. Westergaard, M. L., Hansen, E. H., Glümer, C., Olesen, J., & Jensen, R. H. (2014). Definitions of medication-overuse headache in population-based studies and their implications on prevalence estimates: A systematic review. *Cephalalgia*, *34*(6), 409–425. doi: 10.1177/0333102413512033
164. Winner, P., Landy, S., Richardson, M., & Ames, M. (2005). Early intervention in migraine with sumatriptan tablets 50 mg versus 100 mg: A pooled analysis of data from six clinical trials. *Clinical Therapeutics*, *27*(11), 1785–1794. doi: 10.1016/j.clinthera.2005.11.009
165. Winsvold, B. S., Harder, A. V. E., Ran, C., Chalmer, M. A., Dalmasso, M. C., Ferkingstad, E., Tripathi, K. P., Bacchelli, E., Børte, S., Fourier, C., Petersen, A. S., Vijfhuizen, L. S., Magnusson, S. H., O'Connor, E., Bjornsdottir, G., Häppölä, P., Wang, Y.-F., Callesen, I., & Kelderman, T. (2023). Cluster headache genomewide association study and meta-analysis identifies eight loci and implicates smoking as causal risk factor. *Annals of Neurology*, *94*(4), 713–726. doi: 10.1002/ana.26743
166. Woodyard, C. (2011). Exploring the therapeutic effects of yoga and its ability to increase quality of life. *International Journal of Yoga*, *4*(2), 49–54. doi: 10.4103/0973-6131.85485
167. World Health Organization. (2011). *Atlas of Headache Disorders and Resources in the World* (p. 67).
168. Young, N. P., Ridgeway, J. L., Haddad, T. C., Harper, S. B., Philpot, L. M., Christopherson, L. A., McColley, S. M., Phillips, S. A., Brown, J. K., Zimmerman, K. S., & Ebbert, J. O. (2023). Feasibility and usability of a mobile app–Based interactive care plan for migraine in a community neurology practice: Development and pilot implementation study. *JMIR Formative Research*, *7*, e48372. doi: 10.2196/48372
169. Zhang, X., Yan, Y., Ye, Z., & Xie, J. (2023). Descriptive analysis of depression among adolescents in Huangshi, China. *BMC Psychiatry*, *23*, 176. doi: 10.1186/s12888-023-04682-3

# PART II

# TECHNOLOGICAL ADVANCEMENTS AND INNOVATIONS

## CHAPTER 6

# AI and Machine Learning: Pioneering Frontiers in Women's Health Advancements

NITISH BHATIA

## ABSTRACT

Artificial intelligence (AI) and machine learning (ML) are revolutionizing women's healthcare by harnessing data-driven insights to enhance early disease detection, personalize treatment, and promote holistic well-being. This chapter explores how AI-powered diagnostic tools improve breast and cervical cancer screenings, optimize prenatal care, and help reduce healthcare disparities. It highlights AI's potential in tackling maternal mortality and reproductive health challenges, offering tailored solutions that span fertility, pregnancy, and postpartum support. Chronic conditions such as endometriosis, polycystic ovary syndrome, and menopause also benefit from AI-enabled symptom monitoring and individualized care plans, empowering women to manage their health proactively. Mental health support is another emerging frontier, where AI-driven chatbots and virtual therapists provide accessible, stigma-free platforms to address postpartum depression, anxiety, and related issues. The chapter also explores the ethical considerations, emphasizing the need for data privacy, bias mitigation, and equitable access to ensure these technologies serve all women fairly. By integrating AI and ML responsibly, healthcare professionals, researchers, and policymakers can drive transformative change, fostering a future of precision, inclusivity, and improved outcomes in women's health.

Holistic Approaches for Women's Sustainable Health, Volume 1: Foundations, Innovations, Challenges, and Management. Megh R. Goyal, Anamika Chauhan, and Junaid Ahmad Malik (Eds)


DOI: 10.1201/9781779641632-8

## 6.1 INTRODUCTION

In recent years, the convergence of artificial intelligence (AI) and machine learning (ML) has ushered in an era of transformative possibilities within the domain of healthcare, with particular significance attributed to women's health. The innovative applications of these technologies, as demonstrated in the work of Rony and coworkers, hold the promise of not merely evolving but truly revolutionizing women's health [55]. The capabilities of AI and ML extend across various dimensions, including the delivery of personalized medical interventions, the facilitation of early disease detection, and the enablement of precision treatments [37]. These multifaceted advancements mark a significant paradigm shift in the healthcare sector, where women are provided with the tools to make informed decisions about their health, and healthcare professionals are empowered to deliver more accurate diagnoses and tailor therapeutic strategies [33].

As technology continues to evolve, this chapter is dedicated to delving deeper into the profound implications of AI and ML within the specific context of women's health. It places an emphasis on emerging research and promising developments, pushing the boundaries of what is achievable [2]. The insights presented here draw from an extensive array of scholarly works, incorporating contributions from experts in the field and other accomplished researchers. By synthesizing and expanding upon this body of knowledge, this chapter aims to offer a comprehensive overview of the multifaceted landscape of AI and ML applications in women's health, shedding light on their transformative potential. The advent of AI and ML has disrupted and revolutionized various aspects of the healthcare sector, and women's health stands as a significant beneficiary of these advancements [6]. The applications of AI and ML transcend the boundaries of conventional healthcare, fundamentally altering the way women's health is approached. The profound impact of these technologies span from the delivery of personalized medical interventions, early disease detection, and precision treatments. Personalized medicine, powered by AI, has emerged as a cornerstone of the transformative changes in women's healthcare. It represents a paradigm shift in the way healthcare is delivered. Personalized medicine tailors medical interventions to the unique genetic, environmental, and lifestyle factors of individual patients [37].

AI algorithms, as demonstrated by Hripcsak and Albers, can analyze a patient's genetic data and medical history to predict the most effective treatment options, considering potential risks and side effects [30]. This level of personalization is especially pertinent in women's health, impacting fields such as breast cancer treatment and reproductive health. For instance, AI-driven models can assist in determining the most suitable contraceptive methods for individual women, accounting for their health history, genetic makeup, and personal preferences [17]. This personalized approach not only improves the effectiveness of healthcare but also enhances patient satisfaction and adherence to treatment plans [60]. Moreover, AI and ML offer significant advancements in early disease detection, a critical aspect of women's healthcare [39]. Timely identification of health issues is paramount in this domain, where early intervention can significantly impact outcomes. AI technologies can analyze diverse data sources, encompassing medical records, imaging, and wearable device data, to detect early signs of diseases such as breast cancer, cervical cancer, and preeclampsia [29]. It has been demonstrated how AI-driven models have the potential to identify these conditions in their early stages, greatly increasing the chances of successful treatment [36]. Furthermore, in the field of radiology, AI algorithms have been instrumental in breast cancer screening, where they can analyze mammograms with a high degree of accuracy, reducing the likelihood of false positives and false negatives [43].

In addition to early disease detection, AI and ML have opened the possibility of precision treatments in women's health. Precision medicine, characterized by tailoring treatments based on an individual's specific genetic makeup and the genetic characteristics of their condition, is a game-changer for the treatment of conditions like ovarian and breast cancer [65]. It exemplifies how AI can identify the most appropriate treatment strategies by analyzing a patient's genetic profile and the characteristics of the disease [57]. This approach not only improves the chances of successful treatment but also minimizes the potential side effects and complications associated with generic treatments. AI and ML are not only revolutionizing the medical aspects of women's health but are also empowering women to take control of their healthcare decisions [33]. These technologies provide women with access to a wealth of health-related information, allowing them to make informed choices about their well-being. Mobile apps and wearable devices, driven by AI, enable women to track various aspects of their health, from menstrual cycles to heart rate, and receive personalized insights and recommendations [23]. Such tools can be instrumental in managing conditions like polycystic ovary syndrome (PCOS) and endometriosis, where symptom tracking is essential for both diagnosis and symptom management [11].

AI-driven chatbots and virtual health assistants also play a significant role in educating women about their health and providing them with reliable information and advice [4]. These virtual healthcare providers are available around the clock, answering questions, offering guidance, and helping women understand their symptoms and treatment options [12]. They bridge the information gap and empower women to seek appropriate care when needed. Healthcare professionals, on the other hand, benefit from AI and ML in their daily practice. These technologies provide clinicians with decision support tools that enhance the accuracy of diagnoses and treatment recommendations. Predictive models powered by AI can analyze patient data and suggest potential diagnoses or treatment plans, acting as a valuable second opinion [16]. In the context of women's health, this can be particularly beneficial in the diagnosis of complex conditions like endometriosis, which often involves a lengthy and challenging diagnostic process. AI-driven tools also have the potential to reduce the administrative burden on healthcare providers, allowing them to focus more on patient care [61].

Electronic health records (EHR) systems with AI capabilities can automate tasks such as documentation, appointment scheduling, and billing, streamlining the workflow and increasing the efficiency of healthcare providers. This not only improves the overall quality of care but also reduces burnout among healthcare professionals [58]. As AI and ML technologies continue to advance, the opportunities for further improvements in women's health are boundless. Emerging research is focused on areas such as predicting pregnancy complications, enhancing the accuracy of fertility tracking, and developing novel therapies for gynecological conditions [41].

Additionally, the integration of genomics and AI promises to unlock new insights into genetic contributions to women's health conditions, allowing for more targeted and effective treatments. Furthermore, research is ongoing in the field of ethical considerations related to AI and ML in women's health. Ensuring privacy, security, and informed consent in the use of personal health data is essential, as is addressing potential biases in AI algorithms that can impact underserved populations. Ethical and regulatory frameworks need to evolve in tandem with technological advancements to ensure that women's health is benefited, rather than compromised, by these technologies [20].

This chapter embarks on a comprehensive and in-depth exploration of the pioneering frontiers in AI and ML applications that are rapidly reshaping the landscape of women's healthcare.

## 6.2 ROLE OF AI AND ML IN EARLY DISEASE DETECTION

The integration of AI and ML into the realm of healthcare has ushered in a transformative era, redefining the early detection of diseases affecting women. AI and ML technologies have revolutionized disease detection by offering sophisticated tools that can analyze vast datasets, identify subtle patterns, and provide timely and accurate diagnoses. In this context, they play a pivotal role in transforming women's healthcare by enabling the early detection of diseases such as breast cancer, cervical cancer, and preeclampsia [40]. The contributions of AI and ML in the early detection of women's diseases are paramount, offering the potential to save lives and improve the quality of care.

Breast cancer, one of the most prevalent women's health concerns, has significantly benefited from AI and ML in early detection. Mammography, a traditional method for breast cancer screening, has been enhanced by AI algorithms that can interpret mammograms with remarkable precision [66]. These algorithms, which have been trained on extensive datasets, can identify subtle patterns and anomalies that might be missed by human radiologists. They learn and improve over time, becoming more accurate with each case they analyze [28]. This advancement is particularly valuable for women with dense breast tissue, where traditional mammography can be less effective. The integration of AI in mammography not only enhances early detection but also reduces the incidence of false positives and false negatives, leading to more effective and efficient breast cancer screening [13].

Cervical cancer screening has also witnessed significant progress due to AI and ML. The analysis of Pap smears and human papillomavirus test results can now be automated with AI algorithms, providing highly accurate results [29]. These algorithms can identify abnormal cell patterns with a high degree of sensitivity and specificity, offering early detection of cervical cancer and its precursors [45]. The implementation of AI in cervical cancer screening reduces the rate of false negative results, which is crucial for the early intervention and treatment of this disease. The impact of AI in this context extends beyond individual health; it contributes to the reduction of healthcare costs and the alleviation of the burden on healthcare systems.

Preeclampsia, a serious pregnancy complication, is another condition where early detection is of paramount importance. AI algorithms, when applied to a combination of clinical and biochemical markers, can predict the risk of preeclampsia in pregnant women [63]. Early detection of preeclampsia allows for better management and intervention, potentially reducing the risk of complications for both the mother and the baby. This application of AI and ML is particularly vital in improving maternal and infant health outcomes, underscoring the potential to save lives through early diagnosis [26].

The role of AI and ML in early disease detection is not limited to specific diseases but extends to predictive analytics. By analyzing a diverse array of patient data, including genetic information, medical history, and lifestyle factors, AI can generate risk profiles for individuals [40]. This approach is particularly relevant in women's health, where risk factors for conditions such as breast cancer, ovarian cancer, and cardiovascular diseases can vary significantly among individuals. AI-driven risk assessment models allow healthcare providers to tailor their screening and prevention strategies, ensuring that high-risk individuals receive more intensive monitoring and early interventions [18]. This proactive approach to healthcare plays a pivotal role in preventing diseases or detecting them in their early stages, when treatment outcomes are generally more favorable.

Despite the remarkable progress in early disease detection facilitated by AI and ML, several challenges and considerations require attention. One of the key factors is the quality and diversity of datasets. AI algorithms depend on comprehensive datasets for training and validation, and ensuring the representativeness of the data is crucial to avoid bias and ensure accuracy [28]. Inadequate or biased data can result in algorithmic biases that may disproportionately affect certain demographic groups, including women.

Another crucial aspect is the integration of AI into clinical practice, which necessitates the establishment of clear guidelines and regulatory frameworks. The use of AI in healthcare raises questions about patient privacy, data security, and ethical considerations. As AI algorithms become integral to medical decision-making, transparency and accountability are essential to maintain patient trust and safety [35].

## 6.3 AI AND ML IN REPRODUCTIVE HEALTH ADVANCEMENTS

The field of healthcare has been witnessing remarkable advancements, thanks to the rapid integration of AI and ML technologies. Their role in advancing reproductive health, particularly in the context of women's diseases, has garnered significant attention in recent years [2]. AI and ML technologies have demonstrated remarkable potential in revolutionizing healthcare by offering novel solutions for disease prediction, prevention, and treatment. AI and ML offer a wide array of tools and applications that not only enhance our understanding of women's health but also improve the accessibility and quality of reproductive healthcare services [16].

### *6.3.1 ADVANCEMENTS IN RESEARCH*

AI and ML have emerged as potent tools in the realm of women's reproductive health research. These technologies can efficiently process and analyze vast datasets, enabling researchers to uncover hidden insights and patterns that were previously challenging to discern. The impact of AI and ML on this aspect of healthcare is exemplified by a study conducted by Sivajohan et al., which harnessed AI to analyze genomic data and identify genetic factors associated with endometriosis, a painful and often debilitating condition affecting millions of women worldwide [61].

Endometriosis is characterized by the presence of endometrial tissue outside the uterus, leading to chronic pelvic pain, fertility issues, and a host of other complications. Traditional research methods had made slow progress in understanding the intricate genetic underpinnings of the disease. However, the application of AI and ML has accelerated this process, allowing researchers to identify novel biomarkers, genetic associations, and potential therapeutic targets [51]. By leveraging the power of AI, researchers have uncovered previously elusive genetic factors linked to endometriosis. This not only deepened our understanding of the disease but also holds the promise of developing more effective treatment strategies in the future [10].

Such discoveries exemplify the transformative potential of AI and ML in the field of women's reproductive health. They enable researchers to tackle complex problems, unravel genetic mysteries, and identify key insights that were previously hidden in vast datasets. Moreover, the AI-driven analysis allows for precision medicine approaches, tailoring treatment plans to the individual needs of patients, thus ushering in a new era of personalized healthcare for women.

### *6.3.2 ENHANCING DIAGNOSTIC ACCURACY*

In addition to their role in research, AI and ML are enhancing diagnostic accuracy in women's reproductive healthcare. In many cases, the early detection of conditions is critical for effective treatment and improved outcomes. AI-based algorithms are being developed to interpret various diagnostic data, including medical imaging, clinical tests, and patient history, to aid healthcare providers in making more accurate and timely diagnoses.

For instance, in the context of breast cancer screening, AI-driven mammography analysis has shown great promise in improving early detection rates. AI algorithms can analyze mammograms, identifying subtle abnormalities that might escape the human eye, and can even distinguish between benign and malignant lesions with high accuracy [13]. Such advancements have the potential to significantly reduce false positives and, in turn, decrease unnecessary anxiety and healthcare costs for women undergoing breast cancer screening.

Moreover, AI-based diagnostic tools are being developed for various reproductive health conditions, including PCOS, cervical cancer, and uterine fibroids. These tools are capable of sifting through vast amounts of medical data to identify markers and patterns that may indicate the presence of these conditions, even in their early stages. This early detection is crucial for timely intervention and the prevention of disease progression, improving the overall quality of care for women.

### *6.3.3 PERSONALIZED TREATMENT PLANS*

One of the most promising aspects of AI and ML in women's reproductive healthcare is the ability to create personalized treatment plans. The "one-size-fits-all" approach to healthcare is gradually becoming obsolete as AI technologies enable healthcare providers to tailor treatments to the unique needs and genetic profiles of each patient.

This personalization is particularly beneficial in assisted reproductive technologies (ART), such as *in vitro* fertilization. AI and ML can analyze an individual's medical history, genetic makeup, and reproductive parameters to predict the most effective treatment protocols. These protocols can optimize the chances of successful pregnancy while minimizing the risks and side effects associated with ART procedures [48]. In essence, AI and ML are ushering in a new era of precision medicine in reproductive health, offering women and couples struggling with fertility issues new hope and improved outcomes.

### *6.3.4 PREDICTING PREGNANCY-RELATED COMPLICATIONS*

Another significant contribution of AI and ML in women's reproductive healthcare is the ability to predict pregnancy-related complications. Pregnancy can be a challenging and risky period for women, and early identification of potential issues is crucial for ensuring a safe and healthy pregnancy.

AI-driven predictive models can analyze a wide range of factors, including maternal health, fetal development, and genetic predispositions, to identify women at higher risk for complications such as gestational diabetes, preeclampsia, or preterm birth. By identifying high-risk cases early, healthcare providers can implement preventive measures and offer more vigilant monitoring, ultimately reducing the incidence of complications and improving maternal and neonatal outcomes [53].

Furthermore, AI and ML are being used to enhance the interpretation of prenatal ultrasound and fetal monitoring data. These technologies can identify subtle abnormalities and patterns that may indicate fetal distress, allowing for early intervention and the potential avoidance of adverse outcomes. This level of early detection is a testament to the power of AI and ML in safeguarding the health of expectant mothers and their unborn children.

### *6.3.5 SUPPORTING RESEARCH ENDEAVORS*

In addition to their direct impact on clinical practice, AI and ML are invaluable in supporting research endeavors in women's reproductive health. The sheer volume of data generated in the field of healthcare is vast and ever-expanding, making manual analysis impractical. AI and ML algorithms can quickly sift through massive datasets, identifying trends, correlations, and potential research avenues [31].

Moreover, AI-driven natural language processing algorithms can analyze vast amounts of medical literature and clinical notes, providing researchers with insights and information that might be missed by traditional search methods. This technology not only expedites the research process but also enhances the quality and depth of the findings [47].

Furthermore, AI and ML have enabled the development of predictive models for disease progression and treatment outcomes. For example, in the context of endometriosis research, predictive models can estimate the likelihood of disease recurrence and the effectiveness of different treatment options. These models help researchers and clinicians make more informed decisions about patient care and guide the development of targeted therapies [8].

### *6.3.6 INCREASING ACCESS TO HEALTHCARE SERVICES*

Beyond their contributions to research, diagnosis, and treatment, AI and ML are making significant strides in improving women's access to reproductive healthcare services. The digital age has ushered in telemedicine platforms powered by AI-driven chatbots and virtual health assistants. These platforms offer women easy and convenient access to information and support for a wide range of reproductive health needs, including family planning, prenatal care, and menstrual health [44].

For many women, access to healthcare services can be hampered by geographical constraints, socioeconomic factors, or cultural barriers. Telemedicine, driven by AI and ML, bridges these gaps by providing personalized advice, answers to common questions, and support for women's reproductive health needs [25]. These platforms can assist with birth control choices, provide guidance on fertility awareness, and offer postpartum support. They not only reduce barriers to care but also increase health literacy among women, enabling them to make informed decisions about their reproductive health.

Furthermore, the COVID-19 pandemic accelerated the adoption of telemedicine across the healthcare spectrum. In the context of reproductive healthcare, telemedicine played a pivotal role in maintaining access to essential services while minimizing the risk of viral transmission [49]. This shift toward digital healthcare is likely to persist and expand, making AI and ML-driven telemedicine an integral part of women's reproductive health services in the years to come.

The success stories of AI and ML in women's reproductive health research, exemplified by the groundbreaking work of many researchers in identifying genetic factors associated with endometriosis, demonstrate the potential of these technologies to unlock the mysteries of complex conditions [61]. The development of AI-based diagnostic tools for breast cancer and other reproductive health conditions is making early detection a reality, ultimately improving treatment outcomes.

Furthermore, the era of personalized medicine is upon us, with AI and ML guiding the development of tailored treatment plans for women seeking fertility assistance and other reproductive health interventions. The predictive power of AI models in identifying pregnancy-related complications adds an essential layer of safety and care during the critical period of pregnancy. AI and ML are not only transforming the clinical landscape but also reshaping the research environment [7]. These technologies facilitate the analysis of vast datasets, enhance information retrieval, and support the development of predictive models. In the realm of reproductive health, these capabilities are essential for driving innovation and expanding our understanding of complex conditions.

Finally, AI and ML are fostering a more inclusive healthcare landscape by expanding access to reproductive health services. Telemedicine platforms driven by AI and ML are providing women with convenient, personalized, and informative resources, reducing disparities in access to care. The adoption of digital healthcare, particularly in the wake of the COVID-19 pandemic, is poised to reshape the way women access reproductive health services, making healthcare more accessible and convenient [9].

## 6.4 MANAGING CHRONIC WOMEN'S HEALTH CONDITIONS

AI and ML technologies have made significant strides in enhancing the diagnosis and risk prediction of chronic women's health conditions. These technologies can analyze vast amounts of data to identify patterns and correlations that may not be apparent to healthcare professionals using traditional diagnostic methods. For example, in the case of PCOS, a complex endocrine disorder that affects many women of reproductive age, AI has proven to be a valuable tool in improving diagnosis [62].

A study by Elmannai and coworkers demonstrates how AI can enhance the diagnosis of PCOS by integrating clinical and biochemical variables. The study employed an AI-driven model that combined factors such as age, body mass index (BMI), hormonal profiles, and clinical symptoms. By processing this comprehensive dataset, the AI system achieved high accuracy in identifying PCOS cases, thus facilitating early and accurate diagnosis [19].

Moreover, AI and ML are instrumental in risk prediction for chronic women's health conditions, especially for conditions like osteoporosis. Osteoporosis is characterized by reduced bone density and an increased risk of fractures, particularly in postmenopausal women. AI-based models, such as the one proposed by Fasihi and coworkers, analyze various factors, including age, bone density measurements, and genetic predispositions, to estimate an individual's risk of developing osteoporosis and associated fractures. By identifying high-risk individuals, healthcare providers can implement preventive measures, such as lifestyle changes and medications, to reduce the likelihood of fractures and improve overall patient outcomes [21].

### 6.4.1 PERSONALIZED TREATMENT PLANS

Personalized treatment plans are a cornerstone of effective clinical management for chronic women's health conditions. Each patient may respond differently to treatments, making it crucial to tailor interventions to individual needs. AI and ML have been transformative in developing personalized treatment plans for these conditions.

In the case of PCOS, AI-driven algorithms have been employed to recommend personalized treatment strategies. These algorithms consider a range of factors, such as BMI, insulin resistance, and hormonal profiles, to create tailored lifestyle interventions, medication regimens, and dietary plans. One study described how AI can be utilized to optimize treatment regimens, improve symptom control, and enhance the quality of life for women with PCOS. Personalized treatment approaches empower patients to actively participate in their healthcare and may lead to more favorable outcomes [3].

Similarly, in the context of menopause, the use of AI and ML is gaining momentum for tailoring hormone replacement therapy (HRT) to the individual needs of women. Osteoporosis and cardiovascular health are critical concerns during menopause, and AI-driven models, as proposed by Ryu and coworkers, factor in individual patient characteristics, menopausal symptoms, and bone health to create personalized HRT plans. These plans aim to maximize the benefits of HRT while minimizing associated risks, improving the management of menopausal symptoms, and reducing potential complications [56].

### *6.4.2 CONTINUOUS MONITORING AND INTERVENTION*

The management of chronic women's health conditions often requires continuous monitoring and timely interventions to prevent exacerbation of symptoms and complications. AI and ML provide solutions for remote monitoring and real-time feedback, enabling both patients and healthcare providers to make informed decisions and take necessary actions promptly.

For women with endometriosis, a chronic condition characterized by the presence of endometrial tissue outside the uterus, continuous monitoring of symptoms and pain levels is crucial. AI-powered mobile applications allow women to track their symptoms, menstrual cycles, and pain levels. Using ML algorithms, these apps can detect patterns and triggers related to endometriosis symptoms, providing personalized insights and recommendations for pain management. This technology enables women to actively engage in self-monitoring and facilitates early interventions when symptoms worsen [15].

Furthermore, AI and ML have the potential to facilitate remote monitoring of bone health for women at risk of osteoporosis. Wearable devices and sensors can continuously track physical activity, a crucial factor in maintaining bone density. These devices can alert women and their healthcare providers to changes in activity levels, providing an opportunity for timely interventions to prevent bone loss and fractures. This continuous monitoring represents a significant advancement in the management of osteoporosis, helping to reduce the burden of this chronic condition [5].

### *6.4.3 PATIENT ENGAGEMENT AND EDUCATION*

Engaging patients and providing them with relevant information is vital for the effective clinical management of chronic women's health conditions. AI and ML can enhance patient engagement by delivering personalized information and support, ultimately leading to better treatment adherence and improved outcomes.

AI-driven chatbots and virtual health assistants are being utilized to deliver personalized information and support to women managing chronic conditions. These virtual assistants can answer questions, offer lifestyle advice, provide reminders for medication and appointments, and even engage in interactive conversations with patients. They contribute to patient empowerment and enable women to take an active role in their healthcare management [34].

Moreover, AI and ML are being used to develop predictive models for disease progression and treatment outcomes. In the context of PCOS, predictive models can estimate the likelihood of disease progression and the effectiveness of different treatment options. These models help health-care providers make more informed decisions about patient care and guide the development of targeted therapies [67].

## 6.5 MENTAL HEALTH SUPPORT FOR WOMEN

Mental health is a critical aspect of overall well-being, and it is particularly significant for women who often face unique stressors and challenges. In recent years, the integration of AI and ML in the field of mental health has opened new avenues for providing support and interventions [24]. The role of AI and ML in mental health support for women is multifaceted, offering a range of applications that can improve access to care, personalize treatment plans, enhance early intervention, and provide valuable insights into mental health conditions [6].

### *6.5.1 ENHANCED DIAGNOSIS AND EARLY INTERVENTION*

One of the key strengths of AI and ML in mental health support is the ability to enhance the diagnosis of mental health conditions and enable early intervention. Depression, for example, affects women at a higher rate than men, and timely diagnosis is crucial for effective treatment. AI-powered tools can analyze a wide range of data, including EHRs, social media activity, and even speech and text, to identify signs of depression.

A study has showcased the potential of AI in detecting depression through language patterns in social media posts. By analyzing the linguistic cues and sentiment in individuals' online posts, AI algorithms can identify signs of depression with a high degree of accuracy. This technology allows for early intervention and the provision of support to individuals who may be struggling with their mental health, thus preventing more severe outcomes [50].

AI and ML can also be utilized for early intervention in the context of eating disorders, which disproportionately affect women. These conditions are often challenging to detect, but AI-driven tools can help. For instance, Sharp et al. developed an AI system that can identify eating disorder behaviors by analyzing data from wearable devices, such as heart rate and activity level. Early identification of such behaviors can enable timely intervention and support for individuals at risk of developing eating disorders, ultimately improving their chances of recovery [59].

### *6.5.2 PERSONALIZED TREATMENT PLANS*

AI and ML play a crucial role in personalizing treatment plans for women with mental health conditions. The one-size-fits-all approach to mental health treatment is often insufficient, as individuals may respond differently to various interventions. AI can process a wide array of data, including genetic information, treatment history, and symptoms, to tailor treatment plans to each woman's unique needs [37].

For women with posttraumatic stress disorder (PTSD), personalized treatment plans are particularly essential. AI algorithms can analyze an individual's genetic and environmental factors to predict their likelihood of responding to specific treatments, such as cognitive-behavioral therapy or medication [38]. This enables healthcare providers to choose the most effective treatment for each woman, increasing the chances of successful outcomes [14].

Furthermore, the use of AI and ML in personalized treatment plans extends to the field of women's reproductive mental health. Pregnancy and the postpartum period are vulnerable times for mental health issues. AI-driven predictive models can assess a woman's risk of developing perinatal depression and anxiety based on factors such as pregnancy complications, hormonal changes, and genetic predispositions. This information can guide healthcare providers in developing personalized interventions and providing appropriate support [32].

### 6.5.3 CONTINUOUS MONITORING AND SUPPORT

Continuous monitoring and support are crucial for maintaining mental health and preventing relapse. AI and ML technologies can provide ongoing monitoring of women's mental health conditions, alerting healthcare providers to changes in symptoms or behaviors that may require intervention.

In the case of bipolar disorder, an illness that can have severe consequences if not managed effectively, continuous monitoring is essential. AI-driven mobile apps can track mood fluctuations, sleep patterns, and social activity. By detecting early signs of manic or depressive episodes, these apps enable timely intervention, helping women with bipolar disorder better manage their condition and reduce the risk of severe mood swings [42].

Additionally, AI and ML can enhance continuous support for women with generalized anxiety disorder (GAD). Chatbots and virtual mental health assistants powered by AI can provide women with real-time support and coping strategies. These virtual assistants can engage in conversations, offer relaxation techniques, and provide psychoeducation, helping individuals manage their anxiety and prevent escalation of symptoms. This continuous support contributes to improved mental well-being for women with GAD [4].

### 6.5.4 PATIENT ENGAGEMENT AND EDUCATION

Engaging patients and providing education about their mental health conditions is vital for effective treatment. AI and ML technologies can enhance patient engagement by delivering personalized information and support, ultimately leading to better treatment adherence and improved outcomes.

Virtual mental health assistants can deliver psychoeducation and self-help strategies to women with depression. These assistants can provide information about the nature of depression, treatment options, and strategies for managing symptoms. By engaging patients in their own care and providing them with the tools they need to cope, AI and ML can contribute to better treatment adherence and symptom management [27].

Moreover, AI-driven chatbots can be employed to enhance patient engagement in the context of women's reproductive mental health. Women experiencing infertility or pregnancy-related mental health challenges can access virtual support that offers guidance, answers common questions, and provides coping strategies. This technology empowers women to actively participate in their mental health care and seek help when needed [32].

## 6.6 ETHICAL CONSIDERATIONS IN DETERMINING THE ROLE OF AI AND ML IN WOMEN'S HEALTHCARE

The integration of AI and ML into women's healthcare has ushered in a new era of possibilities, from improving diagnostic accuracy to enhancing patient care. However, as with any technological advancement, the adoption of AI and ML in healthcare, specifically in the context of women's health, raises complex ethical considerations. It is essential to critically examine the ethical implications of AI and ML applications, ensuring that they align with the principles of beneficence, nonmaleficence, autonomy, and justice, while also respecting patients' privacy and confidentiality.

### *6.6.1 DATA PRIVACY AND SECURITY*

One of the foremost ethical concerns in AI and ML applications within women's healthcare is the safeguarding of patient data. AI and ML algorithms rely on vast datasets, often containing sensitive and personal health information. Ensuring the privacy and security of these data are paramount to maintaining trust and compliance with ethical standards [20].

The Health Insurance Portability and Accountability Act in the United States and similar regulations worldwide establish the legal framework for protecting patient data. However, even with these regulations in place, data breaches and misuse of healthcare data are not uncommon. It is crucial to address these challenges to maintain the ethical integrity of AI and ML in women's healthcare.

Additionally, de-identification and aggregation of data can provide a layer of protection for patient privacy, while still allowing AI and ML algorithms to make valuable predictions and recommendations. Advanced encryption techniques and secure data storage solutions must be employed to mitigate the risks associated with data breaches [1].

### 6.6.2 ALGORITHMIC BIAS AND FAIRNESS

Algorithmic bias poses a significant ethical challenge in AI and ML applications. If algorithms are trained on biased data, they may perpetuate and exacerbate existing healthcare disparities. Women from underrepresented or marginalized communities may be disproportionately affected by algorithmic bias.

For example, a study by Ueda et al. revealed that an algorithm used in healthcare significantly underestimated the health needs of Black patients compared to White patients, resulting in unequal access to healthcare resources. Addressing and rectifying algorithmic bias is a fundamental ethical responsibility. AI and ML algorithms should be rigorously tested for fairness and bias, and appropriate measures should be implemented to mitigate disparities and ensure equal access to quality healthcare for all women [64].

### 6.6.3 TRANSPARENCY AND EXPLAINABILITY

The "black box" nature of some AI and ML algorithms presents ethical challenges. Many of these algorithms are highly complex, making it difficult to understand how they arrive at specific decisions or recommendations. For women, who may be seeking explanations for healthcare decisions that affect their well-being, this lack of transparency is concerning [22].

Efforts to enhance the transparency and explainability of AI and ML models are underway. This includes the development of interpretable ML techniques and the establishment of clear guidelines for explaining AI-based decisions to patients. Ensuring that women have access to understandable information about their healthcare, even when AI and ML technologies are involved, is an ethical imperative.

### 6.6.4 INFORMED CONSENT

Informed consent is a fundamental ethical principle in healthcare. Women have the right to make informed decisions about their healthcare, including whether AI and ML technologies are involved in their diagnosis and treatment. This necessitates that patients receive clear and understandable information about the role of these technologies in their care.

The informed consent process should encompass discussions about data usage, the involvement of AI and ML algorithms, the potential benefits and limitations, and the patient's right to refuse AI-driven recommendations or diagnoses. Ensuring that women can make choices about their healthcare that align with their values and preferences is a key ethical consideration [52].

### *6.6.5 CLINICAL ACCOUNTABILITY AND LIABILITY*

Another ethical concern is establishing accountability and liability when AI and ML systems are integrated into healthcare. Who is responsible if an AI-driven diagnosis is incorrect or if a patient experiences harm due to algorithmic recommendations? This ethical question extends to healthcare professionals, institutions, and developers of AI and ML technologies.

Legislation and ethical guidelines must address these concerns and clarify the roles and responsibilities of all parties involved. Balancing innovation with accountability is essential to ensure that women's healthcare is not compromised by the integration of AI and ML technologies [46].

### *6.6.6 PATIENT AUTONOMY AND HUMAN OVERSIGHT*

While AI and ML can greatly enhance the efficiency and accuracy of healthcare processes, it is important to maintain a balance between automation and human oversight. Ethical considerations must prioritize patient autonomy and the role of healthcare professionals in the decision-making process.

Women should have the right to opt for human-led diagnosis and treatment when they prefer it. In situations where AI and ML are used, there should always be the option for patients to consult with healthcare professionals and seek their expertise. A patient-centric approach that respects individual preferences is at the core of ethical women's healthcare [54].

## 6.7 SUMMARY

The role of AI and ML in the early detection of women's diseases represents a remarkable advancement in healthcare. These technologies offer the potential to enhance the accuracy and efficiency of disease screening, enabling timely interventions and improving patient outcomes. From breast cancer and cervical cancer screening to preeclampsia prediction and risk assessment for various conditions, AI-driven solutions are making a tangible difference in women's health. However, as the field continues to advance, it is imperative to address challenges related to data quality, bias, privacy, and ethical considerations to ensure that the promise of early disease detection is realized without compromising patient safety and equity.

The integration of AI and ML technologies is catalyzing a transformative shift in women's reproductive healthcare. These technologies enhance early disease detection, improve diagnostic accuracy, enable personalized treatment plans, predict pregnancy-related complications, support research endeavors, and increase access to healthcare services. Women's reproductive health has historically been plagued by challenges and disparities, but AI and ML offer the promise of addressing these issues, ultimately leading to better outcomes and an improved quality of life for women around the world. AI and ML are ushering in a new era in women's reproductive healthcare, marked by increased knowledge, improved diagnostics, personalized care, predictive safety, and expanded access. As these technologies continue to evolve and become more integrated into clinical practice and research, the future holds great promise for the well-being and health of women, bringing us closer to a world where every woman can access the high quality, personalized reproductive healthcare she deserves.

AI and ML are playing a pivotal role in the clinical management of chronic women's health conditions. These technologies enhance diagnosis, predict risks, and facilitate the development of personalized treatment plans. Continuous monitoring and real-time interventions help manage symptoms and prevent complications. Additionally, AI-driven patient engagement and education empower women to actively participate in their healthcare, improving treatment adherence and overall outcomes.

AI and ML play a pivotal role in providing mental health support for women. These technologies enhance early diagnosis, facilitate personalized treatment plans, enable continuous monitoring and support, and engage patients with relevant information and coping strategies. Mental health conditions can have a significant impact on women's lives, and AI and ML offer innovative solutions that can improve their mental well-being.

AI and ML have the potential to revolutionize women's healthcare by improving diagnostic accuracy, treatment outcomes, and access to care. However, the integration of these technologies also raises important ethical considerations that must be addressed. Data privacy, algorithmic bias, transparency, informed consent, clinical accountability, patient autonomy, and the role of human oversight are all essential aspects of ensuring ethical AI and ML applications in women's healthcare. By carefully navigating these ethical challenges, healthcare providers and technologists can harness the full potential of AI and ML while upholding the highest standards of patient care and well-being.

The advancements in AI and ML offer immense potential to revolutionize early disease detection in women's health, encompassing a wide range of conditions from cancer to pregnancy-related complications. By leveraging these technologies, healthcare providers can enhance patient care, reduce disease burdens, and ultimately save lives. However, addressing challenges related to data quality, bias, and ethical considerations is essential to ensure the responsible and equitable integration of AI into clinical practice. As we continue to push the boundaries of AI and ML applications in women's health, it is crucial to maintain a strong commitment to patient well-being, privacy, and the ethical use of technology in healthcare.

## ACKNOWLEDGMENTS

The author would like to thank Faculty and Staff of Vishwakarma University, Pune for their valuable inputs and support in development of the book chapter.

## KEYWORDS

- **artificial intelligence**
- **healthcare**
- **mental health**
- **personalized treatment**
- **women healthcare advancements**

## REFERENCES


1. Ahmed, Z., Mohamed, K., Zeeshan, S., & Dong, X. (2020). Artificial intelligence with multi-functional machine learning platform development for better healthcare and precision medicine. *Database: The Journal of Biological Databases and Curation, 2020*, baaa010. doi: 10.1093/database/baaa010
2. Ahuja, A. S. (2019). The impact of artificial intelligence in medicine on the future role of the physician. *PeerJ, 7*, e7702. doi: 10.7717/peerj.7702
3. Akre, S., Sharma, K., Chakole, S., & Wanjari, M. B. (2022). Recent advances in the management of polycystic ovary syndrome: A review. *Cureus, 14* (8), e27689. doi: 10.7759/cureus.27689
4. Alanzi, T., Alsalem, A. A., Alzahrani, H., Almudaymigh, N., Alessa, A., Mulla, R., AlQahtani, L., Bajonaid, R., Alharthi, A., Alnahdi, O., & Alanzi, N. (2023). AI-powered mental health virtual assistants' acceptance: An Empirical Study on Influencing Factors Among Generations X, Y, and Z. *Cureus, 15*(11), e49486. doi: 10.7759/cureus.49486
5. Alhussein, G., & Hadjileontiadis, L. (2022). Digital health technologies for long-term self-management of osteoporosis: Systematic review and meta-analysis. *JMIR mHealth and uHealth, 10*(4), e32557. doi: 10.2196/32557
6. Bajwa, J., Munir, U., Nori, A., & Williams, B. (2021). Artificial intelligence in healthcare: Transforming the practice of medicine. *Future Healthcare Journal, 8*(2), e188–e194. doi: 10.7861/fhj.2021-0095
7. Bertini, A., Salas, R., Chabert, S., Sobrevia, L., & Pardo, F. (2022). Using machine learning to predict complications in pregnancy: A systematic review. *Frontiers in Bioengineering and Biotechnology, 9*, 780389. doi: 10.3389/fbioe.2021.780389
8. Blass, I., Sahar, T., Shraibman, A., Ofer, D., Rappoport, N., & Linial, M. (2022). Revisiting the risk factors for endometriosis: A machine learning approach. *Journal of Personalized Medicine, 12*(7), 1114. doi: 10.3390/jpm12071114
9. Bohr, A., & Memarzadeh, K. (2020). The rise of artificial intelligence in healthcare applications. *Artificial Intelligence in Healthcare*, 25–60. doi: 10.1016/B978-0-12-818438-7.00002-2
10. Bouaziz, J., Mashiach, R., Cohen, S., Kedem, A., Baron, A., Zajicek, M., Feldman, I., Seidman, D., & Soriano, D. (2018). How artificial intelligence can improve our understanding of the genes associated with endometriosis: Natural language processing of the PubMed database. *BioMed Research International, 2018*, 6217812. doi: 10.1155/2018/6217812
11. Brady, C., Mousa, S. S., & Mousa, S. A. (2009). Polycystic ovary syndrome and its impact on women's quality of life: More than just an endocrine disorder. *Drug, Healthcare and Patient Safety, 1*, 9–15. doi: 10.2147/dhps.s4388
12. Burton, L., Rush, K. L., Smith, M. A., Davis, S., Rodriguez Echeverria, P., Suazo Hidalgo, L., & Görges, M. (2022). Empowering patients through virtual care delivery: Qualitative study with micropractice clinic patients and health care providers. *JMIR Formative Research, 6*(4), e32528. doi: 10.2196/32528
13. Cè, M., Caloro, E., Pellegrino, M. E., Basile, M., Sorce, A., Fazzini, D., Oliva, G., & Cellina, M. (2022). Artificial intelligence in breast cancer imaging: Risk

stratification, lesion detection and classification, treatment planning and prognosis-a narrative review. *Exploration of Targeted Anti-Tumor Therapy*, *3*(6), 795–816. doi: 10.37349/etat.2022.00113
14. Chekroud, A. M., Bondar, J., Delgadillo, J., Doherty, G., Wasil, A., Fokkema, M., Cohen, Z., Belgrave, D., DeRubeis, R., Iniesta, R., Dwyer, D., & Choi, K. (2021). The promise of machine learning in predicting treatment outcomes in psychiatry. *World psychiatry: Official Journal of the World Psychiatric Association (WPA)*, *20*(2), 154–170. doi: 10.1002/wps.20882
15. Chen, L. H., Lo, W. C., Huang, H. Y., & Wu, H. M. (2023). A lifelong impact on endometriosis: Pathophysiology and pharmacological treatment. *International journal of Molecular Sciences*, *24*(8), 7503. doi: 10.3390/ijms24087503
16. Davenport, T., & Kalakota, R. (2019). The potential for artificial intelligence in healthcare. *Future Healthcare Journal*, *6*(2), 94–98. doi: 10.7861/futurehosp.6-2-94
17. de Santiago, I., & Polanski, L. (2022). Data-driven medicine in the diagnosis and treatment of infertility. *Journal of Clinical Medicine*, *11*(21), 6426. doi: 10.3390/jcm11216426
18. Dileep, G., & Gianchandani Gyani, S. G. (2022). Artificial intelligence in breast cancer screening and diagnosis. *Cureus*, *14*(10), e30318. doi: 10.7759/cureus.30318
19. Elmannai, H., El-Rashidy, N., Mashal, I., Alohali, M. A., Farag, S., El-Sappagh, S., & Saleh, H. (2023). Polycystic ovary syndrome detection machine learning model based on optimized feature selection and explainable artificial intelligence. *Diagnostics (Basel, Switzerland)*, *13*(8), 1506. doi: 10.3390/diagnostics13081506
20. Farhud, D. D., & Zokaei, S. (2021). Ethical issues of artificial intelligence in medicine and healthcare. *Iranian Journal of Public Health*, *50*(11), i–v. doi: 10.18502/ijph.v50i11.7600
21. Fasihi, L., Tartibian, B., Eslami, R., & Fasihi, H. (2022). Artificial intelligence used to diagnose osteoporosis from risk factors in clinical data and proposing sports protocols. *Scientific Reports*, *12*(1), 18330. doi: 10.1038/s41598-022-23184-y
22. Gerke, S., Minssen, T., & Cohen, G. (2020). Ethical and legal challenges of artificial intelligence-driven healthcare. *Artificial Intelligence in Healthcare*, 295–336. doi: 10.1016/B978-0-12-818438-7.00012-5
23. Goodale, B. M., Shilaih, M., Falco, L., Dammeier, F., Hamvas, G., & Leeners, B. (2019). Wearable sensors reveal menses-driven changes in physiology and enable prediction of the fertile window: Observational study. *Journal of Medical Internet Research*, *21*(4), e13404. doi: 10.2196/13404
24. Graham, S., Depp, C., Lee, E. E., Nebeker, C., Tu, X., Kim, H. C., & Jeste, D. V. (2019). Artificial intelligence for mental health and mental illnesses: An overview. *Current Psychiatry Reports*, *21*(11), 116. doi: 10.1007/s11920-019-1094-0
25. Habib, S. S., Jamal, W. Z., Zaidi, S. M. A., Siddiqui, J. U., Khan, H. M., Creswell, J., Batra, S., & Versfeld, A. (2021). Barriers to access of healthcare services for rural women-applying gender lens on TB in a rural district of Sindh, Pakistan. *International Journal of Environmental Research and Public Health*, *18*(19), 10102. doi: 10.3390/ijerph181910102
26. Hackelöer, M., Schmidt, L., & Verlohren, S. (2023). New advances in prediction and surveillance of preeclampsia: Role of machine learning approaches and remote

monitoring. *Archives of Gynecology and Obstetrics*, *308*(6), 1663–1677. doi: 10.1007/s00404-022-06864-y

27. Haque, M. D. R., & Rubya, S. (2023). An overview of chatbot-based mobile mental health apps: Insights from app description and user reviews. *JMIR mHealth and uHealth*, *11*, e44838. doi: 10.2196/44838
28. Hosny, A., Parmar, C., Quackenbush, J., Schwartz, L. H., & Aerts, H. J. W. L. (2018). Artificial intelligence in radiology. *Nature Reviews. Cancer*, *18*(8), 500–510. doi: 10.1038/s41568-018-0016-5
29. Hou, X., Shen, G., Zhou, L., Li, Y., Wang, T., & Ma, X. (2022). Artificial Intelligence in Cervical Cancer Screening and Diagnosis. *Frontiers in Oncology*, *12*, 851367. doi: 10.3389/fonc.2022.851367
30. Hripcsak, G., & Albers, D. J. (2013). Next-generation phenotyping of electronic health records. *Journal of the American Medical Informatics Association: JAMIA*, *20*(1), 117–121. doi: 10.1136/amiajnl-2012-001145
31. Iftikhar, P., Kuijpers, M. V., Khayyat, A., Iftikhar, A., & DeGouvia De Sa, M. (2020). Artificial intelligence: A new paradigm in obstetrics and gynecology research and clinical practice. *Cureus*, *12*(2), e7124. doi: 10.7759/cureus.7124
32. Inkster, B., Kadaba, M., & Subramanian, V. (2023). Understanding the impact of an AI-enabled conversational agent mobile app on users' mental health and wellbeing with a self-reported maternal event: A mixed method real-world data mHealth study. *Frontiers in Global Women's Health*, *4*, 1084302. doi: 10.3389/fgwh.2023.1084302
33. Iqbal, J., Cortés Jaimes, D. C., Makineni, P., Subramani, S., Hemaida, S., Thugu, T. R., Butt, A. N., Sikto, J. T., Kaur, P., Lak, M. A., Augustine, M., Shahzad, R., & Arain, M. (2023). Reimagining healthcare: Unleashing the power of artificial intelligence in medicine. *Cureus*, *15*(9), e44658. doi: 10.7759/cureus.44658
34. Jadczyk, T., Wojakowski, W., Tendera, M., Henry, T. D., Egnaczyk, G., & Shreenivas, S. (2021). Artificial intelligence can improve patient management at the time of a pandemic: The role of voice technology. *Journal of Medical Internet Research*, *23*(5), e22959. doi: 10.2196/22959
35. Jeyaraman, M., Balaji, S., Jeyaraman, N., & Yadav, S. (2023). Unraveling the ethical enigma: Artificial intelligence in healthcare. *Cureus*, *15*(8), e43262. doi: 10.7759/cureus.43262
36. Jhee, J. H., Lee, S., Park, Y., Lee, S. E., Kim, Y. A., Kang, S. W., Kwon, J. Y., & Park, J. T. (2019). Prediction model development of late-onset preeclampsia using machine learning-based methods. *PLoS One*, *14*(8), e0221202. doi: 10.1371/journal.pone.0221202
37. Johnson, K. B., Wei, W. Q., Weeraratne, D., Frisse, M. E., Misulis, K., Rhee, K., Zhao, J., & Snowdon, J. L. (2021). Precision Medicine, AI, and the Future of Personalized Health Care. *Clinical and Translational Science*, *14*(1), 86–93. doi: 10.1111/cts.12884
38. Kar, N. (2011). Cognitive behavioral therapy for the treatment of post-traumatic stress disorder: A review. *Neuropsychiatric Disease and Treatment*, *7*, 167–181. doi: 10.2147/NDT.S10389
39. Krishnan, G., Singh, S., Pathania, M., Gosavi, S., Abhishek, S., Parchani, A., & Dhar, M. (2023). Artificial intelligence in clinical medicine: Catalyzing a sustainable global

healthcare paradigm. *Frontiers in Artificial Intelligence*, *6*, 1227091. doi: 10.3389/frai.2023.1227091

40. Kumar, Y., Koul, A., Singla, R., & Ijaz, M. F. (2023). Artificial intelligence in disease diagnosis: A systematic literature review, synthesizing framework and future research agenda. *Journal of Ambient Intelligence and Humanized Computing*, *14*(7), 8459–8486. doi: 10.1007/s12652-021-03612-z
41. Liu, B., Shi, S., Wu, Y., Thomas, D., Symul, L., Pierson, E., & Leskovec, J. (2019). Predicting pregnancy using large-scale data from a women's health tracking mobile application. *Proceedings of the International World-Wide Web Conference. International WWW Conference*, *2019*, 2999–3005. doi: 10.1145/3308558.3313512
42. Liu, J. Y., Xu, K. K., Zhu, G. L., Zhang, Q. Q., & Li, X. M. (2020). Effects of smartphone-based interventions and monitoring on bipolar disorder: A systematic review and meta-analysis. *World Journal of Psychiatry*, *10*(11), 272–285. doi: 10.5498/wjp.v10.i11.272
43. Marinovich, M. L., Wylie, E., Lotter, W., Lund, H., Waddell, A., Madeley, C., Pereira, G., & Houssami, N. (2023). Artificial intelligence (AI) for breast cancer screening: BreastScreen population-based cohort study of cancer detection. *EBioMedicine*, *90*, 104498. doi: 10.1016/j.ebiom.2023.104498
44. Mills, R., Mangone, E. R., Lesh, N., Mohan, D., & Baraitser, P. (2023). Chatbots to improve sexual and reproductive health: Realist synthesis. *Journal of Medical Internet Research*, *25*, e46761. doi: 10.2196/46761
45. Mustafa, W. A., Ismail, S., Mokhtar, F. S., Alquran, H., & Al-Issa, Y. (2023). Cervical cancer detection techniques: A chronological review. *Diagnostics (Basel, Switzerland)*, *13*(10), 1763. doi: 10.3390/diagnostics13101763
46. Naik, N., Hameed, B. M. Z., Shetty, D. K., Swain, D., Shah, M., Paul, R., Aggarwal, K., Ibrahim, S., Patil, V., Smriti, K., Shetty, S., Rai, B. P., Chlosta, P., & Somani, B. K. (2022). Legal and ethical consideration in artificial intelligence in healthcare: Who takes responsibility. *Frontiers in Surgery*, *9*, 862322. doi: 10.3389/fsurg.2022.862322
47. Niazi, S. K. (2023). The coming of age of AI/ML in drug discovery, development, clinical testing, and manufacturing: The FDA perspectives. *Drug Design, Development and Therapy*, *17*, 2691–2725. doi: 10.2147/DDDT.S424991
48. Oinas-Kukkonen, H., Pohjolainen, S., & Agyei, E. (2022). Mitigating Issues With/of/for True Personalization. *Frontiers in Artificial Intelligence*, *5*, 844817. doi: 10.3389/frai.2022.844817
49. Omboni, S., Padwal, R. S., Alessa, T., Benczúr, B., Green, B. B., Hubbard, I., Kario, K., Khan, N. A., Konradi, A., Logan, A. G., Lu, Y., Mars, M., McManus, R. J., Melville, S., Neumann, C. L., Parati, G., Renna, N. F., Ryvlin, P., Saner, H., Schutte, A. E., … Wang, J. (2022). The worldwide impact of telemedicine during COVID-19: Current evidence and recommendations for the future. *Connected Health*, *1*, 7–35. doi: 10.20517/ch.2021.03
50. Owusu, P. N., Reininghaus, U., Koppe, G., Dankwa-Mullan, I., & Bärnighausen, T. (2021). Artificial intelligence applications in social media for depression screening: A systematic review protocol for content validity processes. *PLoS One*, *16*(11), e0259499. doi: 10.1371/journal.pone.0259499

51. Parasar, P., Ozcan, P., & Terry, K. L. (2017). Endometriosis: Epidemiology, diagnosis and clinical management. *Current Obstetrics and Gynecology Reports*, *6*(1), 34–41. doi: 10.1007/s13669-017-0187-1
52. Quinn, T. P., Senadeera, M., Jacobs, S., Coghlan, S., & Le, V. (2021). Trust and medical AI: The challenges we face and the expertise needed to overcome them. *Journal of the American Medical Informatics Association*, *28*(4), 890–894. doi: 10.1093/jamia/ocaa268
53. Ramakrishnan, R., Rao, S., & He, J. R. (2021). Perinatal health predictors using artificial intelligence: A review. *Women's Health (London, England)*, *17*, 17455065211046132. doi: 10.1177/17455065211046132
54. Richardson, J. P., Smith, C., Curtis, S., Watson, S., Zhu, X., Barry, B., & Sharp, R. R. (2021). Patient apprehensions about the use of artificial intelligence in healthcare. *NPJ Digital Medicine*, *4*(1), 140. doi: 10.1038/s41746-021-00509-1
55. Rony, M. K. K., Kayesh, I., Bala, S. D., Akter, F., & Parvin, M. R. (2024). Artificial intelligence in future nursing care: Exploring perspectives of nursing professionals - A descriptive qualitative study. *Heliyon*, *10*(4), e25718. doi: 10.1016/j.heliyon.2024.e25718
56. Ryu, K. J., Yi, K. W., Kim, Y. J., Shin, J. H., Hur, J. Y., Kim, T., Seo, J. B., Lee, K. S., & Park, H. (2021). Machine learning approaches to identify factors associated with women's vasomotor symptoms using general hospital data. *Journal of Korean Medical Science*, *36*(17), e122. doi: 10.3346/jkms.2021.36.e122
57. Schork, N. J. (2019). Artificial intelligence and personalized medicine. *Cancer Treatment and Research*, *178*, 265–283. doi: 10.1007/978-3-030-16391-4_11
58. Shah, T., Kitts, A. B., Gold, J. A., Horvath, K., Ommaya, A., Frank, O., Sato, L., Schwarze, G., Upton, M., & Sandy, L. (2020). Electronic health record optimization and clinician well-being: A potential roadmap toward action. *NAM Perspectives*, *2020*, 10.31478/202008a. doi: 10.31478/202008a
59. Sharp, G., Torous, J., & West, M. L. (2023). Ethical challenges in AI approaches to eating disorders. *Journal of Medical Internet Research*, *25*, e50696. doi: 10.2196/50696
60. Simmons, L. A., Drake, C. D., Gaudet, T. W., & Snyderman, R. (2016). Personalized health planning in primary care settings. *Federal Practitioner: For the Health Care Professionals of the VA, DoD, and PHS*, *33*(1), 27–34.
61. Sivajohan, B., Elgendi, M., Menon, C., Allaire, C., Yong, P., & Bedaiwy, M. A. (2022). Clinical use of artificial intelligence in endometriosis: A scoping review. *NPJ Digital Medicine*, *5*(1), 109. doi: 10.1038/s41746-022-00638-1
62. Stafie, C. S., Sufaru, I. G., Ghiciuc, C. M., Stafie, I. I., Sufaru, E. C., Solomon, S. M., & Hancianu, M. (2023). Exploring the intersection of artificial intelligence and clinical healthcare: A multidisciplinary review. *Diagnostics (Basel, Switzerland)*, *13*(12), 1995. doi: 10.3390/diagnostics13121995
63. Sufriyana, H., Wu, Y. W., & Su, E. C. (2020). Artificial intelligence-assisted prediction of preeclampsia: Development and external validation of a nationwide health insurance dataset of the BPJS Kesehatan in Indonesia. *EBioMedicine*, *54*, 102710. doi: 10.1016/j.ebiom.2020.102710
64. Ueda, D., Kakinuma, T., Fujita, S., Kamagata, K., Fushimi, Y., Ito, R., Matsui, Y., Nozaki, T., Nakaura, T., Fujima, N., Tatsugami, F., Yanagawa, M., Hirata, K., Yamada,

A., Tsuboyama, T., Kawamura, M., Fujioka, T., & Naganawa, S. (2024). Fairness of artificial intelligence in healthcare: Review and recommendations. *Japanese Journal of Radiology*, *42*(1), 3–15. doi: 10.1007/s11604-023-01474-3

65. Wang, R. C., & Wang, Z. (2023). Precision medicine: Disease subtyping and tailored treatment. *Cancers*, *15*(15), 3837. doi: 10.3390/cancers15153837
66. Yoon, J. H., & Kim, E. K. (2021). Deep learning-based artificial intelligence for mammography. *Korean Journal of Radiology*, *22*(8), 1225–1239. doi: 10.3348/kjr.2020.1210
67. Zad, Z., Jiang, V. S., Wolf, A. T., Wang, T., Cheng, J. J., Paschalidis, I. C., & Mahalingaiah, S. (2024). Predicting polycystic ovary syndrome with machine learning algorithms from electronic health records. *Frontiers in Endocrinology*, *15*, 1298628. doi: 10.3389/fendo.2024.1298628

## CHAPTER 7

# Robotic Surgery for Women

SOWNDARIYA PERUMAL* and CHITRA GUNASEKAR

*Corresponding author

## ABSTRACT

Gynecologic robotic surgery represents the latest innovation in minimally invasive techniques. Utilizing a slender, lighted scope and miniature instruments managed via a robotic system, gynecological surgeons can address various conditions affecting a woman's reproductive organs. Gynecologic robotic surgery allows for the treatment of various conditions, including abdominal and pelvic pain, endometriosis, gynecologic cancers such as cervical, ovarian, and uterine cancer, painful periods and heavy bleeding, pelvic organ prolapse, and uterine fibroids. The adoption of conventional laparoscopy (CL) in gynecological surgery has resulted in significant benefits for women and health providers in terms of shorter hospital admission and a more rapid recovery and return to normal activity. Because of the limited space and intricate anatomy of the pelvis, CL has only been used in few difficult pelvic surgeries where higher precision is required. By offering more dexterity, intuitive movement, 3D-vision, enhanced ergonomics, autonomy of camera control, and a shorter learning curve, the advent of robots as supplemental tools in laparoscopic procedures has addressed several of these shortcomings. Due to varying surgical experience, there is no consensus on the definition of complex surgical operations and no standard surgical complexity matrix. By minimizing blood loss and intra- or postoperative problems, robotic-assisted keyhole surgery reduces the need for repeat abdominal surgery while improving surgical performance without lengthening the

Holistic Approaches for Women's Sustainable Health, Volume 1: Foundations, Innovations, Challenges, and Management. Megh R. Goyal, Anamika Chauhan, and Junaid Ahmad Malik (Eds)


DOI: 10.1201/9781779641632-9

operating time. Additionally, less skeletal damage occurs to surgeons who use robots.

## 7.1 INTRODUCTION

More control, precision, and flexibility are available to surgeons performing a wide range of intricate procedures with robotic surgery, also known as robot-assisted surgery [4], when compared to traditional methods. Minimally invasive surgical techniques involving microscopic incisions are typically linked with robotic surgery [5]. Additionally, in some conventional open surgical procedures, it is occasionally utilized.

Traditionally, vaginal or laparoscopic approaches have been used to teach gynecologic surgery. Depth perception and haptic input from tissue resistance are useful tools for surgeons during laparotomies. Surgical suturing within the abdomen is possible with six degrees of freedom on the human wrist.

When laparoscopy became available, there was a less invasive option to laparotomy for situations when it was not possible to operate vaginally. Over the past few decades, laparoscopy has undergone tremendous evolution thanks to advancements in hand instruments, electrosurgical devices, and high-intensity light sources. Low blood loss improved cosmetic outcomes, a quicker return to regular activities, reduced postoperative pain, and a shorter hospital stay are some of the benefits of laparoscopy over laparotomy.

Robotic surgery provides patients with several advantages over traditional open surgery, such as less extensive cuts mean a lower chance of infection; less need for transfusions and blood loss; less time spent in the hospital; pain and discomfort are lessened; returning to regular activities and healing more quickly; and very little scarring.

This chapter focuses on the scope of robotic surgery in female objects.

## 7.2 ROBOTIC SURGERY [1, 2–4, 8, 10]

### *7.2.1 SCOPE OF ROBOTIC TECHNOLOGY*

- **Gynecological robotic surgery has a wide range of applications and is expanding quickly:** The da Vinci Surgical System is utilized for malignancies, such as ovarian cancer, cervical cancer, endometrial cancer, and fibroids, and benign indications include treatment for fibroids, irregular periods, endometriosis, pelvic prolapse, and ovarian growths.

- The robotic technology could help the gynecological surgeon with lymph node biopsies, oophorectomies, salpingectomies, hysterectomies, and myomectomies. Thus, it is possible that abdominal surgery will become outdated in the future—science fiction, as we mentioned.
- Numerous medical facilities worldwide have conducted in-depth research on the application of robotic surgery and discovered that it reduces the morbidity and death rates of patients suffering from gynecologic malignancies.

### 7.2.2 APPLICATIONS OF COMMON ROBOTIC SURGERY

- Cervical cercalage
- Endometriosis
- Rectovaginopexy
- Repair of genitourinary injuries
- Robotic hysterectomy
- Robotic myomectomy
- Sacrocolpopexy
- Tubal reanastomosis

### *7.2.3 USES OF ROBOTIC SURGERY*

- Delicate and sophisticated surgeries that would have been challenging or impossible with traditional methods are now achievable because of robotic surgery.
- In conclusion, the surgical team will find it more comfortable as the robot will perform the bending and stretching required to reach challenging surgical locations.
- Surgeons may successfully access difficult-to-reach locations with less disruption to surrounding tissues because of the robotic arms' higher range of motion than that of the human wrist.

- This can lower the chance of injuries and prolong a surgeon's working life.
- This helps the patient recuperate more quickly and causes less pain throughout the procedure.
- When compared to traditional approaches, a surgical robot improves an operator's precision, flexibility, and control while also improving their visibility of the operating site.

## 7.3 ROBOT-ASSISTED REPRODUCTIVE GYNECOLOGICAL SURGERY [4, 6–8, 10]

### *7.3.1 DA VINCI® SURGICAL SYSTEM*

- For gynecological surgery in 2005, the da Vinci Surgical System was used. It has been well embraced and has already taken up a significant role in the centers where it is accessible. This system comprises three main components: a high-definition three-dimensional (3D) vision system, a patient-side cart with four robotic arms, and a surgeon's console.
- To identify patients who may benefit from robot-assisted surgery and to identify potential dangers, well-designed randomized controlled trials or similarly rigorous nonrandomized prospective trials are required.
- Selection of robot-assisted instances ought to be based on expert judgement and the data at hand. Repetition is the key to competency in any surgical technique. For any new technology, in addition to the didactic and practical training required, continuous quality assurance is crucial to guarantee optimal technology use and, most importantly, patient safety.

### *7.3.2 PROCEDURE OF ROBOTIC-ASSISTED REPRODUCTIVE GYNECOLOGICAL SURGERY*

The patient-side robot, a vision cart, and a robotic master console make up the fundamental robotic configuration [5, 10]. Similar to a traditional laparoscopy, the patient is positioned and set up in an Allen stirrup with their arms tucked and cushioned for the dorsal lithotomy. The robotic surgeon operates from a remote master console using a combination of hand controllers and foot pedals. Our top choices for trocar locations during conventional and hybrid robotic myomectomy.

Following trocar implantation, the patient is put in the Trendelenburg position, and docking is started. One trocar is linked to each robotic arm on a patient-side cart that is moved either beyond the left Allen stirrup or between the patient's legs. The bedside assistant uses the undocked trocar in the right lower quadrant as a standard laparoscopic port for tissue retraction, suction/irrigation, needle passage, and morcellation. Additionally, the bedside assistance uses the robotic arms to exchange instruments. For this surgery, the harmonic shears, the big and mega needle drivers, the Maryland bipolar forceps, and the tenaculum forceps are our favorite robotic instruments.

## 7.4 DA VINCI SURGICAL SYSTEM [10]

### *7.4.1 COMPONENTS*

The da Vinci Surgical System consists of a patient-side cart with four robotic arms that the surgeon can manipulate (three for manipulating tools and one for managing the camera), a high-definition 3D vision system, and a surgeon's station.

#### *7.4.1.1 SURGEON CONSOLE*

During the process, your surgeon sits at a console that houses the equipment and provides an incredibly clear 3DHD image of your anatomy. Like a human hand but with a significantly wider range of motion, the tiny instruments are "wristed."

#### *7.4.1.2 PATIENT CART*

The patient-side cart is placed on the operating table next to the patient. It is the part of the procedure where the instruments react in real time to the movements made by your surgeon's hand at the surgeon console.

#### *7.4.1.3 VISION CART*

In addition to offering a screen so the care team may see the procedure, the vision cart facilitates communication between the system's components.

### *7.4.2 TYPES OF CONDITIONS CAN BE TREATED WITH DA VINCI ROBOTIC SURGERY*

- Endometriosis resection
- Hysterectomy
- Myomectomy
- Pelvic organ prolapse surgery

## 7.5 ROBOTIC-ASSISTED LAPAROSCOPIC HYSTERECTOMY

During a robotic-assisted hysterectomy, robotic arms are used to aid surgeons in removing the uterus. Compared to conventional treatments, it promises reduced scarring and shorter recovery durations. Robotic surgery enables doctors to have a more precise and extended range of motion than the human hand, along with a high-definition, 3D vision of the operating area.

Using robotic arms, your surgeon creates tiny incisions in the belly to remove the uterus from its surrounding tissue during the hysterectomy. Using a controller and a screen to view the operation, a surgeon operating over the body controls the robotic arms during a robotic hysterectomy. With the robotic arms, the surgeon always has total control.

### *7.5.1 INDICATIONS*

- Advanced endometriosis stage.
- Fibroids in utero.
- Severe and ongoing pelvic discomfort.
- Strong or unusual vaginal bleeding.
- Uterine cancer [9]
- Uterine prolapse.

### *7.5.2 BENEFITS*

- Faster return to previous activities and a shorter recuperation period.
- Less scarring from smaller incisions. Large incisions are not used during surgery; rather, tiny incisions are made.
- Less time spent in the hospital.
- Postoperative pain was reduced.
- Reduction in the chance of infection.
- Reduction of blood loss during surgery.

### *7.5.3 RISKS*

Individuals undergoing robotic-assisted hysterectomy frequently report reduced discomfort, decreased blood loss, and quicker recovery times in contrast to those undergoing open abdominal hysterectomy. Using a da Vinci Surgical System, surgeons execute a robotic hysterectomy. This instrument facilitates a range of additional minimally invasive surgical procedures.

### *7.5.4 PREPARATION OF PATIENT FOR SURGERY*

One kind of laparoscopic procedure is robotically assisted hysterectomy. Compared to traditional surgery, laparoscopic surgery involves less disruption to the body. On your belly, your surgeon makes multiple tiny incisions that are no longer than or equal to 1 cm. A laparoscope and other surgical tools are then inserted into the incisions. A laparoscope is a little tube that has a video camera and light on the end.

A high-definition video screen displays the surgical scene as projected by the laparoscope. When performing surgery, your surgeon keeps an eye on the screen. In robotic-assisted surgery, the surgeon uses robotic arms to operate the surgical instruments while seated at a computer console a short distance away.

### *7.5.5 DURING SURGERY*

- A healthcare professional will conduct a physical examination prior to your surgery. In order to assess your general health, they could request blood, urine, and other tests. Your surgeon will go through every step of the operation with the patient, including any potential risks and adverse effects.

- They will also address any concerns you may have regarding your recuperation and what to expect right after surgery. The healthcare provider will conduct a physical exam and may order blood, urine, and other tests to assess overall health.
- Elucidate the detailed process, considering potential problems and side effects. They shall also answer any questions about the recovery and what one can expect immediately after surgery.
- In the evening before and on the morning of the surgery, they will advise when to cease eating and drinking. Before the procedure, they will also advise as to which of the existing drugs one can keep taking and which ones the patient might need to temporarily cease.

### *7.5.6 AFTER SURGERY*

- To empty the bladder, place a urinary catheter in.
- Make sure the patient uses a sterile solution to clean the abdomen.
- Assume the proper posture for the surgery with arms and legs.

## 7.6 ROBOTIC MYOMECTOMY [1–3, 10]

Patients with fewer than 15 myomas in total, and with any single myoma smaller than 15 cm, are considered candidates for robotic myomectomy. Patients who have diffuse adenomyosis on magnetic resonance imaging (MRI), a uterine fundus or a uterine cavity that is not clearly visible on MRI, are not eligible for this operation.

To rule out adenomyosis and ascertain the number, size, and locations of myomas, preoperative MRI is quite beneficial. Choosing between a normal robotic myomectomy and a hybrid robotic myomectomy is another use for this.

The da Vinci robot is used for reconstruction after a traditional laparoscopic myomectomy in the hybrid procedure. Based on the success that endoscopic surgery had already attained, surgeons have developed and adopted robotic myomectomy.

The robotic platform offers several benefits, particularly for surgeons who have little or no expertise in laparoscopic procedures, particularly when it comes to suturing methods. The adoption and popularity of robotic myomectomy can be attributed to the fact that myomectomy is a procedure that requires extensive suturing. Robotic arms streamline and expedite the suturing process, making it quicker and more straightforward compared to traditional methods.

A robotic myomectomy ensures an operation that is just as successful as traditional open myomectomy. Like laparoscopic surgery, robotic-aided surgery is equally acceptable and safe. Poor incision closure or overuse of diathermy can result in future uterine rupture, which has postoperative repercussions for myomectomy surgery.

## 7.7 SACROCOLPOPEXY

Women who experience pelvic organ prolapse often experience morbidity because of it, and more and more of them choose surgical relief over living with discomfort and humiliation. Vaginal vault prolapse has been observed to occur in between 0.2% and 45% of cases. The surgeon's experience will determine the best course of action. The procedure that is recommended for the patient also depends on her age at presentation, degree of prolapse, and expectations regarding her surgical outcome. The longest success rates have been found with abdominal scarocolpopexy using mesh. For otherwise healthy patients with pelvic organ prolapse, robotic-assisted laparoscopy allows for a speedy recovery.

### *7.7.1 GENERAL*

Pelvic organ prolapse is treated surgically with a sacrocolpopexy. One or more pelvic organs slipping down into the vagina is known as pelvic organ prolapse. The usual support system for the pelvic organs is compromised by weakening or damage to muscles and tissues. The adverse effects of prolapse (such as bulging, pelvic pressure, and urine incontinence) can be relieved by realigning your pelvic organs to their natural positions. Sacrocolpopexy is typically done laparoscopically by use of tiny incisions and a camera. A robot assists certain surgeons during laparoscopic sacrocolpopexy procedures.

### *7.7.2 PREPARATION*

A high-definition 3D vision system, a patient-side cart with four robotic arms, and a surgeon's station make up this system. We have covered several robotic-assisted laparoscopic benign gynecological procedures in this review, including tubal anastomosis, myomectomy, hysterectomy, and sacrocolpopexy. Additionally, surgeries are discussed that may find use in the future. For benign gynecological diseases, most trials conducted to date do not show a discernible benefit over traditional laparoscopic surgery. Robotics does, however, offer a benefit in more intricate surgery. Compared to laparoscopy, there is a lower conversion rate to open surgery with robotic aid.

### *7.7.3 DURING SURGERY*

During a sacrocolpopexy treatment, a surgeon creates a synthetic ligament or bridge by attaching a unique kind of surgical mesh from the upper vagina to your sacrum (tailbone). To make room for the mesh, the bladder and rectum must first be removed from the vagina. The top and bottom walls of your vagina are then covered with surgical mesh by the surgeon. Lastly, they secure it to the sacrum-covering ligament. The mesh provides a lift since your sacrum is higher than your vagina.

During a sacrocolpopexy, a surgeon may remove the ovaries, fallopian tubes, and/or uterus (hysterectomy). The risk of acquiring ovarian or fallopian tube cancer [9] is decreased, and the risk of uterine cancer is eliminated when these organs are removed. The surgeon considers the medical history, risk of cancer, and personal preference when deciding whether or not to remove the uterus.

### *7.7.4 AFTER SURGERY*

Using tape or adhesive, the surgeon will seal the incisions on the body. The wounds need to be kept dry and spotless. The skin will naturally heal over any stitches underneath. When treating the wounds or replacing bandages, especially, make sure that the patient often washes the hands. How to take care of the incisions will be discussed with the patient by the healthcare professional.

For most patients, recuperation from surgery takes six to eight weeks on average. Postoperative instructions that cover things like changing daily activities, taking care of oneself, or taking medicine recommended by the physician.

Within two weeks of surgery, the healthcare practitioner will arrange a follow-up consultation to ensure that everything went well and that the patient is recuperating well.

### *7.7.5 RISK*

- Contamination.
- Excessive bleeding because of an artery or vein injury.
- Hemorrhages.
- Harm to the bladder, rectum, intestines, or other organs.
- Inability to consistently urinate or defecate.
- Pelvic discomfort or pain during sexual intercourse.
- Problems with the mesh the surgeon is using, like erosion (when the mesh wears through the tissue in the vagina).
- Prolapse symptoms that are still bothering or are not getting better.

## 7.8 CERVICAL CERCALAGE

A cervical cerclage is a medical procedure in which the cervix is temporarily sutured shut. This could aid in the cervix's ability to retain a pregnancy inside the uterus. To prevent premature birth, a cerclage is performed during the second trimester of pregnancy. Surgery is typically performed at a hospital. Usually, patients do not have to stay the night. Two types of cerclage exist:

- **Transvaginal cerclage**: Obstetricians and gynecologists typically perform a cerclage by reaching through the vagina to place stitches in the cervix.

- **Transabdominal cerclage**: To place stitches in the cervix, an incision is made in the abdomen, or belly. A laparoscopy, which involves making a tiny incision and using a camera, or open surgery, can be used to do this. Interstitious cerclage is occasionally performed if the patient has undergone cervical surgery in the past and had a prior transvaginal cerclage that failed to save their pregnancy.

## 7.9 COMMON BENEFITS OF ROBOTIC-ASSISTED REPRODUCTIVE GYNECOLOGICAL SURGERY

- Decreased chance of infection
- More accurate surgery
- Quicker recuperation and resumption of employment
- Reduced injuries
- Reduced need for transfusions and less blood loss
- Reduced pain and suffering following surgery
- Shortened hospital stay.

## 7.10 RISK OF ROBOTIC SURGERY [10]

- Additionally, at surgical centers with lower robotic volume or with fewer experienced surgeons, robotic surgery may take longer to complete compared to nonrobotic surgery.
- For instance, components of the system that are prone to failure include binocular lenses, instruments, robotic arms, cameras, and robotic towers.
- Besides the possibility of mechanical failure, there is a risk of human error when using the robotic system during robot-assisted surgery.
- In other instances, electrical current from the robotic instrument may inadvertently escape the robotic arm and cause unintended thermal injury to nearby tissues.
- Similarly, improper body positioning or direct compression of nerves during robotic surgery may lead to nerve palsies.

## 7.11 SUMMARY

Robotics helps medical procedures go better, but they are not always the best option. Before having surgery, it is crucial to talk with the urologist about the benefits and necessity of robot-assisted procedures, as they differ depending on the specifications of each case. In robotic surgery, tiny devices are affixed to a robot's arm to perform surgical operations. The robotic arm is operated by a highly competent and qualified surgeon, who uses it to improve surgical precision. Contrary to popular assumption, the surgeon operating the robot does the actual surgery—not the robot itself. Using minuscule incisions and unparalleled precision, the robot enhances surgical results and augments patient safety.

## KEYWORDS


- **adenomyosis**
- **endometriosis**
- **gynecologic cancer**
- **gynecologic robotic surgery**
- **myomectomy**
- **sacrocolpopexy**
- **uterine bleeding**
- **uterine prolapse**


## REFERENCES


1. Alexander, M. Q., Einarsson, J. I., Srouji, S., & Gargiulo, A. R. (2010). Robotic myomectomy: A review of indications and techniques for National Library of Medicine. *Reviews in Obstetrics and Gynecology*, *3*(4), PMC3046743. https://www.ncbi.nlm.nih.gov/pmc/articles/PMC3046743/
2. Chia-Yi, L., Hui, C., & Pao-Ling, T. (2018). Robotic myomectomy for large uterine myomas. *Taiwanese Journal of Obstetrics and Gynecology*, *57*(6), 796–800. doi: 10.1016/j.tjog.2018.10.004
3. Einarsson, Brigham and Women's Hospital's (BWH). (n.d.). Robotic myomectomy: Overview (Online). https://www.brighamandwomens.org/obgyn/robotic-gynecologic-surgery/robotic-myomectomy
4. Hongqian, L., Lawrie, T. A., Lu, D., Song, H., Wang, L., & Shi, G. (2014). Robot-assisted surgery in gynecology. *The Cochrane Database of Systematic Reviews*, *2014*(12), online, CD011422. doi: 10.1002/14651858.CD011422 published in National Library of Medicine. https://www.ncbi.nlm.nih.gov/pmc/articles/PMC6457792/
5. Imrich, K., Pavla-Svobodov, P., Lubos-Karasek, L., & Bohuslav-Svoboda, B. (2021). The status on robotic assisted myomectomy. *Mini-invasive Surgery*, *5*, 55 (Open access). doi: 10.20517/2574-1225.2021.70

6. Joao, S. N., Siufi, D. F., & Magrina, J. F. (2014). *Robotics in Gynecologic Surgery*. The Global Library of Women's Medicine (GLOWM) online. https://www.glowm.com/sectionview/heading/Robotics%20in%20Gynecologic%20Surgery/item/541
7. Marielle, A. E., Nobbenhuis, N. G., Smith, P. B., O'Sullivan, O., Moss, E., & Thomas, E. J. (2022). Robotic surgery in gynaecology. *International Journal of Obstetrics and Gynecology* (Scientific Impact Paper No. 71), online, ID 17242. doi: 10.1111/1471-0528.17242
8. Randolph, C. W. (2001). Robotic surgical training in an Academic Institution. *Annals of Surgery*, *234*(4), 475–486.
9. Robot-assisted surgery for noncancerous gynecologic conditions: ACOG committee opinion 810 (2020). *Obstet. Gynecol. (American College of Obstetricians and Gynaecologists, ACOG)*, *136*, e22–e30, online. https://journals.lww.com/greenjournal/fulltext/2020/09000/robot_assisted_surgery_for_noncancerous.47.aspx;
10. Smith, R. (2013). Fundamentals of robotic surgery: Outcomes measures and curriculum development: Preventing unintended retained foreign objects. https://www.jointcommission.org/

## CHAPTER 8

# Contribution of Embryonic Stem Cells into Fetal Development: The Monkey Model

MAITRAYEE GHOSH, PITAM GHOSH, and DEBAJYOTI ROY*

*Corresponding author

## ABSTRACT

This chapter delves into the nuanced and pivotal relationship between embryonic stem cells (ESCs) and fetal development, with a focused lens on the utilization of a primate model, specifically the monkey. Unraveling the mysteries of ESCs, known for their pluripotent potential and self-renewal capabilities, is essential for understanding the intricate processes that guide fetal development. This chapter navigates through the fundamental properties of ESCs, exploring their molecular characteristics and significance in the context of normal embryonic development. The choice of a monkey model is carefully considered, emphasizing its biological relevance to humans and its unique position as a bridge between preclinical investigations and potential clinical applications. This exploration extends to the mechanisms governing the integration of ESCs into developing fetal tissues. This chapter might serve as a comprehensive guide to the contribution of ESCs to fetal development, employing a monkey model as a tool to unlock nature's blueprint. With a careful blend of scientific rigor and ethical awareness, this chapter aims to contribute valuable insights that transcend disciplinary boundaries, fostering a deeper appreciation for the intricacies of ESCs in shaping the remarkable journey from embryo to fetus.

Holistic Approaches for Women's Sustainable Health, Volume 1: Foundations, Innovations, Challenges, and Management. Megh R. Goyal, Anamika Chauhan, and Junaid Ahmad Malik (Eds)


DOI: 10.1201/9781779641632-10

## 8.1 INTRODUCTION

Human embryonic stem cells (hESCs) were first derived 20 years ago, marking the beginning of a new era in regenerative medicine. Since then, significant technological advances have brought us closer to clinical therapies derived from hESCs, including the production of "spare parts" for treating degenerative conditions, the study of early embryonic development, and revolutionizing drug screening and development. The pluripotency of hESCs, which allows them to differentiate into any cell type of the human body, has made them a valuable tool for studying human development and potential applications in regenerative medicine [6].

The contribution of embryonic stem cells (ESCs) to fetal development, particularly in the context of primate models, has been a topic of significant scientific interest in recent years. The unique pluripotency of ESCs allows them to differentiate into various cell types, making them a valuable tool for studying fetal development and potential applications in regenerative medicine. The derivation of hESCs from human preimplantation embryos was a significant milestone in the field of stem cell research, and the subsequent development of techniques for maintaining and differentiating these cells has led to a better understanding of human development and disease. Recent studies have demonstrated the generation of chimeric fetuses using ESCs in primate models, such as the cynomolgus monkey, shedding light on the potential of these cells to contribute to the development of various tissues and organs in the fetus [8].

Additionally, advancements in stem cell-derived embryo models, including monkey blastoids, have provided new experimental tools to study postimplantation primate development and have implications for understanding human embryonic development [13]. Furthermore, the use of domesticated cynomolgus monkey ESCs has allowed for the generation of interspecies chimeric pigs, highlighting the potential of primate ESCs in the context of xenogenous grafts and organ generation [8]. These recent findings underscore the significance of primate ESCs, particularly in understanding fetal development and their potential applications in various fields, including regenerative medicine and assisted human reproduction.

This chapter focuses on the contribution of ESCs to fetal development in primate models, with a particular emphasis on the cynomolgus monkey. The chapter will provide an overview of the historical development of the field of stem cell research, including the derivation of hESCs, and will discuss recent advancements in the use of primate ESCs for studying fetal development and potential applications in regenerative medicine. The chapter will also explore the ethical considerations surrounding the use of primate ESCs and the challenges that must be overcome to translate these findings into clinical therapies.

## 8.2 ESCS: NATURE'S VERSATILE ARCHITECTS

ESCs are renowned for their versatility, as they can differentiate into virtually any cell type in the human body [14]. This unique property is a result of their pluripotency, which allows them to contribute to the development of the entire organism [6].

Recent research has expanded our understanding of ESCs' versatility, revealing that they possess a more complex landscape of developmental potential than previously thought. For example, ESCs can give rise to self-renewing progenitor cells with some degree of lineage restriction, and they can also transition between different pluripotent states, such as naïve ESCs, primed ESCs, and intermediate states like Epiblast-like cells [9].

The molecular versatility of pluripotency progression is a key feature that makes ESCs valuable for medical research and potential therapeutic applications. The molecular mechanisms underlying this versatility involve the repurposing of molecules, such as signaling pathways, transcription factors, and epigenetic regulators, which can exert different, sometimes opposite, functions in closely related stem cell configurations. The ESCs help in the formation of various cells within the body like cardiac muscle, fat cells, RBCs, etc. (Figure 8.1).

One study has reported the successful isolation of two ESC lines from cloned embryos made using cells from the skin of an adult rhesus macaque. This research demonstrated that therapeutic cloning of primates was possible, although the efficiency of the process needed to be improved before it could be applied in the clinic using human cells [16].

In a more recent study published in Nature Communications, the molecular versatility of pluripotency progression was explored, revealing that

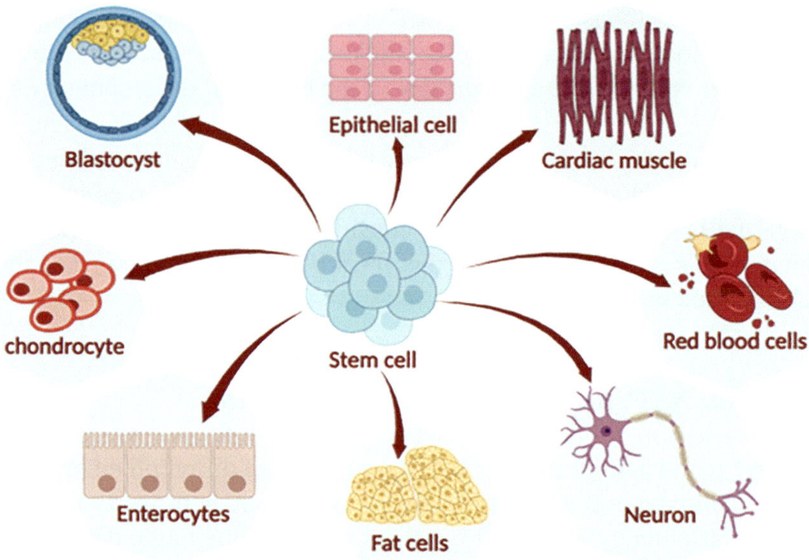


**FIGURE 8.1** Stem cell acts as an architect to form various cells within the body.

molecules are repurposed to exert different, sometimes opposite, functions in closely related stem cell configurations [9]. Research has also explored the use of gene editing to generate versatile human pluripotent stem cell reporter lines for analysis of differentiation and lineage tracing [1].

Additionally, studies have investigated the use of ESCs in generating chimeric fetuses in nonhuman primates. It is important to note that the term "versatility" does not imply that ESCs can differentiate into any cell type without limitations. For example, they cannot form extraembryonic structures like the placenta. Additionally, the versatility of ESCs is not exclusive to ESCs, as induced pluripotent stem cells can also exhibit a similar range of differentiation potential [27].

## 8.3 THE MONKEY MODEL: A BRIDGE TO HUMAN BIOLOGY

### *8.3.1 BEHAVIORAL SIMILARITIES*

Behavioral similarities between monkey models and human biology have been extensively studied in scientific research. Monkeys, particularly nonhuman primates like rhesus macaques, share numerous behavioral traits with humans due to their evolutionary proximity. These similarities extend to social behaviors, cognitive abilities, emotional responses, and even certain neurological processes. Studies have shown that monkeys exhibit complex social structures like humans, including hierarchical relationships, cooperation, and communication through gestures and vocalizations [2]. They also display cognitive abilities such as problem-solving, tool use, and memory functions that parallel those observed in humans [7].

Furthermore, monkeys demonstrate emotional responses like fear, anxiety, and empathy that are comparable to human emotions [18]. Neurologically, monkeys share brain structures and functions with humans that underlie various behaviors. For example, the prefrontal cortex in monkeys is involved in decision-making and executive functions like its role in human cognition [15]. Additionally, studies using monkey models have provided valuable insights into neural mechanisms underlying behaviors related to addiction, stress response, and social interactions [4]. By leveraging the behavioral similarities between monkeys and humans, researchers can gain a deeper understanding of human biology and behavior. Monkey models serve as valuable tools for studying a wide range of conditions such as neurodevelopmental disorders, addiction, and social cognition. Their relevance in biomedical research is underscored by the shared behavioral traits that offer insights into the underlying mechanisms of human behavior.

### *8.3.2 COMPLEX SOCIAL STRUCTURES*

Complex social structures in monkey models offer valuable insights into human biology, reflecting similarities in social organization, communication, and relationships. Nonhuman primates, such as macaques, exhibit intricate social behaviors that parallel aspects of human societies due to shared evolutionary origins. Research has shown that monkeys form complex social hierarchies characterized by dominance relationships, alliances, and kinship bonds [20]. These structures influence access to resources, mating opportunities, and social support within the group. Communication plays a crucial role in maintaining these social dynamics, with monkeys using vocalizations, gestures, and facial expressions to convey information about status, intentions, and emotions [23].

Moreover, studies have highlighted the presence of affiliative behaviors in monkeys that mirror human social interactions. Altruism, cooperation, and reciprocity are observed among primates, indicating a capacity for empathy and prosocial behavior [5]. These behaviors contribute to the cohesion of social groups and facilitate cooperation in tasks such as foraging or defending against threats. The study of complex social structures in monkey models provides a foundation for understanding the evolutionary roots of human sociality. By examining the parallels between primate societies and human communities, researchers can elucidate the biological underpinnings of social behavior, cooperation, and communication in both species.

### *8.3.3 BRAIN CIRCUITRY HOMOLOGY*

The homology of brain circuitry between monkey models and humans underscores the similarities in neural organization and function across species. Nonhuman primates, particularly macaques, share comparable brain structures and connectivity patterns with humans, providing a valuable framework for studying cognitive processes, behavior, and neurological disorders. Studies have revealed that the prefrontal cortex in monkeys exhibits homologous regions to those found in the human brain, such as the dorsolateral prefrontal cortex involved in executive functions and decision-making [19]. This similarity extends to other cortical areas responsible for sensory processing, motor control, and higher cognitive functions, highlighting the conservation of neural circuits across primate species.

Furthermore, research using neuroimaging techniques has demonstrated overlapping functional connectivity patterns between monkey and human brains. Resting-state Functional Magnetic Resonance Imaging studies have identified shared networks involved in attention, memory, and social cognition, indicating a common neural architecture underlying these cognitive processes [24]. These findings support the use of monkey models to investigate neural mechanisms relevant to human brain function and behavior. By leveraging the homology of brain circuitry between monkeys and humans, researchers can gain insights into the neural basis of complex Behaviors and cognitive functions. Monkey models serve as valuable tools for studying neurological disorders, such as Alzheimer's disease or autism spectrum disorders, by elucidating the underlying neural circuits and potential therapeutic targets.

### 8.3.4 GENETIC MANIPULATION

Genetic manipulations in nonhuman primate models, specifically macaques, have significantly advanced our understanding of human genetics and biology. Through targeted gene editing, transgenesis, and genetic knockout strategies, scientists can explore the effects of specific genes on development, physiology, and behavior, thereby shedding light on the molecular basis of diseases and informing potential therapies. One prominent technique used for genetic manipulation in monkey models is CRISPR/Cas9, a powerful gene-editing system derived from bacteria. Studies employing this method have enabled researchers to create animal models carrying mutations associated with human diseases, allowing them to examine the consequences of these alterations at the cellular, organismal, and behavioral levels [17]

Transgenesis, another approach, involves introducing foreign DNA sequences into the germline cells of monkeys to generate animals expressing novel proteins or regulatory elements. Transgenic monkeys have contributed to our knowledge of gene regulation, protein structure–function relationships, and the pathogenesis of inherited disorders [22, 28]. Genetic knockouts represent yet another strategy employed to understand gene function. Using this approach, researchers can delete or disrupt specific genes in monkey models to determine their roles in normal physiological processes and disease states. Knockout monkeys have provided critical insights into the molecular bases of several human diseases, including cardiovascular disorders, metabolic syndromes, and neuropsychiatric illnesses [21]. These genetic manipulation methods have facilitated the creation of monkey models that closely mimic human genetic variations and diseases, thus serving as valuable platforms for investigating the causes, progression, and treatment options for a variety of medical conditions.

### 8.3.5 BRIDGE TO HUMAN DISORDERS

Genetically modified monkey models serve as a crucial link between basic research in rodents and understanding human genetic disorders, enabling scientists to test innovative therapies before clinical trials [26].

## 8.4 MECHANISMS OF ESC INTEGRATION INTO FETAL TISSUES

ESC integration refers to the process whereby ESCs are incorporated into developing fetal tissues during organogenesis and differentiation. These

ESCs further help in the development of different types of cells like kidney cells, neurons, blood cells, germ cells, as illustrated in Figure 8.2. This phenomenon is crucial because it offers potential applications in regenerative medicine, disease modeling, and understanding fundamental aspects of developmental biology [10]. ESCs play a pivotal role in embryonic development through several key mechanisms:

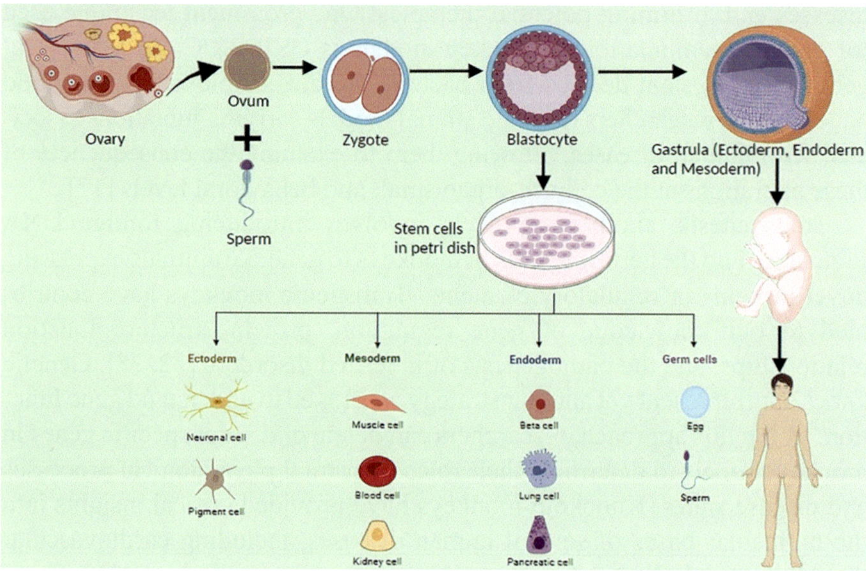


**FIGURE 8.2** Development of different cells from isolated stem cells.

- **Self-renewal and Pluripotency**: ESCs possess the remarkable capability to maintain their population size via symmetric division while retaining their full developmental potential. They can give rise to all three germ layers—ectoderm, mesoderm, and endoderm—and ultimately produce every type of cell found in the adult body [10].
- **Contribution to Germ Layer Specification**: During gastrulation, ESCs begin to differentiate and organize themselves into distinct germ layers, setting up the foundation for subsequent organogenesis and tissue development [10].
- **Generation of Diverse Cell Types**: ESCs serve as a source of cells for studying early developmental processes and generating

specific cell types for experimental purposes and future therapeutic applications [10].

- **Interaction with Extracellular Matrix (ECM)**: ESCs sense and respond to signals from the ECM, which influences their behavior, such as attachment, migration, and differentiation [10].
- **Influencing Epigenetic Modifications**: ESCs are sensitive to changes in chromatin structure and histone modification, which can affect their developmental potential and differentiation capabilities [25].
- **Establishing Spatial Patterning**: ESCs participate in creating the initial molecular blueprint for the formation of specific structures and patterns in developing tissues [10].

## 8.5 ETHICAL CONSIDERATIONS AND TRANSLATIONAL IMPLICATIONS

Studying the contribution of ESCs to fetal development in monkeys holds significant importance for several reasons:

- **Cross-Species Insights:** Research using monkey models provides valuable insights into human embryogenesis and developmental processes shared across species. For instance, a study showed that human ESCs treated with bone morphogenetic proteins (BMPs) exhibit transcriptional similarities with amnion cells in monkey embryos, shedding light on the unique abilities of human ESCs in forming diverse trophoblast subtypes [3].
- **Disease Modeling:** Utilizing monkey ESCs, such as in a Huntington's disease (HD) monkey stem cell model, allows for the investigation of genomic instability and CAG repeat expansion during spermatogenesis. This model provides a platform to study genetic anticipation and related disorders, offering new avenues for understanding disease mechanisms [11].
- **Translational Potential:** Studies involving domesticated cynomolgus monkey ESCs have enabled the generation of neonatal interspecies chimeric pigs, showcasing the translational potential of such research for applications in regenerative medicine and organ development [8].

- **Ethical Considerations:** Despite the scientific advancements facilitated by studying ESCs in monkeys, ethical considerations regarding animal welfare and responsible research conduct are paramount due to the close evolutionary relationship between humans and nonhuman primates.

The ethical implications and translational potential of ESCs derived from nonhuman primates, such as monkeys, in understanding fetal development are multifaceted. Research utilizing monkey models has provided valuable insights into the developmental processes shared across species, particularly regarding human embryogenesis. For example, a study demonstrated that human ESCs treated with BMPs share transcriptional characteristics with amnion cells rather than trophectoderm cells in the monkey embryo, suggesting that human ESCs may be capable of forming diverse trophoblast subtypes via an amnion-like transcriptional state [3].

Another study reported the use of a HD monkey stem cell model to investigate genomic instability and CAG repeat expansion during spermatogenesis, providing a novel *in vitro* system to study the underlying mechanisms of genetic anticipation and related disorders [11]. Additionally, research involving domesticated cynomolgus monkey ESCs allowed the generation of neonatal interspecies chimeric pigs, demonstrating the potential for cross-species organ development [8].

However, it should be noted that the use of nonhuman primate ESCs raises important ethical concerns due to the close evolutionary relationship between humans and great apes. While the benefits of such research include improved understanding of human biology and potential therapeutic applications, there must be careful consideration given to animal welfare and the principles of responsible conduct in research involving animals.

Moreover, the role of Y chromosome genes in the spontaneous differentiation of human ESCs into embryoid bodies has been investigated using a monkey model, revealing that specific genes play roles in the development of neural structures [12].

## 8.6 CHALLENGES IN STUDYING THE CONTRIBUTION OF ESCS TO FETAL DEVELOPMENT IN MONKEYS

Studying the contribution of ESCs to fetal development in monkeys presents several challenges, including:

- **Ethical Considerations:** The use of nonhuman primate models raises ethical concerns due to the close evolutionary relationship between humans and great apes. Researchers must carefully consider animal welfare and responsible research conduct.
- **Availability of Samples and Comparability to Humans:** Obtaining monkey embryos and ESCs for research purposes can be challenging due to limited availability and ethical considerations. While monkey models provide valuable insights into human embryogenesis, there are inherent differences between monkey and human development that must be considered when interpreting results.
- **Technical Limitations:** The use of ESCs in monkey models requires specialized techniques and expertise, and the derivation and maintenance of monkey ESCs can be technically challenging.

Despite these challenges, studying ESCs in monkey models offers significant opportunities for advancing knowledge about human development and disease, and for developing new therapeutic approaches. However, it is important to address these challenges with careful consideration and responsible research practices.

## 8.7 FUTURE DIRECTIONS AND UNEXPLORED AVENUES

Future directions and unexplored avenues in studying the contribution of ESCs to fetal development in monkeys include:

- **Single-Cell Analysis:** The application of single-cell omics technologies (such as RNA sequencing, Assay for Transposase-Accessible Chromatin-sequencing, and Chromatin Immunoprecipitation Sequencing can provide a detailed view of the molecular landscape at the individual cell level within monkey ESC populations and during their differentiation toward various lineages relevant to fetal development. These methods offer several advantages, such as (1) Identification of rare cell types or states that might otherwise go unnoticed in bulk analyses; (2) Quantitative assessment of gene expression levels and regulatory elements activity; (3) Revealing heterogeneity among cells within a population; and (4) Uncovering dynamic changes in gene regulation throughout development. These insights can help researchers better understand the molecular basis of fetal development and identify key regulators involved in the process [3].

- **Gene Editing:** The advent of gene editing tools like CRISPR/Cas9 enables researchers to make targeted mutations in monkey ESCs, generating disease models and providing new avenues for studying human disease and development. Some examples of how gene editing technology can be applied in this context include: (1) Generating monkey models carrying specific genetic mutations associated with human diseases, thereby enabling the study of disease progression and testing of potential therapies; (2) Investigating the function of candidate genes implicated in human development and disease through loss-of-function experiments; and (3) Exploring the effects of multiple genetic alterations simultaneously, which would be difficult if not impossible to achieve through traditional breeding strategies. By applying gene editing technologies to monkey ESCs, researchers can generate a wide range of disease models and gain deeper insights into the molecular mechanisms underlying human development and disease [12].
- **Organoid Culture:** Organoid culture involves the generation of three-dimensional structures that mimic the organization and function of organs from stem cells. The use of organoid culture with monkey ESCs presents an exciting avenue for advancing our understanding of fetal development, disease modeling, and drug discovery. In the context of studying the contribution of ESCs to fetal development in monkeys, organoid culture using monkey ESCs can offer several advantages: (1) Modeling Organ Development: Monkey ESC-derived organoids can recapitulate the complex cellular interactions and tissue organization seen during organ development, providing a valuable tool for studying the processes involved in fetal development; (2) Disease Modeling: Organoids derived from monkey ESCs can be used to model developmental disorders or diseases, offering insights into disease mechanisms and potential therapeutic interventions; (3) Drug Screening: Monkey ESC-derived organoids can serve as a platform for drug screening and toxicity testing, enabling the evaluation of drug effects on organ development and function [8].

- **Comparative Studies:** Comparative studies between monkey and human ESCs involve examining similarities and differences in their behavior, differentiation potential, and gene expression profiles. These studies are crucial for several reasons: (1) Understanding Evolutionary: By comparing monkey and human ESCs, researchers can identify conserved developmental pathways and regulatory mechanisms that are shared across species, providing insights into evolutionary conservation of developmental processes; (2) Modeling Human Development: Monkey ESCs can serve as a valuable model for studying human development due to their closer phylogenetic relationship to humans compared to other animal models. Comparative studies help bridge the gap between nonhuman primate research and human biology; (3) Validating Human Disease Models: Comparative analysis of monkey and human ESCs can help validate disease models generated using monkey ESCs, enhancing their relevance to human conditions.

## 8.8 SUMMARY

This chapter has endeavored to shed light on the intricate relationship between ESCs and fetal development, employing a primate model, specifically the monkey, as a key investigative tool. Through a meticulous exploration of ESC properties, mechanisms of integration into fetal tissues, and their profound influence on cellular differentiation, we have aimed to unravel the complexities of nature's blueprint guiding embryonic to fetal transitions. The careful consideration of the monkey model in this context has allowed us to bridge the gap between preclinical research and potential clinical applications. The biological parallels to humans make the monkey model an invaluable resource, offering insights that may have translational implications for regenerative medicine and our understanding of developmental disorders. Ethical considerations have been a cornerstone of our discussion, recognizing the importance of responsible research practices. By navigating the ethical dimensions of primate research, we strive to ensure a conscientious approach that respects the welfare of the subjects involved.

Moreover, this chapter not only summarizes key findings but also outlines potential future directions and unexplored avenues in ESC research within the primate model. Emerging research areas, technological advances, and the ongoing evolution of scientific methodologies are poised to shape the field, presenting new opportunities for innovative discoveries. As we navigate the complexities of ESCs in fetal development, it is our hope that this chapter sparks further inquiry, interdisciplinary collaboration, and a heightened appreciation for the multifaceted contributions of ESCs. In doing so, we aim to inspire future research endeavors that will unlock additional layers of understanding, paving the way for transformative applications in regenerative medicine and reproductive health.

## KEYWORDS

- **embryonic stem cells**
- **epigenetic regulators**
- **ethical considerations**
- **fetal development**
- **genetic manipulations**
- **primate model**
- **regenerative medicine**
- **signaling pathways**
- **transcription factors**

## REFERENCES

1. Bao, X. (2019). Gene editing to generate versatile human pluripotent stem cell reporter lines for analysis of differentiation and lineage tracing. *Stem Cells*, *37*(12), 1556–1566.
2. Cheney, D. L., & Seyfarth, R. M. (2019). *Baboon Metaphysics: The Evolution of a Social Mind*. University of Chicago Press.
3. Chhabra, S., & Warmflash, A. (2021). BMP-treated human embryonic stem cells transcriptionally resemble amnion cells in the monkey embryo. *Biology Open*, *10*(9), bio058617.
4. Czoty, P. W. (2017). Effects of social reorganization on dopamine D2/D3 receptor availability and cocaine self-administration in male cynomolgus monkeys. *Psychopharmacology (Berl)*, *234*(18), 2673–2682.

5. de Waal, F. B. M., & Preston, S. D. (2017). Mammalian empathy: Behavioral manifestations and neural basis. *Nature Reviews Neurosciences*, *18*(8), 498–509.
6. Eguizabal, C. (2019). Two decades of embryonic stem cells: A historical overview. *Human Reproduction Open*, *2019*(1), 24–28.
7. Fagot, J., & Bonté, E. (2010). Automated testing of cognitive performance in monkeys: Use of a battery of computerized test systems by a troop of semi-free-ranging baboons *(Papio papio)*. *Behavior Research Methods*, *42*(2), 507–516.
8. Fu, R. (2020). Domesticated cynomolgus monkey embryonic stem cells allow the generation of neonatal interspecies chimeric pigs. *Protein Cell*, *11*(2), 97–107.
9. Furlan, G. (2023). Molecular versatility during pluripotency progression. *Nature Communications*, *14*(1), 68.
10. Ho, A. D., Hoffman, R., & Zanjani, E. D. (2006), *Stem Cell Transplantation: Biology, Processes, Therapy*. John Wiley & Sons: New York.
11. Khampang, S. (2021). CAG repeat instability in embryonic stem cells and derivative spermatogenic cells of transgenic Huntington's disease monkey. *Journal of Assisted Reproduction and Genetics*, *38*(5), 1215–1229.
12. Khani, F. (2022). Y-chromosome genes may play roles in the development of neural rosettes from human embryonic stem cells. *Stem Cell Reviews and Reports*, *18*(8), 3008–3020.
13. Kobayashi, N., & Fu, J. (2023). Stem cell-derived embryo models: A frontier of human embryology. *Medical Reviews*, *3*(4), 343–346.
14. Martello, G., & Smith, A. (2014). The nature of embryonic stem cells. *Annual Review of Cell and Developmental Biology*, *30*, 647–675.
15. Miller, E. K., & Cohen, J. D. (2001). An integrative theory of prefrontal cortex function. *Annual Review of Neuroscience*, *24*, 167–202.
16. Mitalipov, S. (2006). Isolation and characterization of novel rhesus monkey embryonic stem cell lines. *Stem Cells*, *24*(10), 2177–2186.
17. Park, J. E., & Silva, A. C. (2019). Generation of genetically engineered non-human primate models of brain function and neurological disorders. *American Journal of Primatology*, *81*(2), e22931.
18. Parr, L. A., Waller, B. M., & Fugate, J. (2005). Emotional communication in primates: Implications for neurobiology. *Current Opinion in Neurobiology*, *15*(6), 716–720.
19. Petrides, M., & Pandya, D. N. (1999). Dorsolateral prefrontal cortex: Comparative cytoarchitectonic analysis in the human and the macaque brain and corticocortical connection patterns. *European Journal of Neuroscience*, *11*(3), 1011–1036.
20. Sapolsky, R. M. (2005). The influence of social hierarchy on primate health. *Science*, *308*(5722), 648–652.
21. Sato, A. (2023). Generation of a familial hypercholesterolemia model in non-human primate. *Scientific Reports*, *13*(1), e15649.
22. Seita, Y. (2020). Generation of transgenic cynomolgus monkeys overexpressing the gene for amyloid-β precursor protein. *Journal of Alzheimer's Disease*, *75*(1), 45–60.
23. Slocombe, K. E., & Zuberbühler, K. (2005). Agonistic screams in wild chimpanzees (Pan troglodytes schweinfurthii) vary as a function of social role. *Journal of Comparative Psychology*, *119*(1), 67–77.
24. Vincent, J. L. (2007). Intrinsic functional architecture in the anaesthetized monkey brain. *Nature*, *447*(7140), 83–86.

25. Warkentin, T. E. (2022). Platelet-activating anti-PF4 disorders: An overview. *Seminars in Hematology*, *59*(2), 59–71.
26. Watson, K. K., & Platt, M. L. (2012). Of mice and monkeys: Using non-human primate models to bridge mouse- and human-based investigations of autism spectrum disorders. *Journal of Neurodevelopmental Disorders*, *4*(1), 21–23.
27. Zakrzewski, W. (2019). Stem cells: Past, present, and future. *Stem Cell Research & Therapy*, *10*(1), 68–72.
28. Zelensky, A. N. (2017). Inactivation of Pol θ and C-NHEJ eliminates off-target integration of exogenous DNA. *Nature Communications*, *8*(1), 66–70.

# CHAPTER 9

# Vaginal Speculum: Balancing Safety, Property, and Practicality

SUMANA SAHA

*Corresponding author

## ABSTRACT

A speculum is a medical instrument for better visualization of hollow parts of the body. A vaginal speculum is an instrument used for visual examination of the lower part of the uterus, cervix, and vagina during gynecological examination. In this chapter, the author narrates a brief history of the use of vaginal speculums from ancient times to the present day. This review chapter comprehensively illustrates the properties of vaginal speculum, which includes functions of vaginal speculum and different types of vaginal speculum used in different healthcare settings, like Cusco's bivalve self-retaining speculum, Sims' double-bladed vaginal speculum, Huffman speculum, pediatric speculum, Pederson speculum, graves speculum, and so on. This chapter also focuses on different parts of the vaginal speculum with their illustration. It also explains how to sterilize and terminate this instrument after use. Additionally, this chapter also highlights the practicality of the vaginal speculum, which includes indications like cervical screening, Pap smear test, any gynecological examination, and so on, and specific contraindications of using this instrument. Additionally, the chapter explores the importance of balancing safety and Ethical considerations while using a vaginal speculum. It explains the detailed steps of pelvic examination used by the healthcare professionals, using a vaginal speculum.

Holistic Approaches for Women's Sustainable Health, Volume 1: Foundations, Innovations, Challenges, and Management. Megh R. Goyal, Anamika Chauhan, and Junaid Ahmad Malik (Eds)


DOI: 10.1201/9781779641632-11

## 9.1 INTRODUCTION

### *9.1.1 BRIEF INTRODUCTION OF VAGINAL SPECULUM*

Vaginal speculum is a widely used obstetrical instrument in the field of obstetrics and gynecology (Figure 9.1). It is one of the oldest instruments used for surveillance and early diagnosis, which has created serious conflicts about its power, propriety, and effectiveness in assessing women's health issues. During the 19th century, the vaginal speculum made its own place in the wide practice of obstetrics and gynecology, and it has established its visual dominance property and interpretive control regarding women's health issues in the 20th century. Compared to the modern visualization methods of patient assessment, speculum examination has sparked some robust discussions about politics, morality, and epistemology of examining women from the inside out. Therefore, in a long line of spectacular medical devices used to treat health issues of women, the vaginal speculum is the first that has been controversial and dramatic in the chronicles of women's healthcare [18].

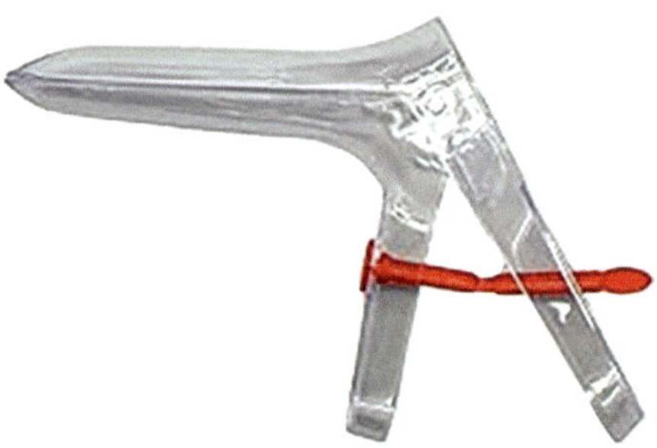

**FIGURE 9.1** Cusco's disposable vaginal speculum (Freely available on https://www.amazon.in/Cusco-Speculum-Vaginal-Disposable-MEDIUM/dp/B0B7DY1XSB).

**Pelvic examination:** A doctor or nurse inserts one or two lubricated, gloved fingers of one hand into the vagina and presses on the lower abdomen with the other hand. This is done to feel the size, shape, and position of the uterus and ovaries. The vagina, cervix, fallopian tubes, and rectum are also checked. A vaginal speculum is used to open the opening between the cervix and uterus.

### *9.1.2 IMPORTANCE OF ADDRESSING THIS ISSUE*

Nowadays, the care of women or diagnosis of any obstetrical or gynecological condition is largely influenced by the advancement of surveillance technology, such as bone density scans, CTG, mammography, cervical screening, intrapartum monitoring, and prenatal diagnosis. However, vaginal examination or speculum examination has its own place in this world of medical diagnosis, due to its clinical importance and choice of obstetricians and midwives for their routine and regular practice, while caring for women [7, 24].

Before the development of a self-retaining model, nurses or medical students were required to assist during the use of Sims' speculum. They used it to retract or pull back the vagina so the treating physician could perform their examination with other devices [20].

Vaginal speculum is a crucial yet troublesome tool in the arena of female healthcare, which is the most common reasons why women experience unexplainable fear, worry, and anxiety before a pelvic examination. Even though the speculum examination can create trauma-related scenarios, it is essential for adequate visualization and assessment of the cervix and uterus [21].

Therefore, while discussing different aspects of vaginal speculum in this chapter, the author wishes to contribute to the safety, improved quality of life, and well-being of women undergoing vaginal examination.

## 9.2 VAGINAL SPECULUM

### *9.2.1 WHAT IS A SPECULUM?*

"The speculum is for the diseases of the womb precisely what the stethoscope is for the diseases of the chest. Without either, there is no accurate diagnosis. Without these important aids to practical medicine, there is no exact appreciation of the pathological condition of the organs in question. Without these indispensable devices, we are often forced to grope entirely and literally in the dark."

Vaginal speculum is a medical instrument made of heavy metal or plastic that enables a better visualization of the cervix and vaginal orifice during a gynecological examination. This is most commonly used during pelvic examinations, Pap smears, and many other gynecological procedures (Figure 9.1).

### 9.2.2 BRIEF HISTORY OF USE OF VAGINAL SPECULUM

*Hippocrates* (432 BC) described the speculum first, as an instrument, the catopter, which was undoubtedly used as an anal speculum; and *Haussmann* explained that the uterine tubes of tin and lead mentioned in his books were intended to dilate the cervix uterus for the treatment of the interior of the uterus, and they were not called a vaginal speculum.

*Alen* (died about 200 AD) made the first vaginal speculum, as distinguished from the anal speculum. At that time, bivalve and trivalve speculums were in use, among which, the bivalve type was apparently intended for the anus, as it corresponds to the descriptions of such instruments given by ancient authors in different books. The trivalve was undoubtedly a vaginal speculum, as evidenced by its size and its use, as it corresponds to the figures and descriptions given by Albucasis (1085) and Scultetus (1666) in their documents [16].

*Rolfe* explained the trivalve speculum with three valves, which are positioned at an angle to the remainder of the instrument, and are mutually dependent on one another, but only one of them receives the expansion during examination. During insertion, its circumference is around an inch when all three valves are in contact. A gradual, consistent, and progressive dilatation, to which extent it is necessary, is created by rotating the screw of this instrument to move one valve closer to the operator and push the other two to open sideways. The examiner can use the left hand to hold the instrument by its two curving handles, while the right hand cranks/ rotates the screw [16].

It is very evident that the vaginal speculum was in use for more than a century across Western and Eastern countries across the globe by the physicians who treat the diseases of the womb (Table 9.1). During the period of Arabian ascendency, the diseases of the female genital organs were given over entirely to midwives, as the Mohammedan religion strictly forbade the examination of women by male practitioners. During this period, speculums were limited in use.

After that, Fergusson's speculum was recognized widely and used extensively due to the shape of this instrument for easy adjustment, its simplicity, and its capability of being used in a poor light, with minimal hazards.

But, this is very surprising that an instrument which was originally made for the diagnosis of different diseases of the womb was used as a uterine dilator for almost a hundred years. This was probably due to that

**TABLE 9.1** Developmental Milestones of Speculum Use [16]

| | |
|---|---|
| 1587 | Jacob Rueff in De Conceptu el generatione Hominis, explained that this trivalve speculum was only used to dilate the cervix and uterus in difficult labor. |
| 1603 | Roderic a Castro identified that the use of the speculum was for the examination of the vagina and operations on the vagina. |
| 1620 | Hieronymus Fabricius explained a three-bladed speculum, which was used for dilating the cervix and uterus in labor. |
| 1627 and 1640 | Galbelshoner and Ambroise Par figured a vaginal speculum, and a tubular speculum (Haussmann's plate) and which was intended to permit fluids to reach the cervix uteri while providing injection. |
| 1650 | Scultetus, in his Armamenta Chirurgica, figured a bivalve speculum and a trivalve speculum and explained that the previous speculum may be used either for the anal examination or vaginal examination, but the trivalve speculum will be used for the vaginal examination only. |
| 1657 | Wierus modified the three-bladed speculum by flattening the blades of the speculum for better visualization and to prevent the vaginal walls from falling into the lumen of the canal during examination. |
| 1766 | Levret in Lart des Accouchemens first proposed to use the vaginal speculum for the treatment of recto-vaginal and vesico-vaginal fistulae. |
| 1768 | Arnaud discovered a six-bladed speculum with a complicated structure, and he was the first to suggest applying artificial light in its use. |
| 1821 | Recamier introduced his tubular speculum, which was improved by Fergusson, and after that, its use has been widespread. |

during medieval times, physicians were called in to see women only during difficult labors, but other diseases were attended by the midwives solely.

Later, the speculum was invented, rather reinvented by Marion Sims, and is widely known as Sims' speculum in 1845, but it was published in the January issue of the American Journal of Medical Sciences in 1852, which is used widely during the retraction of the perineum and many gynecological operations.

However, Sims' speculum has certain drawbacks, which considerably restricted its use in everyday practice as it required a skilled assistant. If the uterine adhesions are present or if the vaginal walls are loose, to hold the base of the bladder forward and to explore the cervix, a second instrument is necessary, though its general excellence remained undoubted [16, 20].

After that, many times these Fergussons', Cusco's, and Sims' speculums were modified for better and hassle-free use during the diagnosis and treatment of different gynecological and obstetrical conditions in women's health. Various types of vaginal speculums are presented in Figures 9.1–9.7.

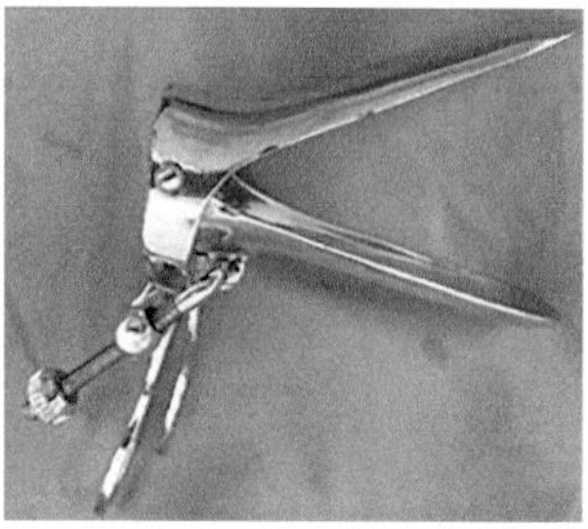

**FIGURE 9.2** Cusco's self-retaining (Duck's) vaginal speculum.

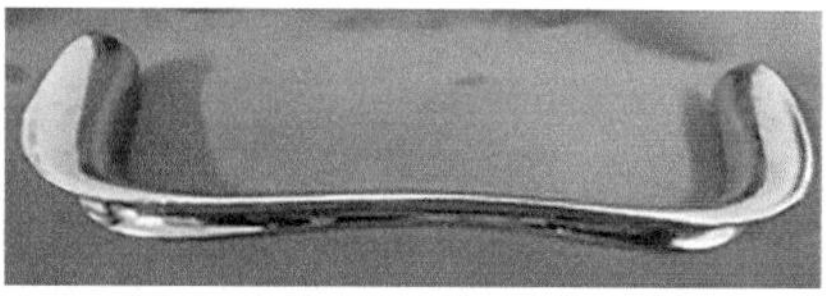

**FIGURE 9.3** Sims' double-bladed vaginal speculum.

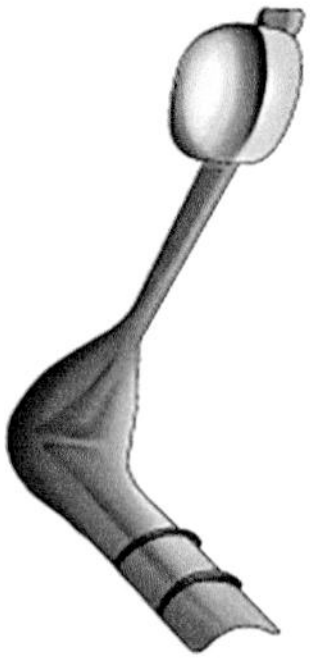

**FIGURE 9.4** Auvard speculum.

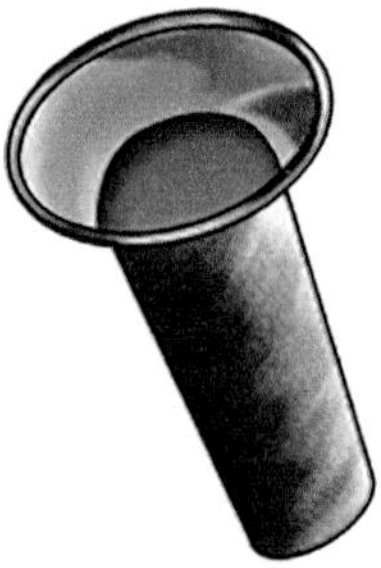

**FIGURE 9.5** Fergusson's speculum.

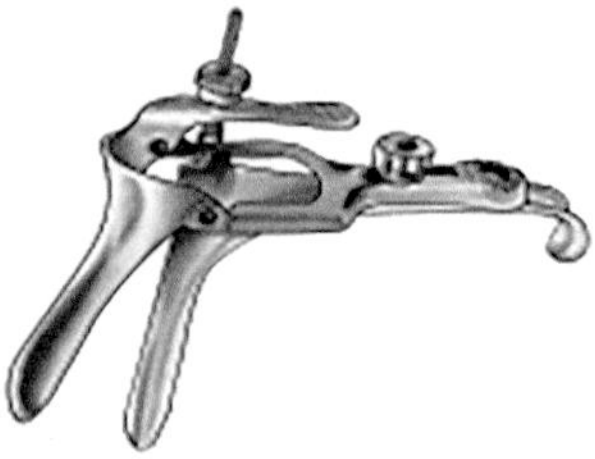

**FIGURE 9.6** Graves' vaginal speculum.

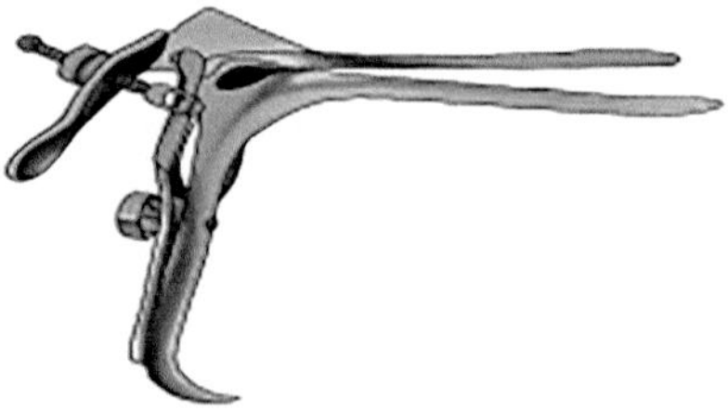

**FIGURE 9.7** Pederson's vaginal speculum.

## 9.3 PROPERTIES

### *9.3.1 FUNCTIONS OF VAGINAL SPECULUM*

Functions of vaginal speculum are listed below.

- To assess and examine the vagina and cervix for surveillance and diagnosis.
- To assist in different obstetric and gynecological surgeries.

- To collect the cervical specimen for screening (Pap smear test).
- To use during pelvic examination and different gynecological procedures.

### 9.3.2 *TYPES OF VAGINAL SPECULUM*

Speculum is made from heavy metals like stainless steel or plastic. Metal instruments are reusable after proper disinfection and sterilization. Plastic speculums are disposable and for single use. Different types of vaginal speculums may be found, and their use may vary as per their functional activities (Figures 9.1 to 9.7). The following are the different types, which are clinically used [1, 8, 17]:

- Auvard speculum
- Cusco's self-retaining vaginal speculum
- Fergusson's speculum
- Graves speculum
- Huffman speculum
- Pederson speculum
- Pediatric speculum
- Sims' double-bladed vaginal speculum

In general, the majority of the speculums consist of two blades that have a groove for easy drainage of fluids, one joint that is hinged and has a lockable position of the blades, allowing self-retaining hands-free access during performing internal examination (see Figures 9.1–9.7). These tools are generally made of heavy metal (reusable) or plastic (disposable). The Graves or Cusco speculum is widely used in clinical practice, but compared to the Graves speculum, having smaller blades in the Pederson speculum, which is used to examine a narrower vagina or for younger children (pediatric patients).

#### 9.3.2.1 *CUSCO'S SELF-RETAINING VAGINAL SPECULUM*

Cusco's bivalve self-retaining vaginal speculum is the most common gynecological instrument widely used in the assessment of the vagina and cervix. Its jaw opens up like a duckbill. That is why it is also known as "Duck's speculum." The device was named after Sir Édouard-Gabriel Cusco (1819–1894) [11]. Cusco's speculum has two blades and a groove in between, typically measures 22 mm (0.87 inches) in width and 80 mm

(3.1 inches) in length. But still, different small and large sizes are clinically available and are used as per the patient's need. Usually, a small size is used for nulliparous, virgins, and adolescent women, while a medium to large size is used for parous women.

**Applications [11]:**

- Cervical screening for the presence of any erosion, any development, or growth
- Collection of Pap smear for cytological study
- During any gynecological diagnostic procedures
- During colposcopy
- During vaginal examinations, as a routine obstetric and gynecological procedure
- Introducing an intrauterine contraceptive device (IUCD), follow-up and removal
- Used in minor surgeries like polypectomy, cryosurgery, etc. As it shields the anterior and posterior sections of the vaginal wall
- Vaginal erosion cauterization

**Advantages:**

- Cusco's speculum is beneficial due to its self-retaining property. Thus, assistance is usually not required in maintaining the speculum in position during vaginal examination.
- It acts as a vaginal wall retractor.
- It is easy to use, as it is designed to accommodate a wide range of patients comfortably while maintaining optimal visibility and good access during examinations
- It is made of long-lasting metal, high-grade stainless steel, which provides durability and corrosion resistance.
- It is reusable and autoclavable after each use.
- This is a cost-effective instrument.

**Limitations:**

The only limitation is, this vaginal speculum is not recommended during vaginal operations, as it has such a small vulvar orifice, which constricts the vaginal cavity and covers the majority of the vaginal wall with the blades of the speculum, thereby hiding minor lesions on the vaginal wall [17].

### *9.3.2.2 DOUBLE BLADED SIMS' SPECULUM*

Sims' double-bladed vaginal speculum is a non-self-retaining gynecological instrument, which is used in the vaginal and cervical examination. It is an "S"-shaped instrument, first developed with a pewter spoon by Sir J. Marion Sims [20], and presently it is made from polymer plastic (disposable) or high-grade stainless steel.

Disposable Sims' speculum is made of plastic material; however, the stainless steel Sims' speculum is reusable after proper disinfection. The metallic speculum requires a light source during examination, but the plastic speculum may or may not require a light source during examination.

Different sizes of Sims' speculum are available, and it is selected as on the vaginal length and cavity. Usually, a small size is used for nulliparous, virgins, and adolescent women, while a medium to large size is used for parous women.

**Applications:**

- During any diagnostic procedures like hysteroscopy, hysterosalpingography, sonosalpingography, tubal inflation, etc.
- During any uterine procedures like dilatation and curettage (D and C), endometrial biopsy, IUCD insertion, etc.
- During performing minor surgical procedures like cervical biopsy, conization of cervix, cervical tear repair, polypectomy, etc.
- During pregnancy, to assess for any discharge, amount of bleeding in APH, abortions, PPH, or to diagnose traumatic PPH, and repair tears after delivery.
- For vaginal cytology, culture, swab test, etc., diagnostic procedure purposes.
- To retract the posterior vaginal wall during major gynecological operations like, vaginal hysterectomy, Mc. Donald stitch, Shirodkar stitch, or Fothergill's operation, anterior colporrhaphy, posterior colpoperiniorrhaphy, VVF repair, etc.
- Used during any pelvic speculum examinations of obstetric and gynecological procedures.
- Used during MTP, D and E, and D and C.
- Used during vaginal examinations of vaginitis, cystocele, rectocele, enterocele, VVF, as it provides better visualization.
- Used in cervical screening for any growth, erosion, or any discharge.

**Advantages:**

- It is preferred because it exposes the vaginal walls more than Cusco's speculum does during different gynecological procedures.
- It keeps the area dry by allowing blood and secretions to flow freely outside through the grooves of the speculum during any procedure or surgery.
- Sims' speculum is used in retracting the vaginal wall posteriorly.
- This is simple to insert to allow better visibility of the vaginal wall, due to its shape.

**Limitations:**

- If the uterine adhesions are present, or if the vaginal walls are loose, it is necessary to apply Sims' speculum in conjunction with an anterior wall retractor to hold forward the base of the bladder and for improved cervical visualization [17].
- It is not self-retaining.
- It requires a skilled assistant.

#### *9.3.2.3 AUVARD SPECULUM*

Auvard vaginal speculum is a single-ended self-retaining vaginal instrument manufactured to keep the surgeon's hands free by opening the vaginal canal during any obstetrical and gynecological procedures. It is made of heavy metal, a right-angled half-tube that has a hefty ball or spherical weight on the handle. This instrument is available in different weights and blade diameters, suitable for various cases.

**Applications:**

- It is also used in anterior colporrhaphy, VVF repair, etc.
- It is used to retract the posterior vaginal wall during vaginal, cervical, or uterine surgeries, vaginal hysterectomy.

**Advantages:**

- Better visualization of the posterior vaginal wall
- It is reusable after appropriate disinfection.
- Self-retaining property of the instrument.

**Limitations:**

- Prolonged use can cause postoperative perineal pain
- Requires anesthesia, as it is a painful one.

#### *9.3.2.4 FERGUSSON SPECULUM*

The Fergusson speculum is undoubtedly the best instrument used for internal vaginal examination, was found at the demolished Roman city of Pompeii in 79 AD [23].

It was a simplified design of a tube speculum, which was invented by Recamier in 1821. In 1870, Sir William Fergusson modified the tubular speculum and referred to this device as "the speculum that I devised" in his writings. In 1855, the first obstetric medicine professor, Dr. Robert Fergusson (1799–1865) from King's College, started using a straight glass speculum [23].

The tubular glass speculum was silver-coated inside, as per the evidence available. This instrument has not survived or been used in a practical field for longer [23]. William Fergusson's design was completely lacquered, coated with quicksilver, and covered with India rubber. It has a mirror-like glass inside, which is an elastic gum covering and a great light reflector inside the vaginal canal to enable internal examination after speculum insertion. It is said that no other instrument can be compared in elegance, cleanliness, and utility to this speculum [22].

The surgical instrument company Simpson, London, manufactured the speculum. It was found in different sizes. This instrument is not in use nowadays.

**Applications:**

- Fergusson's speculum was mainly used for the diagnosis and treatment of vaginal and uterine disorders.
- It is extremely practical for applications in the vaginal canal or external cervical os.

**Advantages:**

- Acids and other corrosive substances do not harm it, unlike other substances that frequently destroy metal speculums.
- It can be washed and cleaned easily.
- Its illuminating power during examination is the best advantage.

**Limitations:**

- Sometimes it is difficult to introduce.
- The field of vision is limited due to its shape.
- It is very fragile, as it is made of glass.

### *9.3.2.5 GRAVES VAGINAL SPECULUM*

**Applications:**

- For examination of postpartum women who have recently or subsequently given birth, the Graves speculum may be used to adapt to the postpartum physiological change in the reproductive canal.
- It is available in various sizes and providers' preferences for biopsies or colposcopies.
- These are excellent choices for patients with an increased elasticity in the vaginal walls or a longer birth canal, as in older or multigravida women.

**Advantages:**

- Graves' speculum is expanded and transformed into a Sims' speculum, yet it results in terrible Sims' speculum, when considered as cost effectiveness.

**Limitations:**

- Graves' speculum serves its purpose well enough, as a simple bivalve. However, it fails as a base expander and as a Sims in both cases. It is advisable that, better to avoid the disadvantage of an unsatisfactory Sims in a practical situation.

### *9.3.2.6 HUFFMAN VAGINAL SPECULUM*

A Huffman speculum is the ideal choice for women who have not yet experienced intercourse or childbirth. This speculum is larger than a pediatric variation but much smaller than the commonly used Pederson or Graves. This long, thin speculum is narrower than a regular Sims' or

Cusco's speculum. It is used for adolescent girls who have not yet been sexually active.

**Applications:**

- The Huffman speculum is commonly used for the vaginal examinations of adolescent girls with guardians' consent.

### *9.3.2.7 PEDIATRIC SPECULUM*

The pediatric speculum is made for children, but among children it is shorter in length and narrower in width.

- Because of the sensitivities and structural changes of the vaginal canal, it is easy to use among adolescent girls and postmenopausal women.
- Patients/adolescent girls who have not experienced intercourse or childbirth, or postmenopausal women, will require a pediatric speculum because of its size and shape.

### *9.3.2.8 PEDERSON SPECULUM*

This is used for the examination of patients/women who have not given birth but are sexually active, and it is a good choice for them. This is another widely used vaginal speculum choice in care for obstetrics and gynecological patients, and is also available in different sizes. Its blades are narrower in size than those of the regular adult vaginal speculums, but larger than the blades of a Huffman speculum.

- It is applicable for the adult-elderly women, given their sexual history and childbearing experiences. It is essential to ensure the speculum is appropriate and comfortable for the patient.
- Sometimes a Pederson speculum is used in teenage girls who have been sexually active for the easy insertion and examination.

Usually, two types of speculums are available: plastic or disposable speculums and metal speculums.

Plastic or disposable speculums are usually for single one-time use. It should be discarded after each use. It should be disinfected properly and disposed of in a blue bag, as per the Bio-Medical Waste Management policy.

*Metal speculums* are generally reusable. After each use, three basic steps are used for disinfection after any diagnostic procedures, any surgery, or any treatment.

### 9.3.3 STEPS FOR STERILIZATION AFTER USE

- **Decontamination** [2, 19]: (1) It comprises a series of steps used to reduction of contamination with microorganisms or other harmful substances after use of any instrument, which causes the majority of organisms, including HIV and hepatitis B, to become inactive. To make sure that the speculum is cleansed and sterilized, additional processing is required properly before next use. (2) Immediately after use, soak the used speculum for ten minutes with 0.5% hypochlorite solution. A 0.5% chlorine solution is prepared by adding one part concentrated bleaching powder to nine parts of water.
- **Cleaning**: (1) A thorough cleaning is done manually under running water with liquid soap or detergent, which eliminates all organic products including tissue remnants, vaginal fluids, vaginal secretions and blood, etc. (2) Speculums should be washed immediately after use, to prevent any organic material from drying out and adhering to the equipment. (3) Scrub with a brush to clean the grooves, joints of the speculum properly.
- **High-level disinfection (HLD) or Sterilization** [19]: The process of sterilization involves subjecting the used speculum to physical or chemical agents to eradicate any bacteria. All types of germs, including bacterial spores, are eliminated by this process. (1) In the context of clinical practice, if there is survival chance of a microorganism is less than one in a million in an instrument, it is considered sterile. (2) It is advised to sterilize using autoclaves and high-pressure saturated steam. Unwrapped metal tools, such as a speculum, should be subjected to temperatures between 121 and 132°C for 20 minutes while maintaining 106 kPa (15 $lb/inch^2$) pressures. (3) Where autoclaving is not available, the boiling

method can also be used for sterilization. Boiling plain tap water is a very cost-effective and easily accessible form of HLD. In this method, speculums should be immersed in boiling water, at least for 20 min after commencement of boiling. The sterilizer should be washed and the water changed daily, and kept dry.

- **Decontamination of surfaces** [19]: In OPD, examination table, labor table, procedure clinic, trolley, floor of the clinic, etc., which might be contaminated by bodily fluids, secretions, vaginal blood, purulent discharge-like substances. Also necessary, along with the sterile instrument, for achieving an optimum level of sterility. These surfaces should be cleaned with 60–90% ethyl alcohol or isopropyl alcohol, 0.5% chlorine (hypochlorite) solution, or other available disinfectants regularly.

## 9.4 PRACTICALITY AND CONTRAINDICATION

### *9.4.1 INDICATION/USE/PRACTICALITY FOR USING VAGINAL SPECULUM*

The purpose of the gynaecological examination is to evaluate the urethra and rectum as well as the external and internal genitalia (Figure 9.1). When treating extremely unstable patients—either mentally, emotionally, or physically—providers should use caution [26]. Informed verbal consent must be obtained before the examination. Gynaecological screening should be done at 21 years onwards and subsequently and regularly after the first screening, and for patients having gynaecological disorders [15]. The following are the indications for any vaginal speculum examination [5]:

- Abnormalities of menstruation
- Acute pain in the lower abdomen
- After any sexual abuse or physical trauma
- Any vaginal discharge
- Bleeding per vagina
- Diagnostic examinations among females for screening purposes
- Disorders of pelvic floor muscles
- Neurological disorders
- Pregnancy or postpartum

- Presence of any signs of infection
- Screening of sexually transmitted infection/disease
- Sexual developmental abnormalities
- Swelling of glands
- Urinary incontinence

### *9.4.2 CONTRAINDICATIONS FOR SPECULUM EXAMINATION*

The absence of consent is the absolute contraindication of any speculum examination [26].

## 9.5 BALANCING SAFETY

### *9.5.1 PELVIC ASSESSMENT*

It usually consists of inspection and systematic internal examination, which includes a speculum examination of female reproductive organs, to assess the lower part of the abdomen, followed by external genital organs; vagina and cervix; uterus with adnexa; anal orifice and rectum, as well as cervical cytology, by a registered obstetrician or a registered practitioner, or a registered midwife. It may be for gynecological or obstetrical purposes.

Gynaecological examination usually consists of an external and internal genitalia assessment. However, a rectal examination may be required sometimes, along with the gynaecological examination, to rule out the underlying disease. The examination is helpful for early detection of space-occupying lesions, Pap smear (used for screening of cervical cancer), and to evaluate lower abdominal pain, bleeding per vagina, and/or features of infection in genitalia [21]. In the case of obstetrical examination, it helps to assess the cervical dilatation and the progress of labor.

### *9.5.2 MATERIALS, TOOLS, AND EQUIPMENT FOR PELVIC EXAMINATION*

- One examining table, preferably one with foot supports, to perform pelvic examination.
- Vaginal speculum for internal examination.
- Two pairs of sterile gloves for speculum examination and for recto-vaginal examination (as required).

- Good light source for better visualization, as room light may be inadequate for the procedure.
- Lubricant: may be a gel or sterile water.
- A sterile cervical spatula, if the cervical cytology specimen is required.
- A screen and a sheet to maintain the privacy of the women during examination.

### *9.5.3 PREPARATION OF PATIENT BEFORE VAGINAL SPECULUM EXAMINATION*

- A good interpersonal relationship should be established with the client before proceeding to reduce her fear and anxiety about the examination.
- Steps of the examination should be explained to the women in their local language, avoiding any medical jargon, prior to it being done. A thorough explanation of the steps of the examination should be provided.
- Informed verbal consent should be obtained from the patient.
- Environmental preparation should be done. The room should be clean, comfortable temperature, and well-lit.
- The privacy of the patient should be assured by putting up a screen.
- Advise the client to empty her bladder before examination.
- After positioning the client on the examination table, she should be instructed to rest in dorsal lithotomy position, while lying on her back comfortably. She should then move down to the bed herself, until her legs are nearly perpendicular (almost perfectly parallel) to the floor by placing her feet in the stirrup.
- Patient should be advised to remove the clothes down to the waist, as required during examination, and maintain her privacy by covering with a sheet.
- To enhance mobility and usability of the speculum and improve visibility during the examination, it is recommended to position the client's buttocks near the edge of the examination table or a little bit further away.

### 9.5.4 STEPS OF PELVIC EXAMINATION

The "RAD technique" is a procedure that involves a bimanual examination before the speculum is inserted. This helps to select the best speculum size and provides adequate visualization of the cervical canal, allowing quicker examination and reduced discomfort to the client [6].

The RAD technique corrects the misconceptions, including doing the speculum examination before the bimanual examination, assessment of multiparous women with a large size speculum, and inclining the table and patient by thirty degrees [6]. This technique is widely used in the field of obstetrics and gynecology. The steps in the pelvic examination are as follows, according to current medical textbooks:

- **Inspection of external genitalia**: Assessment of the external vulva for fundamental anatomy, development, its symmetry, distribution of pubic hair, any swelling, rashes, redness, bruising, any secretions, lesions, abnormal growths, and presence of acute pain and tenderness or abnormalities should be the first step in the examination. After that, place the thumb of the examiner over the perineal region and put the index finger into the vaginal introitus and palpate the labia for any soreness or presence of any growths. Next, assess for the presence of nodules, any abscesses, cysts, pain, or soreness in both labia with the fingers [13].
- **Internal speculum examination**: At first, lubricant should be applied to the tips of the speculum, holding it in the right hand by using the middle and index fingers to keep both blades close together at their base. Then both labia should be slightly spread with the left hand and gently insert the speculum at a 0–90° angle. After immediate insertion of the speculum, rotate it to point down the handle by pressing the rear perineum throughout the vaginal wall posteriorly. It is important to angle the speculum tip away from the vaginal wall anteriorly, since it is more sensitive there. Although it is easier to adjust a handle straight, which is downward-angled but in patients with a narrow vaginal canal, a slanted insertion of the speculum may be required. This is very important to use a properly sized speculum for examination. For examining older women and young girls, a narrow, small-sized speculum may be useful, and a medium-sized Graves or Cusco's speculum may be satisfactorily used for adult parous women.

But occasionally a large speculum may be required [5, 6]. Place the inferior blade in the posterior vaginal fornix before opening the speculum. In the case of nulliparous women, this is required significantly. After that, the cervix is opened like a duckbill and examined for color, lesions, eversion, erosion, polyps, cysts, any lacerations, ulcerations, enlargement of the cervix, bleeding per vagina, any discharge, and whether the external os is closed or open. In case of improper visualization of the cervix, subsequent bimanual examination may be required. At this point in time, a cervical specimen is collected. Specimens for cervical cytology should be obtained for different cytological examinations by using different techniques [13]. After that, the speculum blades are released loosely and withdrawn slowly to prevent squeezing the cervical and vaginal walls. During the removal of the speculum, vaginal walls should be examined for any irregularities or abnormalities, like symptoms of vaginal discharge, presence of foreign bodies, vaginitis, and any other lesions.

- **Bimanual examination with lubricated and gloved fingers**: The next step is bimanual examination, which includes internal insertion of one hand while the nondominant other hand should be placed externally across the abdomen to press down the cervix and vice versa. The first two fingers are then lubricated and gently placed into the vagina. After that, the cervix is located and the consistency of the cervix is assessed with either finger of the other hand, to bring it closer to the inferiorly placed abdomen. By inserting one finger, assess for the external os and internal os, whether open or closed. Then any motion tenderness in the cervix is identified. Palpate the uterus by the other hand over the abdomen by pushing it between the hands for its shape, dimension, position, consistency, symmetry, or mobility; either adnexa, including the uterine tubes, ovaries, the small intestine, recto-sigmoid, urinary bladder, and ureters, are also assessed for any masses and tenderness. After that, fingers are withdrawn gently [13].
- **Performance of recto-vaginal examination**: Sometimes, a recto-vaginal assessment is required to evaluate the recto-vaginal septum and cul-de-sac posteriorly, to identify any hemorrhoids, the presence of polyps, and any growths. In this step, the third

digit is inserted slowly and gently after lubrication in the rectum, through the anal orifice by using another sterile glove, and the patient is asked to strain down. This allows relaxing the anal sphincter muscles to minimize patient discomfort. Then, introduce the index finger into the vaginal canal to assess any recto-vaginal septum tenderness with both fingers [13].

### 9.5.5 CONSEQUENCES/COMPLICATIONS OF USING VAGINAL SPECULUM

Complications generally are not associated with speculum examination, but iatrogenic effects may be encountered, such as acute pain, traumatic experiences, and anxiety, in some special circumstances are discussed below [14]:

- The speculum examination can be quite painful for women who have atrophic vaginitis, and generous lubrication is necessary to reduce the pain. Certain medical standards of care recommend performing the manual exam first to reduce the fear and anxiety of the patients and not to use lubricant on the speculums, as the chance of contamination of collected specimens increases during the examination. But some studies suggest adopting a small amount of lubricating gel as the standard practice when performing speculum examinations [12].
- One of the most common sexual pain disorders is vaginismus among women, which is characterized by intense dread and avoidance of any vaginal penetration, and is a common consequence of pelvic examinations. In this case, 7–8 minutes of deep breathing exercise was found to be helpful to ease the pain [27].
- A pelvic assessment may provoke acute anxiety and/or post-traumatic stress disorder in a woman who has had past sexual trauma or abuse. In these cases, counselling and, use of anxiolytics is found to be effective.

### 9.5.6 CONSIDERATIONS FOR WOMEN'S SAFETY DURING SPECULUM EXAMINATION

Before the use of the vaginal speculum for pelvic examination, doctors used to avoid vaginal or rectal examination of their patients. Even in the field of medical practice, the women's body was a contentious topic [3, 18].

To maintain the respect and virtue of women, the doctors used to assess the vagina blindly, without taking off the patient's clothing in any way. He would intentionally refrain from making eye contact with the patient or purposefully keep her eyes open to reassure her that he was not focusing on her genital organs, ensuring preservation of her virtue, as the field of medical profession was predominated by several male physicians [18, 25].

After the Second World War, when psychosomatic medicine and Freudian psychology were established, women's understanding of their reproductive organs changed, but still, nowadays, women feel an unexplained fear and anxiety toward speculum examination [16]. The following considerations should be followed by the examiner/obstetrician/midwife during speculum examination:

- The level of women's comfort during pelvic assessment is the targeted compliance in the field of obstetrics and gynecology. Obstetrician, physician assistants, nurse practitioners, or midwives must be familiar and thorough with the procedure of pelvic examinations and must be experienced enough in providing psychological support and ensuring patient privacy during providing "patient-centered" examination.
- Communication is the key to establishing an interpersonal relationship between the patient and the examiner before starting a procedure. Explain the procedure in her understandable language, which will help to ease her fear and anxiety and make comfortable during the examination. Encourage a conversation with the patient throughout the examination. The attitude of the examiner can greatly influence patient experience and the performance of the physician simultaneously.
- Liberal use of lubrication and careful selection and insertion of the proper size of speculum can ease this unexplained fear and anxiety. It is especially essential for adolescent girls and women who are menopausal, women who belong to sexual minority groups, women with some disabilities or obesity, as well as those who have a history of sexual traumatic experience, before any pelvic procedure.
- Examine gently otherwise, the patient may become frustrated and put up involuntary muscular resistance to it. If the steps are properly explained before examinations are gently performed with adequate concern for the level of comfort and privacy of the patient, accurate and adequate information can be explored.

- Patients must be undressed that much only, which is necessary for the examination, and proper draping is required to prevent unnecessary exposure. This is very helpful for the patients, who are embarrassed to undress or who are going for their first vaginal examination [4].
- Generally, moderate sedation or general anesthesia is not essential for a pelvic examination, but may be required in some unusual circumstances.
- Pelvic examination should not be postponed if the woman is menstruating, as pelvic examination is not contraindicated by menstruation, and the patient will not be harmed anyway [4].
- In case of Pap smear test, pelvic examination should be done when the woman does not have her menstrual cycle, since a Pap smear yields a more accurate result when menstrual blood is absent.
- The presence of a chaperone during examination is essential, and usually a nurse or a midwife, or any female healthcare provider acts as a chaperone during pelvic examination. Between 1946 and 1956, different gynecology textbooks for nurses were suggesting that nurses should be present in order to reassure the client and to shield the doctor from any unwanted issues during vaginal examinations [4, 9, 10].
- In a few cases, clinical counseling must be done, or anxiolytics may be helpful if the patient is psychologically not stable.
- Patient must be informed that the procedure can be discontinued or stopped whenever she feels any pain or discomfort [4].
- Different alternatives could be recommended, like only taking off the underwear during examination, insertion of a speculum by the patient herself, presence of a female healthcare provider or any family member, or an accompanying friend in the examination room to enhance the level of comfort during examination, as necessary for the women [4].

## 9.6 CONCLUSION

The three major factors—unexplained fear and anxiety, traumatic painful experiences, and acute discomfort—are identified to avoid the speculum examination by women. In the healthcare industry, ensuring a female patient's maximum comfort during a pelvic examination is crucial to compliance. Though it is unattainable to some extent, under some circumstances, using present standards of care. This is very necessary to enhance the positive experience of women during speculum examination, by improving new designs of speculum which are easy to use; frequent training of the physicians/midwives; adoption of patient centered care approach to improve patient participation; before performing speculum examination, do bimanual examination as a standard of care, and selection of suitable sized speculum to establish the ideal ratio of high-tech monitoring to high-touch treatment.

This chapter dealt with importance of discussing the topic, history of use of different vaginal speculum, detailed description, including their indication for use, advantages and limitations of various types of vaginal speculum with their diagram, how to disinfect and sterilize speculum after use, detailed steps of pelvic and speculum examination, including indication and contraindication of speculum examination and examiner's responsibility while performing a speculum examination.

## KEYWORDS

- **bimanual examination**
- **gynecological assessment**
- **Pap smear test**
- **pelvic examination**
- **vaginal speculum**
- **women's health screening**

## REFERENCES

1. Agarwal, K. (2022). *Instruments and Procedures in Obstetrics and Gynecology*, 2nd edn., Jaypee Brothers Medical Publishers, India: Delhi.
2. Altschäffl, J. (1976). Sterilization of the vaginal specula. *ZFA (Stuttgart—Germany)*, *52*(25), 1286. https://pubmed.ncbi.nlm.nih.gov/983243/
3. Balbirnie, J., & Lond, A. M. (1837). The speculum applied to diagnostic and treatment of the organic diseases of the womb. *Medico-Chirurgical and Review. (London)*, *26*(51), 105–124.

4. Bates, C. K., Carroll, N., & Potter, J. (2011). The challenging pelvic examination. *Society of General Internal Medicine, 26*(6), 651–657.
5. Bialy, A., Kondagari, L. & Wray, A. A. (2024). Gynecologic examination. In: *StatPearls Treasure Island (FL)*. StatPearls Publishing: Miami, FL.
6. Carter, S., Rad, M., Schwarz, B., Van Sell, S., & Marshall, D. (2013). Creating a more positive patient experience of pelvic examination. *Journal of the American Association of Nurse Practitioners, 25*(11), 611–618.
7. Cartwright, E. (1998). The logic of heartbeats: Electronic fetal monitoring and biomedically constructed birth. In: *Cyborg Babies*: *From Techno-sex to Techno-tots* (pp. 240–254). Routledge: New York.
8. Cowperthwait, A. C. (1888). *A Text Book of Gynecology Designed for the Student and General Practitioner*. Ann Intern Med.
9. Crossen, R. J., & Campbell, A. J. (1956). *Gynecologic Nursing*, 5th edn., C. V. Mosby: St. Louis.
10. Crossen, R. J., & Hoffert, F. W. (1946). *Gynecologic Nursing*, 3rd edn., C. V. Mosby: St. Louis, MO.
11. Dorland, J., & Newman, *W. A. (1917). The American Illustrated Medical Dictionary (p. 272). W.B. Saunders Company.*
12. Hill, A., & Lamvu, G. (2012). Lubricating gel for vaginal speculum insertion. *The American College of Obstetricians and Gynecologists* (Lippincott Williams & Wilkins), *119*(2), part 1.
13. Long, W. N. (1990). Pelvic examination. In: Walker, H. K., Hall, W. D., & Hurst, J. W. (Eds.), *Clinical Methods: The History, Physical, and Laboratory Examinations,* 3rd edn., (Chapter 177). Butterworths: Boston.
14. Millstein, S. G., Adler, N. E., & Irwin, C. E. (1984). Sources of anxiety about pelvic examinations among adolescent females. *Journal of Adolescent Health Care, 5*, 105–111.
15. Qaseem, A., Humphrey, L. L., Harris, R., Starkey, M., & Denberg, T. D. (2014). Screening pelvic examination in adult women: A clinical practice guideline from the American College of Physicians. *Clinical Guidelines Committee of the American College of Physicians*, *161*(1), 67–72.
16. Reid, W. L. (1986). The history, forms, and theories of the vaginal speculum. *The Glasgow Medical Journal*, *46*(3), 161–173.
17. *Salhan, S. (2011). Textbook of Gynaecology (p. 848). Jaypee Medical Publishers Ltd.: New Delhi.*
18. Sandelowski, M. (2000). This most dangerous instrument: Propriety, power, and the vaginal speculum. *Journal of Obstetric, Gynecologic, and Neonatal Nursing (JOGNN/NAACOG)*, *29*(1), e7382.
19. Sellors, J. W., & Sankaranarayanan, R. (Eds.) (2022). Decontamination, cleaning, high-level disinfection and sterilization of /instruments used during the diagnosis and treatment of cervical neoplasia. In: *Colposcopy and Treatment of Cervical Intraepithelial Neoplasia: A Beginners' Manual* (Chapter 14). International Agency for Research on Cancer (WHO).
20. Sims, M. (1885). *Story of My Life*. Appleton and Company.

21. Taylor, G. A., Donagh, D., & Hansen, M. J. (2017). Improving the pelvic exam experience: A human-centered design study. *The Design Journal*, *20*(suppl. 1), S2348–S2362.
22. Thomas, T. G. (1880). *A Practical Treatise on the Diseases of Women* (pp. 93–94). LEA: Philadelphia, PA.
23. Thompson, C. J. S. (1938). The vaginal dilator or speculum. *British Journal of Surgery*, *102*(XXXVI), 232.
24. Treichler, P. A., & Cartwright, L. (1992). *Imaging Technologies, Inscribing Science* (Special issue, pp. 28–29). Camera Obscura.
25. Whatley, M. H., & Worcester, N. (1989). The role of technology in the co-optation of the women's health movement: The cases of osteoporosis and breast cancer screening. In: *Healing Technology: Feminist Perspectives* (pp. 199–220). University of Michigan Press: Ann Arbor.
26. Williams, A. A., & Williams, M. (2013). *A Guide to Performing Pelvic Speculum Exams: A Patient-centered Approach to Reducing Iatrogenic Effects*, *Teaching and Learning in Medicine, 25*(4), 383–391.
27. Zinnante, M. (2024). Interview at Methodist Mansfield Medical Center (Mansfield, TX) on the article, Improving the pelvic exam experience: A human-centered design study. *The Design Journal*, 20(suppl. 1), S2348–S2362.

# PART III

# CHALLENGES AND MANAGEMENT IN FEMALE HEALTH

## CHAPTER 10

# Impact of Certain Medical Conditions and Substance Abuse on Health of Women and Fetuses

KHURSHEED AHMAD WANI, JAVID MANZOOR, HEENA QADIR, and JUNAID AHMAD MALIK*

*Corresponding author

## ABSTRACT

This chapter indicates how early childhood represents a time of remarkable immune development and heightened vulnerability to infectious illness. It also presents how maternal HIV infections expose uninfected kids to numerous infections such as HIV and AIDS. How our inability to develop and execute effective treatments stems from our incomplete mechanistic knowledge of how prenatal factors impact baby outcomes. This chapter will also discuss how common sexually transmitted infections (STIs) are in developing countries among infants who have contracted them from their mothers and how the lack of easy and cheap diagnostic tests has complicated the management of STIs in pregnancy in many developing countries. One of the classic issues in medicine is the potential danger that certain medications pose to an unborn child. This chapter will focus on this issue. This chapter will also explain how prenatal alcohol use may lead to significant birth defects such as fetal alcohol spectrum disorder or its more severe form, fetal alcohol syndrome.

Holistic Approaches for Women's Sustainable Health, Volume 1: Foundations, Innovations, Challenges, and Management. Megh R. Goyal, Anamika Chauhan, and Junaid Ahmad Malik (Eds)


DOI: 10.1201/9781779641632-13

## 10.1 INTRODUCTION

Miscarriage, stillbirth, and a wide variety of congenital abnormalities and intellectual impairment have all been linked to maternal alcohol use. Fetal alcohol spectrum disorders (FASDs) refer to these impairments. Prenatal opioid exposure has been related to low-birth-weight babies, premature deliveries, stillbirths, certain congenital anomalies, and neonatal abstinence syndrome (NAS) or neonatal opioid withdrawal syndrome [16, 37].

Exposure to secondhand smoke during pregnancy significantly heightens the likelihood of babies being born prematurely, having low birth weight, and being born with cleft lips and palates. The risk of sudden infant death syndrome (SIDS) is increased both while pregnant and after delivery if the mother smokes. The same goes for electronic cigarettes and other tobacco products that contain nicotine (the addictive chemical present in tobacco). Marijuana usage during pregnancy has been associated with a lower birth weight in several studies. Child development issues, such as attention and learning difficulties, may be exacerbated as a result. More study is required to determine the long-term effects of marijuana on pregnant women and their unborn children. Using prescription drugs for recreational purposes raises the danger of negative health effects and accidental overdose [9, 21]. The danger of drug overdose may be further increased by combining drugs such as opioids with benzodiazepines or opioids with alcohol. In low- and middle-income nations, the prevalence of drug use among pregnant women is poorly understood. Some nations have substantially higher maternal rates, up to 15%; yet generally the prevalence of smoking in these regions is 2.6% [34].

Women of reproductive age are likely to use cannabis, amphetamine-type stimulants, and opiates, according to the World Health Organization; however, data on illicit substance use during pregnancy is lacking for most middle- and low-income countries. South African data, which is all that is currently available for Africa, shows that between 3.6% and 8.8% of pregnant women there use illegal drugs, and 19.6% use alcohol during pregnancy. Methamphetamine and cannabis are the two most often used illegal narcotics among South Africans aged 16 and above. There has been a 17% growth in opiate usage worldwide, and it is expected that this trend will continue in regions such as Africa and Asia [7, 18, 50, 73, 75].

Substance abuse during pregnancy is associated with a spectrum of health challenges for both the mother and the developing baby. Some pregnant women may be motivated to reduce their drug and alcohol use out of worry for the health of their unborn child [17]. Women who drank heavily before becoming pregnant had a 96% success rate at abstinence, whereas those who used marijuana had a 78% success rate, those who used cocaine had a 73% success rate, and cigarette smokers had a 32% success rate [33, 55, 58].

The sharp increase in drug abuse between 6 and 12 months postpartum more than makes up for the decline in pregnancy-related usage. Researchers found that during the first three months after giving birth, 58% of women who had stopped smoking, 51% of women who had stopped drinking, 41% of women who had stopped using marijuana, and 27% of women who had stopped using cocaine relapsed. High rates of relapse after giving birth mean that even if abstinence was widespread throughout pregnancy, its effects would be muted. Tragically, relapse among mothers occurs during the critical early months of baby development, when care giving demands are at their highest. It is also worth noting that this research was conducted in the United States, and that women in middle- and low-income countries may face different barriers to abstinence due to factors such as higher rates of socioeconomic stressors, lower levels of education, and fewer treatment options for substance abuse [1, 8, 35].

Drug use, whether legal or illicit, during pregnancy has been shown to have negative effects on the developing baby. Your unborn child shares your susceptibility to the effects of smoking, alcohol use, and caffeine consumption. The effects of substances such as marijuana and crystal meth are felt by the developing baby as well. You endanger the lives of both you and your unborn child if you are addicted to cocaine (also known as coke, snow, or blow). Cocaine use may lead to cardiac arrest, respiratory failure, stroke, and convulsions. These potentially fatal diseases may also be transmitted to an unborn child. Delivery defects, early delivery, low birth weight, and stillbirth are all more likely when medications are used during pregnancy. Prenatal exposure to substances such as marijuana (also known as weed, ganja, dope, or pot) and alcohol has been linked to behavioral issues later in life. The child's memory and focus may be negatively impacted by these medicines as well. Moreover, evidence suggests that the brain structure of children born to mothers who use substances such as cocaine, alcohol, or cigarettes during pregnancy may exhibit noticeable alterations as early as adolescence [3, 11, 27, 29, 58].

Cocaine's effects on an adult are often seen right away, but the long-term consequences on a developing baby may be devastating. "Crack babies," children whose moms used crack during pregnancy, are at increased risk for a variety of health and behavioral issues. The National Institute on Drug Abuse reports that prenatal cocaine exposure may result in slight but substantial developmental delays in offspring. These numbers show that drug abuse during pregnancy is a major public health issue. The objective of this chapter is to provide a concise overview of pregnancy outcomes, the neonatal and long-term developmental effects of prenatal drug use, and the current treatment options for pregnant females who are struggling with such issues [1, 10].

This chapter focuses on the impact of certain medical conditions and substance abuse on health of women and fetus.

## 10.2 ADVERSE EFFECTS OF SUBSTANCE USE IN PREGNANCY

Miscarriage, stillbirth, premature birth, and small-for-gestational age are just some of the adverse birth outcomes linked to heavy alcohol use during pregnancy. Other negative outcomes include reduced gestational age, low birthweight, and congenital anomalies. There is either unclear evidence for low to moderate alcohol consumption during pregnancy (Higgins), or no increased risk for these poor pregnancy outcomes [24]. Pregnancy-related alcohol consumption is linked with an increased risk of FASDs [28, 30, 61] and negative neurodevelopmental outcomes [14, 22]. Furthermore, prenatal alcohol use is linked to long-term impacts, including cognitive and behavioral difficulties [5] poor speech and language outcomes, difficulties with executive functioning [36], and negative psychosocial outcomes [49] among others.

Damage to the umbilical cord structure [66], miscarriage [74], and increased risk of ectopic pregnancy, low birthweight, placental abruption, premature birth, and increased infant mortality are all direct adverse effects of smoking during pregnancy. Higher incidence of respiratory and ear infections, SIDS, behavioral dysfunction, and cognitive impairment are just some of the negative health impacts of secondhand smoking on babies. Furthermore, prepregnant women who smoked may discontinue nursing early to resume smoking [60].

Cannabis use during pregnancy is seen as safe by some expectant mothers; however, it has been related to negative outcomes such as premature delivery, low birth weight, small-for-gestational age, and hospitalization in the neonatal intensive care unit (NICU). Cannabis use during pregnancy has also been associated with negative outcomes for fetal and adolescent brain development, including impaired attention and executive functioning, worse academic performance, and an increase in behavioral issues. Marijuana's negative effects are more pronounced among chronic users and those who use it in combination with other substances [32].

Sometimes the potential dangers of using cocaine while pregnant are exaggerated. Recent large-scale studies, however, have linked cocaine use during pregnancy to several adverse outcomes such as premature membrane rupture, placental abruption, preterm birth, low birthweight, and small-for-gestational age infants. Long-term effects of prenatal cocaine exposure on linguistic, motor, and cognitive development have been reported inconsistently, with some research presenting favorable results and others reporting very little or no effects. This discrepancy may be traced back to the obscuring influences of the postnatal environment such as unstable and chaotic living conditions, dysfunctional parenting, and excessive mother polysubstance use [75]. Methamphetamine use during pregnancy is associated with the same negative outcomes as cocaine use during pregnancy, including premature delivery, low birth weight, fetal loss, developmental and behavioral abnormalities, hypertension, preeclampsia, and fetal mortality [19].

Low birth weight, respiratory difficulties, bleeding in the third trimester, toxemia, and maternal and infant mortality are all increased by opioid use during pregnancy. Prenatal opiate exposure may cause withdrawal symptoms in a newborn, a condition called NAS. Opioid opioids such as methadone and buprenorphine may cause NAS in as many as 94% of exposed newborns. Signs and symptoms of NAS include irritability, feeding problems, tremors, hypertonia, emesis, loose stools, convulsions, and respiratory distress, and the condition is associated with significant newborn morbidity and increased healthcare consumption. Postnatal growth retardation, microcephaly, neurobehavioral disorders, and SIDS have all been linked to maternal opioid use. Poor pregnancy outcomes may not be solely attributable to opioid use, since cigarette smoking is quite prevalent among pregnant women with an opioid use disorder (77–95%) [39].

Consequences of drug abuse during pregnancy are complicated by the high prevalence of concurrent substance abuse and concomitant mental disorders. Women with drug use disorders often experience inadequate prenatal care, poor nutrition, chronic medical issues, poverty, and domestic abuse at higher rates. The deleterious consequences of prenatal drug exposure might be compounded by the fact that substance abuse during pregnancy can lead to an early dysfunctional maternal–infant connection [65].

Substance abuse disorders are a major, avoidable source of illness worldwide. Cannabis is still the most widely used illegal substance in the world, with amphetamines coming in second. This is according to the 2017 report from the United Nations Office on Drugs and Crime. Opioids are the most dangerous, and many individuals are abusing several substances at once. The frequency, patterns, and experiences of drug use vary by gender due to biological, psychological, and cultural variables. While males still have a larger risk of developing a substance use problem, women's use of nicotine, alcohol, and illegal drugs is on the rise. When compared with males, it takes much less time for a woman to develop a drug use problem when she begins using substances. The highest incidences of drug use disorder in women are seen throughout adolescence and early adulthood, when they are most likely to have children [26]. A nationwide study conducted in the United States in 2013 found that 15.4% of women smoked during pregnancy, 9.4% drank alcohol, and 5.4% used illegal drugs. In Australia, 9 out of 10 pregnant women drink alcohol. As many as 27% of Australian women drank in their first trimester of pregnancy, and another 27% drank at least sometimes throughout their pregnancies, according to data collected from a population-based cohort. According to previous research, 13.8% of pregnant Australian women said they smoked cigarettes in the first weeks, and screenings found that 5% of women were using cannabis and 2% were using other illegal substances. In poor and middle-income nations, data on the frequency of drug abuse during pregnancy are scarce. Among pregnant women in South Africa, 19.6% had alcohol in their systems and 8.8% had tested positive for drugs (including methamphetamine, cannabis, and Mandrax). Self-report measures showed that at the time of their first prenatal visit, 36.8% of women smoked cigarettes, 20.2% drank alcohol, and 4% used illegal drugs. Substance-using pregnant women have been observed to use several drugs at high rates. Pregnant women who use drugs have much increased rates of comorbid cigarette smoking, and the rates are substantially higher for polysubstance users.

The first 1000 days of life, starting from conception, are widely acknowledged as critical for future health and development. Knowing how drug use affects pregnancy, lactation, maternal–infant bonding, and child outcomes is critical. This chapter summarizes the current evidence and recommendations on screening and therapies for pregnant women who use drugs, as well as the research on the effects of substances on pregnancy and child outcomes. This chapter is intended for both the ordinary obstetrician and the obstetric medicine expert and provides a comprehensive overview of most drugs used during pregnancy (Figure 10.1) [28, 61].

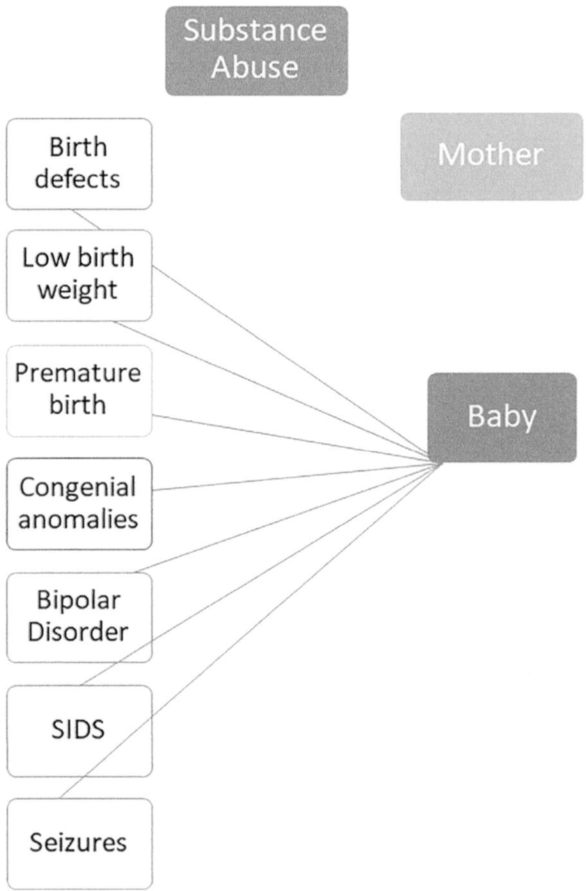


**FIGURE 10.1** Transmission of symptoms of substance abuse from mother top baby.

## 10.3 IMPACT OF SUBSTANCES ON PREGNANCY AND CHILD OUTCOMES

Risk factors for problematic substance use during pregnancy include prior alcohol, nicotine, or illicit drug use, unplanned pregnancy, lower education levels, unemployment, younger age, cooccurring physical and mental health issues, childhood trauma, environmental stress, intimate partner violence, easy access to substances, and insufficient awareness of the effects of substances on fetal development [63].

Unwanted pregnancies account for 41% of births worldwide, and many mothers use drugs or alcohol before they realize they are pregnant. The chance of an unwanted pregnancy rises in tandem with substance use. Pregnancy is a powerful motivator for many women to seek out and participate in harm reduction treatments, such as opioid substitution programs, or to reduce their drug use altogether. Substance use problems are persistent and often relapsing, making it difficult for some pregnant women to abstain. Relapse rates are especially high in the first six months after giving birth, even for women who were able to abstain from substance use during their pregnancies. In prospective research conducted in the United States, 83% of women ($N$=152) abstained from at least one drug throughout pregnancy, but 80% relapsed in the postpartum period [15].

Substance-abusing mothers-to-be are less likely to obtain prenatal care than their sober counterparts. Several factors can hinder women from receiving adequate antenatal care, including medical and psychiatric comorbidities, lack of coping skills, challenges with transportation and childcare, intimate partner violence, incarceration, poor provider communication, stigmatization, fear of legal consequences such as being reported to the police or losing child custody, and negative health beliefs like an external locus of control, skepticism about the effectiveness of healthcare, and lack of social support. Substance-using mothers confront numerous challenges, including inadequate prenatal care, mental and medical comorbidities, and challenging sociocultural environments. In such circumstances, evaluating the impact of medication on both mother and child becomes complex. Factors such as insufficient prenatal care, poor nutrition, medical and psychiatric comorbidities, intimate partner violence, compromised maternal–infant bonding, and chaotic postnatal environments significantly influence pregnancy and child outcomes among substance-using mothers [45]. It is well documented that drug use during pregnancy adversely affects maternal physiology and easily crosses the placenta, thereby impairing fetal cognitive and physical development. Pregnancy and child outcomes are extensively studied concerning substances such as alcohol, nicotine, cannabis, opioids, cocaine, and methamphetamine.

### *10.3.1 MARIJUANA*

Marijuana use during pregnancy has been related to several health issues, including an increased risk of using cigarettes and other drugs that may have negative effects on pregnancy and baby health. The potential effects of marijuana on pregnant women and their unborn children need to be studied further. The Centers for Disease Control and Prevention (CDC) concurs with the American College of Obstetricians and Gynecologists' (ACOG) recommendation against consuming marijuana while pregnant. Talk to your doctor if you use marijuana and are pregnant or trying to become pregnant [71].

### *10.3.2 ALCOHOL*

No quantity of alcohol consumption is considered safe during pregnancy or while attempting to conceive. Additionally, there is never a good moment to drink when pregnant. All wines and beers are created equal when it comes to the damage they cause. It is never too late for a pregnant woman to give up alcohol. You need professional assistance to quit drinking if you are pregnant or trying to conceive. Get in touch with your doctor, the local chapter of Alcoholics Anonymous, or a rehab facility specializing in alcoholism. Alcohol is a proven teratogen, and FASD are the most common avoidable cause of birth abnormalities and developmental delays worldwide. According to the results of a recent meta-analysis, eight out of every 1000 people in the general population suffer from FASD, and one in every 13 pregnant women who drank alcohol during pregnancy gave birth to a kid with FASD. The results of FASD may change depending on how much, when, and how often a person drinks. Other long-term poor child outcomes related with maternal alcohol consumption include growth deficits, behavioral issues, cognitive and motor delays, and low birth weight. Miscarriage, stillbirth, low birth weight, premature birth, and small-for-gestational age are only few of the unfavorable consequences linked with heavy alcohol consumption during pregnancy. Results for low and extremely low alcohol consumption during pregnancy are contradictory. There is a lot of confusion among pregnant women about how much alcohol is safe to consume. The teratogenic effects of alcohol have been shown in animal models at all stages of embryonic development, and even brief exposure to alcohol has been shown to have an influence on brain development, In light of the proven danger of teratogenicity and the possible adverse effects on the child's development and health down the road, no quantity of alcohol use during pregnancy is safe, even at moderate levels. Health professionals should deliver a consistent message about abstinence, which is recommended by most standards [2, 56].

### *10.3.3 NICOTINE*

Premature delivery, low birth weight, and cleft lip and palate are just a few of the many birth abnormalities that may affect a growing baby if the mother smokes throughout pregnancy. The risk of SIDS is increased both while pregnant and after delivery if the mother smokes. Nicotine, the addictive substance present in tobacco, should also be avoided during pregnancy, which includes e-cigarettes and other tobacco products. Pregnant women and their unborn children are more vulnerable to the negative health effects of nicotine, which includes harm to the developing brain and lungs. E-cigarette flavorings have also been linked to birth defects. Research the effects of vaping on pregnancy. Putting down the cigarette is a difficult task, but it can be done. One of the best things you can do for your health and the health of your kid is to kick the habit of smoking. It is ideal to stop smoking before becoming pregnant, but it is never too late to do so. The doctor may be a huge asset in the quest to kick the habit by providing guidance, emotional support, and referrals to other helpful organizations. The coaches at the quit line are there to assist you every step of the way. How to quit and smoking during pregnancy and motherhood are two further resources for helping you kick the habit. The health of children is significantly impacted by smoking cigarettes as well.

The risks of infection, cochlear malfunction, SIDS, and death are all higher for newborns. Poor cognitive development, behavioral issues, childhood obesity, hypertension, diabetes, and respiratory disorders are all detrimental long-term effects for children. According to a recent review by Holbrook, prenatal nicotine exposure negatively affects a child's health, academic performance, and behavior in a variety of ways that cannot be undone. Miscarriage, ectopic pregnancy, premature rupture of membranes, abruption placentae, placenta previa, intrauterine growth restriction, premature delivery, low birth weight, stillbirth, and perinatal death are all adverse outcomes that have been linked to cigarette smoking during pregnancy. These adverse effects may be moderated by the time and quantity of smoking, with longer and heavier exposure during pregnancy leading to more severe effects. Reducing the risk of low birth weight, premature delivery, and intensive care unit (ICU) admissions are only some of the positive pregnancy and child health outcomes linked with quitting smoking during pregnancy [40]. Smoking during pregnancy has a paradoxical protective effect against preeclampsia, but the other risks exceed this one.

Some pregnant women consider electronic nicotine delivery systems (ENDS) to be a safe alternative to cigarettes. However, there is a shortage of studies examining the safety and effectiveness of ENDS when pregnant. Because of possible adverse effects on the developing brain of the fetus, the World Health Organization advises pregnant women to avoid using ENDS. There have been reports of several pregnant women utilizing ENDS to help them quit smoking. Yet, very little data exist on the effect of ENDS on smoking reduction or cessation, according to a recent systematic review and meta-analysis of ENDS in nonpregnant patients [67, 72].

### *10.3.4 CANNABIS*

Due to its lipophilicity, cannabis easily passes the placental barrier, where it might interfere with the brain development of an unborn child. Many expecting mothers believe that cannabis is safe to use. However, cannabis usage is linked to anencephaly and other negative effects on neurodevelopment; thus, it should be avoided if possible. Smaller than average head circumferences, learning and cognitive difficulties (especially executive function impairments), depression, hostility, and behavioral disorders are all negative consequences for children. Cannabinoids in cannabis have been linked to several adverse pregnancy outcomes such as low birth weight, small-for-gestational age, preterm delivery, stillbirth, and admission to NICUs.

Medical marijuana is increasingly being used to treat anything from chronic pain to nausea and vomiting during pregnancy. However, the feasibility of using medicinal cannabis during pregnancy has not been confirmed. Women who are pregnant or who want to become pregnant are urged to stop using medicinal cannabis and switch to agents with superior pregnancy-specific safety evidence by the ACOG [31, 52].

### *10.3.5 OPIOIDS*

Opioids are a type of medications used for pain relief; however, they come with major side effects including dependency. Opioids are available legally and illegally. When dealing with moderate to severe pain, physicians may recommend opioid prescription drugs. Narcotic opioids include heroin. Fentanyl is an opioid pain medication available by prescription. The distribution of fentanyl, however, is on the increase due to its unlawful production. Opioid use disorder refers to a pattern of opioid abuse that causes significant distress and often leads to the inability to carry out essential duties at home, at school, or in the workplace. Medication-assisted treatment for opioid use disorder often combines counseling and behavioral therapy with the use of opioid medicines, including buprenorphine, methadone, and naltrexone [18, 41].

Pregnant women with opioid use disorder are a major public health issue in the United States. A recent CDC study found that the percentage of pregnant women who had an opioid use disorder during labor and delivery more than doubled between 1999 and 2014. Preterm delivery, stillbirth, maternal death, and NAS are only some of the unfavorable health consequences associated with opioid use disorder during pregnancy. Babies born to mothers who used opioids during pregnancy may display a cluster of withdrawal symptoms known as NAS. The CDC advises that pregnant women who use opioid pain drugs consult with their practitioner before beginning or discontinuing treatment (Figure 10.2) [42].

### *10.3.6 COCAINE*

Cocaine use during pregnancy has been linked to severe maternal morbidity, such as hypertensive crisis, myocardial infarction, cerebrovascular accidents, pulmonary edema, aortic dissection, and renal failure, due to the

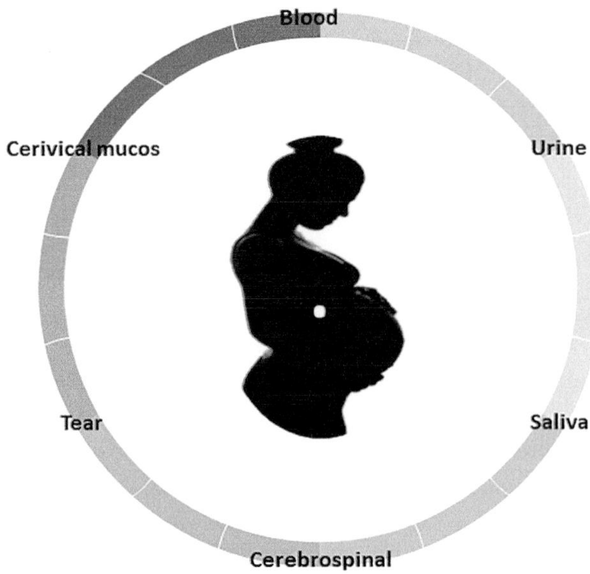


**FIGURE 10.2** Some body floods that may transmit infection from mother to fetus and probably the mother affected by any substance abuse may be transmitted to fetus.

surge of catecholamines that occurs because of cocaine usage. Heart, brain, bladder, intestine, and limb deformities have all been shown in animal and human investigations as having teratogenic potential. Growth restriction, neurodevelopmental and behavioral issues, and cognitive deficiencies in language and executive function are also long-term unfavorable implications for children's health. Cocaine use during pregnancy has been linked to several adverse outcomes, including premature delivery, low birth weight, small-for-gestational age, and even intrauterine mortality [25].

### *10.3.7 METHAMPHETAMINE*

The direct teratogenicity of methamphetamine use has not been established. However, babies that are exposed have a higher risk of having their development stunted, having trouble gaining weight, and requiring ICU hospitalization. Infant and neonatal mortality rates are also higher. The long-term effects of methamphetamine use on children are little understood. Possible cognitive, behavioral, and emotional consequences on children, low birth weight, shorter gestational age, premature delivery, preeclampsia, gestational hypertension, placental abruption, and intra-uterine mortality are among adverse pregnancy outcomes linked to meth-amphetamine use [17].

## 10.4 USE OF PLANTS FOR THE TREATMENT OF DRUG ADDICTION

### *10.4.1 IBOGA (TABERNANTHE IBOGA) AND IBOGAINE*

The use of iboga or ibogaine has been shown to lessen the severity of opioid withdrawal symptoms in animal experiments. It is believed that the effect is due to its metabolite noribogaine [48], and other studies have shown reduced self-administration of morphine, cocaine, alcohol, amphetamine, methamphetamine, and nicotine following iboga/ibogaine treatment. Many people quit taking drugs or have extended periods of abstinence, but there are also examples of relapse [6]. Many publications are case studies that describe the lack of or an improvement of the withdrawal symptoms and desire following the drug abstinence (detoxification phase). Single-dose ibogaine patients maintained abstinence for an average of 5.5 months, whereas those who got repeated doses maintained abstinence for an average of eight months [62].

### *10.4.2 KUDZU (PUERARIA LOBATA)*

Alcohol intake was reduced by more than half when daidzin was administered at a dosage of 150 mg/kg (i.p.). The most common plant *isoflavone, puerarin* also have a significant role in cutting down on drinking [57]. Benlhabib et al. [4] conducted a large-scale research testing three different kudzu concentrations (0.5, 0.75, and 1 g/kg) found in a commercial product. In order to simulate the effects of alcohol tolerance and dependency, rats in this investigation were given alcohol for 30 days prior to receiving kudzu therapy. After day 70, ethanol was taken away for 10 days to cause a withdrawal episode, and then given again between days 80 and 90. While the animals were on kudzu, they consumed less ethanol overall, with the best results coming at a dose of 0.5 g/kg, which reduced alcohol consumption by 50–60% and prevented withdrawal symptoms without significantly impacting body weight.

Although initial research showed that kudzu therapy did not assist sober individuals lessen their alcohol cravings or remain sober, more recent studies have shown that the extract is effective in lowering alcohol intake by a modest amount. After using the extract for a week, both men and women consumed less alcohol. Heavy drinkers' beer intake dropped after being given puerarin (1200 mg) for a week in a controlled study, and they began drinking more slowly and with fewer sips [53].

### 10.4.3 HYPERICUM (HYPERICUM PERFORATUM)

To combat alcoholism and opiate addiction, doctors prescribe naltrexone, an opioid receptor antagonist. Both hypericum and naltrexone were tested at two dosages each, with the former proving effective at a lower level of 125 mg/kg but ineffective at 7 mg/kg and the latter showing similar results at a higher dose of 3 mg/kg but ineffective at 0.5 mg/kg in lowering ethanol consumption. There was no resistance to the antialcohol effect when hypericum 7 mg/kg was combined with naltrexone 0.5 mg/kg, and ethanol consumption was reduced throughout the course of the 12-day assessment period [54]. When the medication was stopped, the animals went back to drinking alcohol, indicating that the effect was not the result of a conditioned avoidance of the substance. These findings suggest that St. John's wort may be useful, particularly as an adjuvant therapy operating synergistically with other drugs and in the treatment of alcoholism in individuals suffering from depression.

One research found that the strength of withdrawal syndrome signals was reduced when hypericum was orally administered in conjunction with morphine injections [23]. Subhan et al. [68] found that hypericum extracts alleviated symptoms of heroin withdrawal, including diarrhea and writhes (abdominal spasms indicating unpleasant feeling).

### 10.4.4 AYAHUASCA (BANISTERIOPSIS CAAPI AND PSYCHOTRIA VIRIDIS)

Most of the clinical research done on ayahuasca is observational and retrospective, and it involves interviewing and assessing adherents to ayahuasca religions. After beginning regular ayahuasca usage, these former drug users were able to permanently abstain from substance abuse. A group of four drug addicts who began attending ayahuasca ceremonies and eventually kicked their habit were studied by Labigalini Jr. [44]. According to different research [20], adolescents who practice ayahuasca religion are less likely to abuse alcohol and other drugs than their nonpracticing peers of the same age.

Communities in Brazil and Peru that utilize ayahuasca to treat addiction were the focus of a research. According to the author, ayahuasca treatment is distinct from replacement therapies like methadone therapy for heroin users since it considers broader societal factors. As a result, this therapy facilitates a psychological and societal shift that lessens the likelihood of recurrence. Qualitative research, including medical practitioners and indigenous healers, investigated ayahuasca's therapeutic potential in the treatment of drug addiction and found promising results [46, 71].

### 10.4.5 DANSHEN OR CHINESE SAGE (*SALVIA MILTIORRHIZA*)

Two models of alcohol self-administration in rats found that self-administration was reduced by an extract containing 4.3% miltirone at dosages of 50–200 mg/kg [47]. Miltirone, either in its pure form or as an extract with varying concentrations, was shown to reduce alcohol consumption in rats in a dose-dependent manner [12]. In addition, both danshen extract and miltirone reduced ethanol absorption and, hence, blood ethanol levels in the mice when delivered intragastrically (but not intraperitoneally).

### 10.4.6 INDIAN GINSENG OR ASHWAGANDHA (*WITHANIA SOMNIFERA*)

Indian ginseng's effectiveness in drug-abuse simulation experiments is limited. It has been observed that the plant mitigates the onset of morphine tolerance and prevents the distinctive leaping behavior of mice seen in the naloxone-induced withdrawal syndrome [43]. The development and manifestation of a conditioned place preference to morphine in mice were blocked by a standardized ashwagandha extract at doses of 50 and 100 mg/kg [59].

*Rhodiolarosea, Piper methysticum, Schizandrachinensis, Rauvolfia serpentine, Thunbergia laurifolia, Carydolis yanhusuo, Oenothera biennis,*

*Scutellaria laterifolia, Hovenia dulcis, Thymus vulgaris, Trigonella foenum-graecum, Paullinia cupana, Turnera diffusa, Passiflora quadrangularis* among others can be helpful in this direction [9, 64, 69].

## 10.5 AYURVEDIC REMEDIES

Ayurveda, with its ancient wisdom and natural medicines, aids in effectively reestablishing the body's balance in drug addicts. Natural herbs have a track record of having no negative side effects. As a result, its inclusion will facilitate efficient recovery. Among the various medicinal plants studied in Ayurvedic medicine, *Silybum marianum* (milk thistle), *Passiflora incarnata* (passionflower), *Panax ginseng* (ginseng), *Capsicum annuum* (cayenne pepper), and *Withania somnifera* (Ashwagandha) have been found particularly beneficial. Ayurvedic medicine has found milk thistle, *Passiflora incarnata* (passionflower), *Panax ginseng* (ginseng), *Capsicum annuum* (cayenne pepper), and Ashwagandha (*W. somnifera*) to be particularly helpful.

## 10.6 ROLE OF NGOS

To assist the impacted people, several nongovernmental organizations (NGOs) have appeared and expanded internationally over the past 10 years. NGOs and associated organizations are currently registered in their thousands worldwide. Most of these NGOs, like Innovations for Poverty Action (a US-based nonprofit expert in intervention research utilizing randomized controlled trials), are dedicated to eradicating poverty and providing social services to rural poor people. Specific target populations are served by Psycho-Mental Health International, MindFreedom, and Friends of Mental Health. Most NGOs are motivated by a passion to help poor groups cultivate or obtain healthy food and water, provide formal and informal education for at-risk children and adults, and give free or reasonably priced health care to at-risk populations [51].

The "Beyond 2008" project was established to conduct a thorough analysis of NGO successes in drug control since the 1998 UNGASS (Special Session of the United Nations General Assembly), as well as to share ideas on promising new strategies, to come to agreements on how to collaborate, and to make suggestions to multilateral organizations and UN member states on future directions for drug control. According to interviews and the survey conducted, NGO activity has significantly increased since 1998, with many new organizations being founded and the number of full-time employees doubling. The UN Conventions, which have mostly concentrated on drug supply and law enforcement, have been met with a variety of measures. Other accomplishments include the growth of knowledge in addictions, the formation of coalitions among NGOs, and a gradual increase in the number of services provided.

**Conclusion:** Since the United Nations General Assembly last met to examine the global drug problem in 1998, NGOs working in the subject of drug reduction have made significant progress, but there is still much work to be done. It is necessary to address issues such as the overemphasis on supply at the expense of demand and the need to address the detrimental social and health effects of criminalization that have been recognized as unintended outcomes of efforts to comply with the Conventions [12]. Additionally, there was a solid consensus among regional groupings that NGOs needed to be more involved in the development of national or UN agency strategies and that there was still potential for consultation and cooperation. There is mounting evidence that NGOs play a crucial role in the development of other countries. There are a sizable number of officially recognized NGOs that support medical treatment, particularly mental health. Due to the documented rising rates of substance abuse and relapse into substance use disorders (SUDs) [13], a coordinated effort is required to address this public health emergency. It is crucial to explore and understand the roles of these organizations in managing recovery among vulnerable groups, including the recovery capital they provide to clients. Health-focused NGOs predominantly work with vulnerable populations, including individuals with SUDs [38].

## 10.7 MEDICAL CARE AND SUPPORT

Prenatal care refers to a woman's medical treatment throughout her pregnancy. During pregnancy, the patient will have many checkups with their doctor. The provider checks on the mother and the developing child regularly. They encourage the parent and aid in the labor and delivery process. When pregnant, some drug abusers put off or forego prenatal care. Those who choose to get prenatal care have additional healthcare resources available to them. They also report a higher rate of favorable delivery outcomes.

## 10.8 BEHAVIOR MODIFICATION

Substance abuse treatment mostly relies on counseling sessions with a therapist. A woman's physical and emotional health both require attention throughout pregnancy. The goals of this kind of counseling are met. Training in self-care is a common topic of therapy. The dynamics of addiction are the subject of investigation by others. Some addictions may be treated with medication, but even these are more effective when combined with psychosocial support. Treatment at the inpatient and residential levels is strenuous. They might go on for a few months and cover a wide range of topics. The same may be said for outpatient treatment centers. They are more flexible in terms of time and money spent. Different plants have been tested that are quite useful for drug deaddictions at various levels. The science of Ayurveda is growing and is still at its infancy stage in this regard. Different NGOs are playing a vital role and has been successful at different stages across the globe.

## 10.9 SUMMARY

More than half of pregnant women use drugs, either legally or illegally, at some point throughout their pregnancies. This includes both prescribed and over-the-counter (OTC) medications, as well as social drugs like cigarettes and alcohol. Many medicines pose risks to the developing baby and should be avoided during pregnancy unless essential. Only 2–3% of birth abnormalities are linked to medications used to treat a condition or symptom. Pregnant women and their unborn children may need to take certain medications in extreme cases. It is recommended that a woman discuss the potential side effects and advantages of the medicine with her doctor in such a situation. A pregnant woman should check with her doctor before taking any medication, including OTC medications and dietary supplements like medicinal herbs. A doctor may advise a pregnant lady to take certain vitamins and minerals.

The placenta is the primary pathway for drug delivery to the fetus, just as oxygen and nutrients are for the baby's growth and development. Fetal injury may occur even if a substance does not reach the placenta if it has an effect on the uterine or the placenta. Women of childbearing age have a higher rate of substance abuse than males. During pregnancy and the postpartum period, women and their families might be negatively impacted by substance use disorders; thus, it is important to see these problems as chronic and relapsing. Substance abuse screenings should be performed on all pregnant and potentially pregnant women. Comorbidities in women's mental health and physical health should also be tested for. Women who use substances throughout pregnancy have a crucial window of opportunity for intervention. The existence of problems, such as intra-uterine growth restriction, should guide the technique and frequency of prenatal surveillance. It is important to start early with individualized, safe, and socially acceptable therapy for drug abuse. First, shorter-term solutions should be tried, and only if they do not work can more extensive, specialized therapies be introduced. Services for mental health and addiction should be provided together wherever possible. Long-term treatment with proactive outreach and relapse prevention measures is necessary because of the high recurrence rates. Pregnant women who use substances need further study of pharmaceutical interventions.

Substance abuse during pregnancy is dangerous for both the mother and the developing child. The combined effects of numerous drugs may be devastating. Substances used during pregnancy may reach the developing embryo via the placenta. During pregnancy, the uterus grows an organ called the placenta. The uterus is a hollow pelvic organ that serves as the baby's carrying space. The placenta acts as a gateway for oxygen and nutrients to reach the fetus from the mother's bloodstream. That unborn child will be exposed to anything you are exposed to throughout pregnancy. Medicine is one example of a drug that may be useful in this context. However, poisonous compounds may also pass through. If a mother smokes cigarettes while pregnant, for instance, nicotine might potentially enter the fetus via the placenta. Alcohol and other substances, including methamphetamine, opiates, and cannabis (marijuana), may have the same effect.

People struggling with opioid addiction might find relief from some drugs. Opioid use disorder medicine is also known as medications for opioid use disorder (MOUD) study therapy. It has the same effect on the body as opioids. MOUD aids in desire management without inducing euphoria or other altered states of consciousness. By removing the ebb and flow of addiction, MOUD aids expecting mothers. This suggests they have stopped actively seeking out and use opioids. The parent thus has more mental bandwidth for things such as prenatal care, proper diet, and substance abuse treatment. Pregnant mothers and their children benefit from MOUD as well. In what ways do pregnant women who struggle with drug abuse require special care? Women under addiction also suffer from depression and anxiety that are outside the scope of this chapter.

## KEYWORDS


- **drugs**
- **fetus**
- **impact**
- **medical interventions**
- **mother**


## REFERENCES


1. Addis, A., Moretti, M. E., Ahmed Syed, F. A., Einarson, T. R., & Koren, G. (2001). Fetal effects of cocaine: An updated meta-analysis. *Reproductive Toxicology*, *15*(4), 341–369.
2. Alvik, A., Heyerdahl, S., Haldorsen, T., & Lindemann, R. (2006). Alcohol use before and during pregnancy: A population-based study. *Acta Obstetriciaet Gynecologica Scandinavica*, *85*(11), 1292–1298.
3. Bakoyiannis, I., Gkioka, E., Pergialiotis, V., Mastroleon, I., Prodromidou, A., Vlachos, G. D., & Perrea, D. (2014). Fetal alcohol spectrum disorders and cognitive functions of young children. *Reviews in the Neurosciences*, *25*(5), 631–639.
4. Benlhabib, E., Baker, J. I., Keyler, D. E., & Singh, A. K. (2004). Kudzu root extract suppresses voluntary alcohol intake and alcohol withdrawal symptoms in P rats receiving free access to water and alcohol. *Journal of Medicinal Food*, *7*(2), 168–179.
5. Benningfield, M. M., Arria, A. M., Kaltenbach, K., Heil, S. H., Stine, S. M., Coyle, M. G., Fischer, G., Jones, H. E., & Martin, P. R. (2010). Co-occurring psychiatric symptoms are associated with increased psychological, social, and medical impairment in opioid dependent pregnant women. *American Journal on Addictions*, *19*(5), 416–421.
6. Brown, T. K. (2013). Ibogaine in the treatment of substance dependence. *Current Drug Abuse Reviews*, *6*(1), 3–16.
7. Caleyachetty, R., Tait, C. A., Kengne, A. P., Corvalan, C., Uauy, R., & Echouffo-Tcheugui, J. B. (2014). Tobacco use in pregnant women: Analysis of data from demographic and health surveys from 54 low-income and middle-income countries. *Lancet Global Health*, *2*(9), e513–e520.

8. Carai, M. A., Agabio, R., Bombardelli, E., Bourov, I., Gessa, G. L., Lobina, C., Morazzoni, P., Pani, M., Reali, R., Vacca, G., & Colombo, G. (2000). Potential use of medicinal plants in the treatment of alcoholism. *Fitoterapia*, *71*(Suppl. 1), S38–S42.
9. Carlini, E. A. (2003). The brain and the nervous system of plants. *Pharmacology, Biochemistry and Behavior*, *75*(3), 501–512.
10. Chaplin, T. M., Freiburger, M. B., Mayes, L. C., & Sinha, R. (2010). Prenatal cocaine exposure, gender, and adolescent stress response: A prospective longitudinal study. *Neurotoxicology and Teratology*, *32*(6), 595–604.
11. Cnattingius, S. (2004). The epidemiology of smoking during pregnancy: Smoking prevalence, maternal characteristics, and pregnancy outcomes. *Nicotine and Tobacco Research*, *6*(Suppl. 2), S125–S140.
12. CND. (2008). Beyond 2008—The contribution of non-governmental organizations to implementation of the political declaration and action plans adopted by the 20th United Nations General Assembly special session. In: *51st Session of the Commission on Narcotic Drugs*, March 10–14. Commission on Narcotic Drugs (CND).
13. Colombo, G., Serra, S., Vacca, G., Orrù, A., Maccioni, P., Morazzoni, P., Bombardelli, E., Riva, A., Gessa, G. L., & Carai, M. A. (2006). Identification of miltirone as active ingredient of *Salvia miltiorrhiza* responsible for the reducing effect of root extracts on alcohol intake in rats. *Alcoholism, Clinical and Experimental Research*, *30*(5), 754–762.
14. Conradt, E., Flannery, T., Aschner, J. L., Annett, R. D., Croen, L. A., Duarte, C. S., Friedman, A. M., Guille, C., Hedderson, M. M., Hofheimer, J. A., Jones, M. R., Ladd-Acosta, C., McGrath, M., Moreland, A., Neiderhiser, J. M., Nguyen, R. H. N., Posner, J., Ross, J. L., Savitz, D. A., & Lester, B. M. (2019). Prenatal opioid exposure: Neurodevelopmental consequences and future research priorities. *Pediatrics*, *144*(3), e20190128.
15. Creeley, C. E., & Denton, L. K. (2019). Use of prescribed psychotropics during pregnancy: A systematic review of pregnancy, neonatal, and childhood outcomes. *Brain Sciences*, *9*(9), 235–240.
16. Degenhardt, L., Whiteford, H. A., Ferrari, A. J., Baxter, A. J., Charlson, F. J., Hall, W. D., Freedman, G., Burstein, R., Johns, N., Engell, R. E., Flaxman, A., Murray, C. J., & Vos, T. (2013). Global burden of disease attributable to illicit drug use and dependence: Findings from the Global Burden of Disease Study 2010. *Lancet*, *382*(9904), 1564–1574.
17. Della Grotta, S., LaGasse, L. L., Arria, A. M., Derauf, C., Grant, P., Smith, L. M., Shah, R., Huestis, M., Liu, J., & Lester, B. M. (2010). Patterns of methamphetamine use during pregnancy: Results from the Infant Development, Environment, and Lifestyle (IDEAL) Study. *Maternal and Child Health Journal*, *14*(4), 519–527.
18. Desai, R. J., Hernandez-Diaz, S., Bateman, B. T., & Huybrechts, K. F. (2014). Increase in prescription opioid use during pregnancy among Medicaid-enrolled women. *Obstetrics and Gynecology*, *123*(5), 997–1002.
19. Dinger, J., Hinner, P., Reichert, J., & Rüdiger, M. (2017). Methamphetamine consumption during pregnancy—Effects on child health. *Pharmacopsychiatry*, *50*(3), 107–113.
20. Doering-Silveira, E., Grob, C. S., De Rios, M. D., Lopez, E., Alonso, L. K., Tacla, C., & Da Silveira, D. X. (2005). Report on psychoactive drug use among adolescents

using ayahuasca within a religious context. *Journal of Psychoactive Drugs*, *37*(2), 141–144.
21. Dotson, J. A. W., Pineda, R., Cylkowski, H., & Amiri, S. (2017). Development and evaluation of an iPad application to promote knowledge of tobacco use and cessation by pregnant women. *Nursing for Women's Health*, *21*(3), 174–185.
22. Ehrmin, J. T. (2001). Unresolved feelings of guilt and shame in the maternal role with substance-dependent African American women. *Journal of Nursing Scholarship*, *33*(1), 47–52.
23. Feily, A., & Abbasi, N. (2009). The inhibitory effect of *Hypericum perforatum* extract on morphine withdrawal syndrome in rat and comparison with clonidine. *Phytotherapy Research*, *23*(11), 1549–1552.
24. Forray, A., Merry, B., Lin, H., Ruger, J. P., & Yonkers, K. A. (2015). Perinatal substance use: A prospective evaluation of abstinence and relapse. *Drug and Alcohol Dependence*, *150*, 147–155.
25. Frank, D. A., Zuckerman, B. S., Amaro, H., Aboagye, K., Bauchner, H., Cabral, H., Fried, L., Hingson, R., Kayne, H., & Levenson, S. M. (1988). Cocaine use during pregnancy: Prevalence and correlates. *Pediatrics*, *82*(6), 888–895.
26. Frusinoiu, P. Ș., & Bănacu, C. S. (2022). The consequences of illicit drug use: Estimation, methods and challenges. *Technium Social Sciences Journal*, *34*, 472–482.
27. Fuglestad, A. J., Whitley, M. L., Carlson, S. M., Boys, C. J., Eckerle, J. K., Fink, B. A., & Wozniak, J. R. (2015). Executive functioning deficits in preschool children with fetal alcohol spectrum disorders. *Child Neuropsychology*, *21*(6), 716–731.
28. Gopman, S. (2014). Prenatal and postpartum care of women with substance use disorders. *Obstetrics and Gynecology Clinics of North America*, *41*(2), 213–228.
29. Green, C. R., Roane, J., Hewitt, A., Muhajarine, N., Mushquash, C., Sourander, A., Lingley-Pottie, P., McGrath, P., & Reynolds, J. N. (2014). Frequent behavioral challenges in children with fetal alcohol spectrum disorder: A needs-based assessment reported by caregivers and clinicians. *Journal of Population Therapeutics and Clinical Pharmacology*, *21*(3), e405–e420.
30. Gyarmathy, V. A., Giraudon, I., Hedrich, D., Montanari, L., Guarita, B., & Wiessing, L. (2009). Drug use and pregnancy—Challenges for public health. *Euro Surveillance*, *14*(9), 33–36.
31. Hayatbakhsh, M. R., Flenady, V. J., Gibbons, K. S., Kingsbury, A. M., Hurrion, E., Mamun, A. A., & Najman, J. M. (2012). Birth outcomes associated with cannabis use before and during pregnancy. *Pediatric Research*, *71*(2), 215–219.
32. Hoch, E., Noack, R., Henker, J., Pixa, A., Höfler, M., Behrendt, S., Bühringer, G., & Wittchen, H. U. (2012). Efficacy of a targeted cognitive–behavioral treatment program for cannabis uses disorders (CANDIS). *European Neuropsychopharmacology*, *22*(4), 267–280.
33. Horne, A. W., Brown, J. K., Nio-Kobayashi, J., Abidin, H. B., Adin, Z. E., Boswell, L., Duncan, W. C., Lee, K. F., Duncan, W. C., & Duncan, W. C. (2014). The association between smoking and ectopic pregnancy: Why nicotine is bad for your fallopian tube. *PLoS One*, *9*(2), e89400.
34. Howell, E. M., Heiser, N., & Harrington, M. (1999). A review of recent findings on substance abuse treatment for pregnant women. *Journal of Substance Abuse Treatment*, *16*(3), 195–219.

35. Hull, L., May, J., Farrell-Moore, D., & Svikis, D. S. (2010). Treatment of cocaine abuse during pregnancy: Translating research to clinical practice. *Current Psychiatry Reports*, *12*(5), 454–461.
36. Hutchins, E., & DiPietro, J. (1997). Psychosocial risk factors associated with cocaine use during pregnancy: A case-control study. *Obstetrics and Gynecology*, *90*(1), 142–147.
37. Huybrechts, K. F., Bröms, G., Christensen, L. B., Einarsdóttir, K., Engeland, A., Furu, K., Gissler, M., Hernandez-Diaz, S., Karlsson, P., Karlstad, Ø., Kieler, H., Lahesmaa-Korpinen, A. M., Mogun, H., Nørgaard, M., Reutfors, J., Sørensen, H. T., Zoega, H., & Bateman, B. T. (2018). Association between methylphenidate and amphetamine use in pregnancy and risk of congenital malformations: A cohort study from the international pregnancy safety study consortium. *JAMA Psychiatry*, *75*(2), 167–175.
38. ICASO/HDN. (2006). *Meaningful Involvement of Civil Society in the UNGASS Review Meeting*, New York.
39. Jones, H. E., Heil, S. H., Tuten, M., Chisolm, M. S., Foster, J. M., O'Grady, K. E., & Kaltenbach, K. (2013). Cigarette smoking in opioid-dependent pregnant women: Neonatal and maternal outcomes. *Drug and Alcohol Dependence*, *131*(3), 271–277.
40. Jones, H. E., Kaltenbach, K., Heil, S. H., Stine, S. M., Coyle, M. G., Arria, A. M., O'Grady, K. E., Selby, P., Martin, P. R., & Fischer, G. (2010). Neonatal abstinence syndrome after methadone or buprenorphine exposure. *New England Journal of Medicine*, *363*(24), 2320–2331.
41. Kaltenbach, K., Berghella, V., & Finnegan, L. (1998). Opioid dependence during pregnancy: Effects and management. *Obstetrics and Gynecology Clinics of North America*, *25*(1), 139–151
42. Kulkarni, S. K., & Ninan, I. (1997). Inhibition of morphine tolerance and dependence by *Withania somnifera* in mice. *Journal of Ethnopharmacology*, *57*(3), 213–217.
43. Labigalini, Jr., E. (1998). *O uso de ayahuascaem um contextoreligiosopor ex dependentes de álcool—Um estudo qualitative.* M.Sc. thesis, Universidad Federal de São Paulo.
44. Lester, B. M., Boukydis, C. F., & Twomey, J. E. (2000). Maternal substance abuse and child outcome, 2nd ed., In: *Handbook of Infant Mental Health* (pp. 161–175). The Guilford Press.
45. Loizaga-Velder, A., & Verres, R. (2014). Therapeutic effect of ritual ayahuasca use in the treatment of substance dependence—Qualitative results. *Journal of Psychoactive Drugs*, *46*(1), 63–72.
46. Maccioni, P., Vargiolu, D., Falchi, M., Morazzoni, P., Riva, A., Cabri, W., Carai, M. A., Gessa, G. L., & Colombo, G. (2014). Reducing effect of the Chinese medicinal herb, *Salvia miltiorrhiza*, on alcohol self-administration in Sardinian alcohol-preferring rats. *Alcohol*, *48*(6), 587–593.
47. Mačiulaitis, R., Kontrimaviciute, V., Bressolle, F. M., & Briedis, V. (2008). Ibogaine, an anti-addictive drug: Pharmacology and time to go further in development. A narrative review. *Human and Experimental Toxicology*, *27*(3), 181–194.
48. Mansoor, E., Morrow, C. E., Accornero, V. H., Xue, L., Johnson, A. L., Anthony, J. C., & Bandstra, E. S. (2012). Longitudinal effects of prenatal cocaine use on

mother–child interactions at ages 3 and 5 years. *Journal of Developmental and Behavioral Pediatrics*, *33*(1), 32–41.

49. O'Leary, C., Jacoby, P., D'Antoine, H., Bartu, A., & Bower, C. (2012). Heavy prenatal alcohol exposure and increased risk of stillbirth. *BJOG*, *119*(8), 945–952.
50. Omofonmwan, S. I., & Odia, L. O. (2009). The role of non-governmental organizations in community development: Focus on Edo State—Nigeria. *Anthropologist*, *11*(4), 247–254.
51. Passey, M. E., Sanson-Fisher, R. W., D'Este, C. A., & Stirling, J. M. (2014). Tobacco, alcohol and cannabis use during pregnancy: Clustering of risks. *Drug and Alcohol Dependence*, *134*, 44–50.
52. Penetar, D. M., Toto, L. H., Farmer, S. L., Lee, D. Y.-W., Ma, Z., Liu, Y., & Lukas, S. E. (2012). The isoflavone puerarin reduces alcohol intake in heavy drinkers: A pilot study. *Drug and Alcohol Dependence*, *126*(1–2), 251–256.
53. Perfumi, M., Mattioli, L., Cucculelli, M., & Massi, M. (2005). Reduction of ethanol intake by chronic treatment with *Hypericumperforatum*, alone or combined with naltrexone in rats. *Journal of Psychopharmacology*, *19*(5), 448–454.
54. Pineles, B. L., Park, E., & Samet, J. M. (2014). Systematic review and meta-analysis of miscarriage and maternal exposure to tobacco smoke during pregnancy. *American Journal of Epidemiology*, *179*(7), 807–823.
55. Popova, S., Lange, S., Probst, C., Gmel, G., & Rehm, J. (2017). Estimation of national, regional, and global prevalence of alcohol use during pregnancy and fetal alcohol syndrome: A systematic review and meta-analysis. *Lancet. Global Health*, *5*(3), e290–e299.
56. Rezvani, A. H., Overstreet, D. H., Perfumi, M., & Massi, M. (2003). Plant derivatives in the treatment of alcohol dependency. *Pharmacology, Biochemistry, and Behavior*, *75*(3), 593–606.
57. Rua, E. D. A. O., Porto, M. L., Ramos, J. P. L., Nogueira, B. V., dos Santos Meyrelles, S., Vasquez, E. C., & Pereira, T. D. M. C. (2014). Effects of tobacco smoking during pregnancy on oxidative stress in the umbilical cord and mononuclear blood cells of neonates. *Journal of Biomedical Science*, *21*, 1–9.
58. Ruiu, S., Longoni, R., Spina, L., Orrù, A., Cottiglia, F., Collu, M., Kasture, S., & Acquas, E. (2013). *Withania somnifera* prevents acquisition and expression of morphine-elicited conditioned place preference. *Behavioral Pharmacology*, *24*(2), 133–143.
59. Sarfi, M., Sundet, J. M., & Waal, H. (2013). Maternal stress and behavioral adaptation in methadone- or buprenorphine-exposed toddlers. *Infant Behavior and Development*, *36*(4), 707–716.
60. Schempf, A. H., & Strobino, D. M. (2009). Drug use and limited prenatal care: An examination of responsible barriers. *American Journal of Obstetrics and Gynecology*, *200*(4), 412.e1–412.e10.
61. Schenberg, E. E., de Castro Comis, M. A., Chaves, B. R., & da Silveira, D. X. (2014). Treating drug dependence with the aid of ibogaine: A retrospective study. *Journal of Psychopharmacology*, *28*(11), 993–1000.
62. Shankaran, S., Lester, B. M., Das, A., Bauer, C. R., Bada, H. S., Lagasse, L., & Higgins, R. (2007, April). Impact of maternal substance use during pregnancy on

childhood outcome. In: *Seminars in Fetal and Neonatal Medicine* (Vol. 12, No. 2, pp. 143–150). W. B. Saunders.
63. Shebek, J., & Rindone, J. P. (2000). A pilot study exploring the effect of kudzu root on the drinking habits of patients with chronic alcoholism. *Journal of Alternative and Complementary Medicine*, *6*(1), 45–48.
64. Stone, R. (2015). Pregnant women and substance use: Fear, stigma, and barriers to care. *Health and Justice*, *3*(1), 1–15.
65. Strathearn, L., & Mayes, L. C. (2010). Cocaine addiction in mothers: Potential effects on maternal care and infant development. *Annals of the New York Academy of Sciences*, *1187*, 172–183.
66. Streissguth, A. P., Barr, H. M., Martin, D. C., & Herman, C. S. (1980). Effects of maternal alcohol, nicotine, and caffeine use during pregnancy on infant mental and motor development at eight months. *Alcoholism, Clinical and Experimental Research*, *4*(2), 152–164.
67. Subhan, F., Khan, N., & Sewell, R. D. (2009). Adulterant profile of illicit street heroin and reduction of its precipitated physical dependence withdrawal syndrome by extracts of St John's wort (*Hypericum perforatum*). *Phytotherapy Research*, *23*(4), 564–571.
68. Tomczyk, M., Zovko-Koncić, M., & Chrostek, L. (2012). Phytotherapy of alcoholism. *Natural Product Communications*, *7*(2), 273–280.
69. Volkow, N. D., Compton, W. M., & Wargo, E. M. (2017). The risks of marijuana use during pregnancy. *JAMA*, *317*(2), 129–130.
70. Whiteman, V. E., Salemi, J. L., Mogos, M. F., Cain, M. A., Aliyu, M. H., & Salihu, H. M. (2014). Maternal opioid drug use during pregnancy and its impact on perinatal morbidity, mortality, and the costs of medical care in the United States. *Journal of Pregnancy*, *2014*, 906723.
71. Wickström, R. (2007). Effects of nicotine during pregnancy: Human and experimental evidence. *Current Neuropharmacology*, *5*(3), 213–222.
72. Williams, P. P. (2014). *Maternal Alcohol and other Drug (AOD) use Among Pregnant Women Attending Midwife Obstetric Units (MOUs) in the Cape Metrople, South Africa*. PhD thesis, University of Cape Town.
73. Wouldes, T. A., & Woodward, L. J. (2010). Maternal methadone dose during pregnancy and infant clinical outcome. *Neurotoxicology and Teratology*, *32*(3), 406–413.
74. Wu, M., Lagasse, L. L., Wouldes, T. A., Arria, A. M., Wilcox, T., Derauf, C., Newman, E., Shah, R., Smith, L. M., Neal, C. R., Huestis, M. A., Dellagrotta, S., & Lester, B. M. (2013). Predictors of inadequate prenatal care in methamphetamine-using mothers in New Zealand and United States. *Maternal and Child Health Journal*, *17*(3), 566–575.

# CHAPTER 11

# Impact of Human Immunodeficiency Virus Infection on Fetal Development and Pregnancy Outcomes

KHURSHEED AHMAD WANI, JAVID MANZOOR, UROOJ NISSAR, and JUNAID AHMAD MALIK*

*Corresponding author

## ABSTRACT

Human immunodeficiency virus infection is among one of the deadliest diseases that is taking toll of many people around the world. There is increasing evidence that the infection is not only restricted to the individual that is infected but gets transmitted to the people by different ways. Similarly, the mother to baby and fetus infection is causing toll to the infants. Different types of natural products have been tested to control this infection as well that have provided a new pathway in restricting this infection from mother to baby. There is a dire need to intervene and search for the possible mechanisms that may restrict the infection.

## 11.1 INTRODUCTION

By the end of 2015, it was projected that 37.1 million individuals throughout the globe were afflicted with human immunodeficiency virus (HIV) [25]. Two-thirds of all new HIV infections occur in sub-Saharan

Holistic Approaches for Women's Sustainable Health, Volume 1: Foundations, Innovations, Challenges, and Management. Megh R. Goyal, Anamika Chauhan, and Junaid Ahmad Malik (Eds)


DOI: 10.1201/9781779641632-14

Africa (SSA), making this area the epicenter of the worldwide epidemic. Pregnant women are particularly vulnerable to this illness, which is a leading cause of maternal morbidity and death. Around 50 women are reportedly infected with HIV per hour throughout the globe. In addition, there are still high rates of HIV transmission from mothers to their children despite the widespread distribution of inexpensive antiretroviral (ARV) medications via the public health system in recent years [31]. In 2014, the number of newly infected children worldwide was 220,000, with the greatest concentration in SSA [25].

Preterm delivery, low birth weight (LBW), small for gestational age (SGA), and stillbirth have all been linked to maternal HIV infection in women who have not received ARV medication, particularly in SSA. Notably, preterm delivery is the second biggest cause of mortality for children less than 5 years old worldwide [63]. In 2010, it was projected that 32.4 million newborns in low- and middle-income countries were born SGA, accounting for 27% of all live births, compared to the anticipated 10.6 million children delivered at term with LBW [32].

Most research on HIV's consequences during pregnancy has been conducted in wealthy nations, where the disease load and healthcare systems are quite different from those in Africa. Multiple studies in SSA have shown that HIV-positive mothers have a higher risk of maternal anemia, as well as of giving birth to LBW and premature infants. Furthermore, independent of their own HIV infection status, infants born to HIV-positive mothers have a higher risk of death [49, 57, 66].

Because of the prevalence of factors such as malnutrition, anemia, and other frequently concurrent infections (such as HIV and adverse pregnancy outcomes), such as syphilis and malaria, it is especially difficult to establish the impact of HIV infection on maternal and infant health in SSA [65]. Coinfection with malaria and HIV is estimated to affect around one million pregnancies annually in SSA. It is possible that the influence of HIV infection on pregnancy outcomes is more pronounced in women from low-income nations than in those from developed areas due to the existence of the aforementioned variables [9, 43, 47, 58]. After a decade of the distribution of ARV medications, this study aims to add to the body of information on how HIV infection during pregnancy affects the health of the newborn.

Highly active ARV medication has greatly improved the quality of life for those living with HIV, but HIV infection is still a serious public health problem across the world [50]. About 1.1 million pregnant women were living with HIV in 2017. Pregnant women living with HIV are a particular demographic because of the risk of vertical HIV transmission to their infants during the duration of their pregnancy, labor, and lactation if no preventative measures are taken [20]. In addition, HIV infection in children less than 15 years of age most often occurs via mother-to-child transmission (MTCT). Prematurity, LBW, and a poor Apgar score, as well as neurodevelopmental issues, have all been linked to HIV infection in pregnant women. Antiretroviral therapy (ART) to prevent HIV transmission from mother to child has been more widely available in recent decades, with 85% of pregnant persons living with HIV receiving ART in 2019 [50].

Pregnancy outcomes for women living with HIV have improved because of worldwide efforts to avoid MTCT, with rates of stillbirth, premature delivery, and LBW decreasing. Moreover, an estimated 14.8 million infants were exposed to HIV before they were born or while they were nursing but did not get the virus. There is mounting evidence that children born to mothers with HIV have stunted growth and development compared to infants born to mothers without HIV [73]. Challenges with treatment adherences or concurrent adversities (such as malnutrition, food insecurity, and low socioeconomic status) may exacerbate poor health outcomes in children, who are HIV-exposed uninfected, but the mechanisms driving these outcomes are not well understood [19].

LBW (defined as birth weight $<2500$ g) and increased perinatal and early neonatal mortality are two examples of the negative pregnancy outcomes linked to maternal HIV infection. Complications during pregnancy and childbirth among HIV-positive women account for the bulk of the negative effects. In 2015, about 20.5 million babies throughout the world were born with a LBW. LBW has been linked to increased rates of infant morbidity and death, according to research [25]. SSA continues to have high rates of infant death and morbidity despite the region's relatively low HIV incidence among pregnant women [28].

Understanding the processes underlying the link between maternal HIV infection and pregnancy outcomes may be aided by the identification of key and modifiable variables that impact LBW and perinatal death in a community with a high HIV burden. In addition, the prevention of mother-to-child transmission (PMTCT) program has access to the scientific knowledge necessary to make informed decisions about prevention and intervention [59].

Evidence for a link between maternal HIV and negative outcomes during pregnancy, such as LBW, is becoming more and more mixed [33]. LBW, intrauterine growth restriction, premature delivery, and stillbirths have all been linked to ART among HIV-infected women, according to some research. However, several studies have shown that HIV-infected mothers who consistently take ART had fewer complications during pregnancy, including fewer stillbirths, smaller babies, and later deliveries. Statistical approaches may be utilized to evaluate the moderating impact of ART on the link between maternal HIV infection and birth weight and perinatal death, notwithstanding the inconsistency of the findings [37].

Most of what we know about how HIV in mothers affects babies comes from observational research. It is difficult to determine whether maternal HIV infection has an effect on birth weight and perinatal death since there may be other claimed variables than maternal HIV infection linked with these outcomes. Since the distribution of confounding variables may vary between women who are HIV infected and those who are not, the existence of these factors misrepresents the effect of maternal HIV infection on pregnancy outcomes [35].

Factors, such as maternal anemia, genitourinary tract infection during pregnancy, hypertension, birth weight during previous pregnancies, and birth order, have all been linked to worse birth outcomes. Maternal education, maternal age, poverty, air pollution, and smoking are additional environmental and socioeconomic variables that are linked to worse pregnancy outcomes [29]. A randomized controlled trial (RCT) would be excellent for ensuring that HIV-infected and HIV-negative mothers get the same treatment. However, as most HIV studies are observational, the same goal of balancing confounder factors across HIV-infected and HIV-uninfected mothers may be accomplished by using techniques proposed by Rosenbaum and Rubin [53, 69]. Propensity score matching is one such strategy; it attempts to simulate the randomization process of RCTs by creating a more uniform distribution of assessed confounders across exposure groups [7].

This chapter summarizes current understanding of the effects of prenatal HIV and ART exposure on baby development and health in the first two years of life and so contribute to a better comprehension of the health requirements of mothers living with HIV and their infants.

## 11.2 IMPACT OF HIV DISEASE PROGRESSION ON PREGNANCY

Both HIV-infected and HIV-negative women experience a suppression of immunological function during pregnancy [15]. Immunoglobulin and complement levels fall in the first trimester of pregnancy, and cell-mediated immunity declines much more dramatically later in pregnancy [4]. Because of these natural alterations, some worry that having a baby might hasten the development of HIV infection. Pregnancy reports among women with HIV at the time appeared to confirm this. To present, prospective follow-up studies have failed to corroborate these results. During a mean of 61 months, researchers in France monitored 114 HIV-negative women who had never conceived and 57 who had [55]. The progression of illness was similar among the groups. Research conducted in Edinburgh on 145 women monitored from 1985 to 1992 found that the progression of HIV disease markers did not change during pregnancy [8].

The disease development of 32 HIV-infected pregnant women with known CD4 cell counts before to conception was compared to that of 416 HIV-infected women who did not get pregnant in separate Swiss research [34]. Women's entrance age and CD4 cell count were matched. The pregnant women were followed for an average of 4.8 years, whereas the controls were followed for an average of 3.6 years [34]. Death rates and rates of progression to AIDS-defining events were similar across the two groups; however, HIV-infected pregnant women were more likely to acquire bacterial pneumonia than their never-pregnant controls.

Identical findings have been found in several additional research studies. The American research found that the viral load did not change much throughout pregnancy. In asymptomatic or early-stage HIV-positive women, pregnancy seems to have no influence on disease progression. However, in women with advanced HIV illness, pregnancy may hasten disease progression [36, 46, 64].

Despite the extra hazards of many pregnancies, other infections, and poor nutrition, pregnant African women do not seem to face a more rapid development of HIV illness. There is no evidence from studies conducted in Africa to suggest that pregnancy and HIV infection have a temporary synergistic impact on the immune system. The CD4+/CD8+ cell ratio did not alter significantly throughout pregnancy in Kenyan research comparing HIV-positive and HIV-negative women. In a study conducted in Malawi, researchers found that the proportion of CD4+ and CD8+ T cells did not change significantly during the third trimester of pregnancy and the postpartum period among HIV-positive women [6].

As the AIDS pandemic has spread, it has become a leading cause of death among pregnant women in various nations in central Africa. This is not likely attributable to a speeding up of HIV-related diseases during pregnancy but rather to an increase in the proportion of pregnancies among women with advanced disease [13].

## 11.3 EFFECT OF HIV INFECTION ON PREGNANCY

In the industrialized world, HIV infection has been documented to have negligible effects on pregnancy outcomes and complications. Adverse outcomes in these women are typically complicated by other factors, including HIV infection, drug use, and insufficient prenatal care [5]. Many studies have shown that African women are more likely to have negative pregnancy outcomes, such as early and late pregnancy problems.

HIV might be a cause of or a marker for a variety of medical and social factors that contribute to prenatal problems. However, contrary findings have been found in other research. These varying rates of complications may reflect the severity of the pandemic and the unique characteristics of HIV-related sickness in various regions [12].

Multiple studies have linked HIV infection to prenatal complications. Infection with both HIV-1 and HIV-2 has been associated to an increase in spontaneous abortions in Africa. Women who tested positive for both HIV and syphilis in Uganda were 1.81 times more likely to have had a prior spontaneous abortion than HIV-negative women [62]. A prospective follow-up study conducted in the United States found that the rate of spontaneous early abortion had increased by a factor of three. Moreover, half of these fetuses who were terminated showed signs of HIV infection, most notably in the thymus gland [22].

HIV-positive women have been shown to have higher incidences of ectopic pregnancy than uninfected women, which may be due to the impact of other sexually transmitted infections (STIs). Women living with HIV have been shown to have an increased risk of contracting genital tract infections, such as *Neisseria gonorrhoeae*, *Chlamydia trachomatis*, *Candida albicans*, and *Trichomonas vaginalis*. African research has shown that HIV-positive women are more likely to get syphilis. Thirty-three percent of HIV-positive pregnant women in South Africa were also infected with syphilis, which is three times the prevalence among HIV-seronegative women. These high syphilis rates may introduce bias into analyses of pregnancy outcomes if the risk is not accounted for [11, 72].

Even in low-income locations, all HIV-positive pregnant women should be tested for syphilis. Seropositive women with HIV are more likely to get bacterial pneumonia, urinary tract infections, and other diseases during pregnancy. Opportunistic infections, including those associated with HIV, may also occur during pregnancy in addition to these illnesses and parasite infestations [11, 35].

Due diligence should be given to the detection of tuberculosis in HIV-positive pregnant women since it is the most prevalent opportunistic illness associated with HIV in the poor countries. Although herpes zoster is not frequent in women of reproductive age who do not have HIV, it is quite common among young HIV-positive women. HIV-positive pregnant women have been documented to develop Kaposi sarcoma [11].

Some studies have shown that the risk of preterm birth in HIV-positive women is as high as double that in uninfected women. In South Africa and Kenya, it has been reported that HIV-positive women had a higher incidence of preterm membrane rupture and abruption placentae [45, 47].

Babies born to HIV-positive mothers in affluent nations often have normal birth weights. HIV positivity was related to a smaller decline in birth weight in Edinburgh than smoking was. Some studies have shown that babies born in poor nations had lower than average birth weight. Researchers in Nairobi found that HIV-positive mothers were three times more likely to have a kid with a LBW. When HIV infection caused noticeable symptoms, this danger increased. Babies born to HIV-positive mothers in Zambia weighed substantially less than those delivered to women with a negative serology. Although the difference in mean birth weight between the two groups was just 120 g in a prospective study conducted in Rwanda, the birth weight of singleton children of asymptomatic mothers was substantially lower. No significant differences in birth weights have been found in other investigations of symptom-free populations [59].

Particularly in long-affected regions, reports of increased stillbirth rates have emerged. Although stillbirth rates have been observed to be more than twice those in HIV-seronegative mothers in several African centers, they seem to be lower in asymptomatic women [62]. Some of the cited studies, however, fail to account for the possibility of syphilis or other conditions that may contribute to stillbirths. HIV infection was shown to be independently associated with both intrauterine and intrapartum mortality [48].

HIV-positive mothers are at increased risk for infectious problems after giving birth. According to one research conducted in Rwanda, cesarean sections (CSs) are linked to an increased risk of death and infectious morbidity. This is especially true for women with low CD4+ levels [51].

## 11.4 MOTHER-TO-CHILD TRANSMISSION OF HIV

Studies in Europe and the United States report transmission rates of 15%–25%, whereas those in Africa and Asia reported between 25% and 40%. Much reduced transmission rates are currently being recorded, because to the widespread use of ARV drugs, in many wealthy nations. After widespread use of ARV medication during pregnancy, the estimated yearly incidence of perinatal infections dropped by 27% in the United States between 1992 and 1995 [71].

In addition to prenatal exposure, HIV-1 may also be transmitted after childbirth and during nursing (Figure 11.1). The design of potential treatments relies on accurate estimates of the anticipated time of transmission. The presence of p24 antigen in fetal serum, the detection of HIV-1 in fetal specimens and placental tissue, viral isolation from 20% to 60% of infected infants at the time of birth, and the bimodal distribution of symptoms in children all point to *in utero* transmission (as early as eight-week gestation) [44].

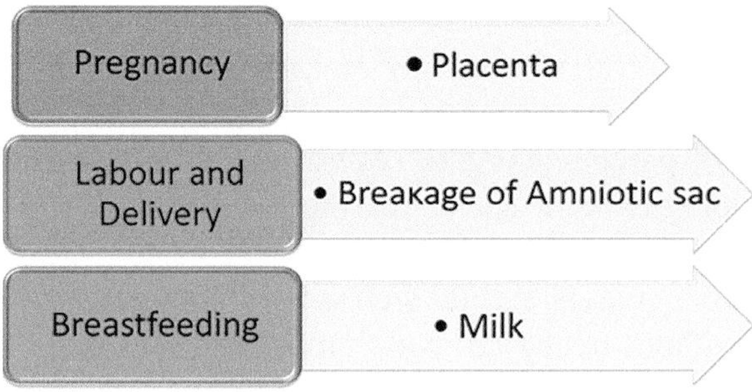


**FIGURE 11.1** Transmission of HIV from mother to baby.

Initial evidence for intrapartum transmission came from a twin registry, which showed that the probability of HIV-1 infection was twice as high for the first-born child compared to the second-born child. It is hypothesized that fetal exposure to the virus via cervicovaginal secretions has a role, yet the same condition is seen in twins delivered after CS. The transmission rate may also depend on the mechanism of distribution, according to recent studies. Some research suggests that the risk of transmission is reduced by elective CSs and increased by protracted membrane rupture. Roughly, half of all affected newborns will test negative for viruses. Breast milk, both the cell-free and cellular fractions, has been shown to contain HIV. The increased prevalence in Africa may be explained by postnatal transmission during nursing [10].

Although it is unclear how much each of these channels contributes to total transmission, yet *in utero* transmission is rare, and that most infections happen around or after birth. This result is supported by data showing that only approximately 50% of infants who are subsequently shown to be infected with HIV-1 have detectable levels of HIV-1 in the first week of life. Based on when HIV is first detected in a newborn, a criterion has been developed for classifying when transmission occurs. *In utero* infection is presumed when virus is detected within 48 hours of delivery; intrapartum infection is presumed when viral investigations are negative during the first week of life but turn positive between days 7 and 90. According to a Markov model of the timing to p24 antigenemia based on data from the French Collaborative Study group, 65% of newborns were infected around the time of childbirth, and 35% were infected while still in the womb. In the Women and Infants Transmission Study in the United States, researchers found that the likelihood of *in utero* transmission was 27%, whereas in Kinshasa, researchers estimated that 23% of newborns were infected *in utero*, 65% intrapartum or early postpartum, and 12% late postpartum [70].

The health of parents is one of several variables that affect children's health. For biological and social reasons, maternal HIV positivity is a particularly powerful factor inequity in child health. Birth to an HIV-positive mother increases a child's chance of contracting the virus from 15% to 45% without treatment, which may lead to a variety of negative health effects, including early death. Children of HIV-positive mothers experience social risks, including malnutrition and parental loss and limited access to health care and education. Both the biological health of the kid (by lowering the rate of HIV transmission from mother to child to below 5%) and the social health of the mother (by increasing maternal health) are enhanced by PMTCT activities [2].

In 2001, Ethiopia launched a program to reduce the likelihood of HIV being passed from mother to child. All pregnant and breastfeeding women, regardless of clinical stage of disease or CD4 count, are recommended to start ART immediately after diagnosis, as per current PMTCT guidelines. As a result, both the mother's risk of HIV transmission to her child and her own risk of HIV-related illness are reduced. ARV prophylaxis, including nevirapine once daily for six weeks, is given to all infants born to HIV-infected mothers (i.e., HIV-exposed infants), and then they are tested using polymerase chain reaction (PCR) at 6 weeks of age or as soon as possible thereafter. If an infant's virological test comes out positive, they will begin ART right away and be followed up on every month for the first 6 months of their lives and then every three months after that. At 18 months, a second test is done to confirm the absence of HIV [74].

In 2009, the Tigray Regional Laboratory began offering HIV testing for infants in the area using PCR. However, the number of new infections in both adults and pregnant women has dropped dramatically. Mother-to-child HIV transmission rates also vary widely across Ethiopia, from 15% in Dire Dawa to 8.2% in Addis Ababa. The current adult HIV prevalence in Ethiopia is considered low, at 1.5% on a national level. Although the overall HIV prevalence rate in Tigray Region is 1.8%, it varies greatly by location (4.2% in urban and 0.6% in rural) and by sex (1.9% in women and 1% in men) [42]. These are due to number of factors, including unequal access to health care as well as poor rates of antenatal care and competent delivery. Though the HIV infection incidence was relatively low in Ethiopia in 2013, an estimated 33,200 pregnant women and over 200,000 children under the age of 15 years were infected. These numbers are consistent with what has been seen in number of other African nations, where HIV is still being transmitted from mother to child despite the availability of PMTCT services. When it comes to health and other areas of development, the post-2015 Sustainable Development Goal (SDG) agenda places an emphasis on equality as a unifying element. The SDG focuses on improving children's health, with goals to reduce infant and under-5 death rates [74]. Ethiopia's current health sector reform plan includes efforts to address the problem of child health disparity. Evaluations of services are necessary to provide an educated decision-making process for healthcare provision based on local circumstances and to assess the impact of policies to minimize child mortality.

An estimated 1.3 million HIV-positive women and girls worldwide get pregnant every year. The risk of HIV transmission from an HIV-positive mother to her child during pregnancy, labor, delivery, or nursing is between 15% and 45% if no preventative measures are taken. As a result, those who test positive for HIV should be offered rapid linkage to lifetime treatment and care, along with the encouragement and resources they need to stay in treatment and maintain viral suppression [75].

ART for the prevention of MTCT was available to 85% of women and girls worldwide in 2019. While high ART coverage is encouraging, it does not account for the ongoing transmission that happens the first treatment. To meet global eradication objectives, preventing new HIV infections among uninfected populations and keeping people in treatment remain top priority. Virtual eradication of MTCT, also known as vertical transmission, has been demonstrated to be achievable since the worldwide change and faster deployment of highly effective, simpler therapies based on lifetime ART for pregnant women living with HIV [44].

Global commitments and the promotion of integrating prevention of MTCT interventions into maternity, newborn, child, and adolescent health care, as well as stronger health systems, provide substantial support for the elimination of MTCT of HIV. Women and girls with HIV are also encouraged to be screened for and get treatment for sexually transmitted diseases, as well as to take use of other sexual and reproductive health services, such as those that aim to prevent unwanted births.

## 11.5 MECHANISM AND TIMING OF TRANSMISSION

Numerous risk factors for HIV transmission have been discovered. MTCT may happen at any time throughout pregnancy, labor, or the postpartum period; however, it is uncommon during the first trimester.

- **Disease of the uterine lining**: Infection of the placenta by HIV may lead to intrauterine infection of the developing fetus. Two peaks of HIV positivity may be observed in the infected neonate, with 38% of HIV-infected newborns testing positive with HIV DNA PCR within 48 h of birth and practically all the remainder at two weeks of age, providing support for this hypothesis [63].
- **Pregnancy-related infection**: Blood and the mother's vaginal secretions may both be vectors for transmission during labor and delivery. That is why, it makes sense that infants whose mothers' membranes ruptured for more than 4 h before delivery were more likely to get infected after birth (25% vs. 14%). The association between infection and the concentration of HIV in cervicovaginal secretions suggests that infection via the maternal genital system may potentially play an essential role [31, 32].
- Transmission occurs postnatally via breast milk. This explains why MTCT is so much more common in underdeveloped nations. At 24 months, the percentage of breast milk transmission in one randomized experiment conducted in Kenya was 16.2% (36.7% in the nursing arm vs. 20.5% in the control arm). When compared to the risk of pediatric HIV infections, the risk of infectious gastro-enteritis owing to less access to clean water and medical services may be greater in underdeveloped nations. Breastfeeding should be avoided by HIV-positive mothers in wealthy nations when safe formula is readily accessible [35].
- **Prenatal testing for HIV**: Strategies for prenatal HIV testing range from mandated testing to optional testing to universal testing with an opt-out option to epidemiological monitoring, which employs techniques, including unlinked, anonymous screening. Unlinked, anonymous screening of newborn cord blood revealed a 0%–0.03% prevalence of HIV antibodies between 1997 and 2000, according to the Department of Health. Researchers in Hong

Kong found 41 pregnancies in which 32 women were exposed to HIV between 1992 and 1999. Only one infant was infected with HIV from one of the 12 pregnancies when the virus was detected before birth. In comparison, 9 out of 14 (64.3%) were infected among those whose diagnosis was obtained after delivery. This highlights the critical significance of an early diagnosis [74].

- **Routine prenatal testing for HIV**: In March 2000, the Scientific Committee on AIDS advocated ways to minimize MTCT of HIV, including universal prenatal HIV testing, to address the issue of missed diagnosis. The acceptance rate for regular HIV testing was quite high (97.5%), and a local prenatal clinic reported an HIV prevalence of 0.05% among pregnant women in the same year [21].

In addition to the standard prenatal blood work, all pregnant women who have their pregnancies scheduled at a public antenatal clinic since September 2001 have been provided a free HIV antibody test. Expectant mothers are provided all the information they need and have the option to decline participation. The Hong Kong College of Obstetricians and Gynecologists issued a similar set of guidelines in November 2001 to spread the practice. After implementing universal prenatal HIV screening in 2003 and again in 2005, two studies were published to assess the program's efficacy. Out of a total of 136,052 pregnant women who visited public prenatal clinics between September 2001 and December 2004, 132,333 (97.26%) were tested for HIV. In the same time frame, HIV was detected in 28 females. Ten mothers-to-be sought termination of their pregnancies, while 14 others took advantage of ARV treatment. There were 15 births in the area, and one of them had an infected baby. The most important factor in preventing MTCT is early diagnosis and treatment.

## 11.6 NEW ISSUES ARISING FROM ANTENATAL HIV SCREENING

Rapid HIV testing is a helpful adjunct method to increase screening coverage when a patient is near term or in labor. It has also been commonplace in several underdeveloped nations when prenatal care and screening are unavailable. There has been a recent drop in the percentage of births in Hong Kong when the mother's HIV status was known. A fast HIV test with reliable sensitivity should be administered to every pregnant woman hospitalized in the third trimester, at the time of birth, and immediately thereafter. Negative test results essentially rule out HIV infection, whereas positive results allow for the provision of prophylaxis while confirmation is sought for a final diagnosis. There is still advantage to the newborn in administering ARV medication at this late gestation, as will be detailed in the section on "Regimens in late presentation" below. The woman may be counseled to have a CS or stop breastfeeding to lessen the likelihood of MTCT. Due to the high volume of unscheduled cases when HIV status is unknown, fast HIV testing may be useful in Hong Kong. Improved infection prevention strategies are also possible. Even if an initial HIV test taken during pregnancy comes out negative, a second test taken near term or during labor may be warranted in locations where HIV is common. Patients at risk of exposure after the first screening may potentially benefit from a repeat screening [16].

## 11.7 CLINICAL MEASURES TO LOWER MTCT PREVALENCE

Depending on variables, including breastfeeding, maternal plasma viral load, clinical condition, and prenatal CD4 T-lymphocyte counts, the probability of MTCT without treatments ranges from 20% to 40%. Transmission is most reliably predicted by the viral load in the mother's plasma. The viral load and associated MTCT risk may be drastically lowered using ARV medications and highly active antiretroviral therapy. The vertical transmission rate is less than 1% when many treatments are used (such as combination ARV therapy, CS, and not nursing). Guidelines for the prevention of perinatal transmission were first created in 2001 by the Scientific Committee on AIDS (later called the Scientific Committee on AIDS and STI) in Hong Kong and amended in 2007 [11, 25, 45, 57].

- **Termination of pregnancy (TOP)**: It is difficult to generally justify TOP based on maternal HIV infection alone, given that roughly 70% of infants delivered without interventions are not affected.
- **ARVs**: The risk of transmission was lowered by 68% with a three-part regimen of zidovudine (ZDV) beginning as early as

14 weeks of pregnancy in the landmark randomized placebo-controlled experiment known as ACTG Protocol 076. Numerous observational studies have corroborated the usefulness of this strategy, which was immediately implemented with notable success in industrialized nations. Therefore, ARV medication should be administered to all HIV-positive pregnant women to avoid MTCT. In the next section, we will discuss taking ARVs while pregnant [3].

- **CS**: In the absence of ARV treatment and with ZDV monotherapy, CS done before to the commencement of labor and/or membrane rupture is linked with reduction in MTCT ranging from 55% to 80%. Recent findings from PACTG 36712 suggested that combination of ART was associated with the lowest rates of transmission in all subgroups of viral load, and that in patients with viral loads of 1000 copies/mL, MTCT rates were significantly lower with multiagent versus single-agent ART (0.6% vs. 2.2%) but did not differ by mode of delivery. Elective CS is beneficial in lowering the risk of MTCT for women with detectable plasma viral load who are not receiving multiagent treatment [43, 49]. Women on multiagent treatment who have a viral load in their plasma that is undetectable at the time of birth may benefit from an elective CS, although the evidence is mixed. The most up-to-date advice for using CS is summarized as follow, when:
    - The mother is unable to take ARV prophylaxis, elective CS may be considered.
    - It is too late in the pregnancy for the woman to get effective prophylaxis.
    - The viral load is undetermined.
    - ARV medications not reducing viral load to an acceptable level.
    - Pregnancy-related indications.
    - Stopping nursing altogether.

Breastfeeding is associated with a slight increase in perinatal transmission risk (5–20%). Hong Kong has safe drinking water and a well-developed healthcare system; therefore, the benefits of formula feeding outweigh the hazards.

## 11.8 PLANT-BASED PRODUCTS AS ANTI-HIV AGENTS

Several plant-based substances, such as coumarins, terpenes, flavonoids, alkaloids, phenolics, lignans, and quinones, are utilized as medicines to prevent or treat HIV infection [61]. Coumarins, a pyrocoumarin derivative that may be isolated from the fruits of *Angelica morii* and *Lomatium suksdorfii* of the Apiaceae family, exhibit inhibitory effects on the replication of the virus in the T-cell line [68]. Similar to maslinic acid, which is produced from the *Geum japonicum*, terpenes have been shown to have a potent inhibitory effect against HIV-1 protease. Additionally, flavonoids such as xanthohumol, a prenylchalcone derived from hops *Humulus lupulus*, have shown to suppress HIV-1 [61, 76].

Alkaloids such as papaverine, an alkaloid derived from the Papaveraceae family's *Papaver somniferum*, can prevent HIV replication. Harmine, which is produced from *Symplocos setchuensis*, has been demonstrated to inhibit HIV replication in H9 cells [77, 79]. *Leitneria floridana* produces anti-HIV compound 1-methoxycanthinone. These are phenolics. In H9 cells, lithospermic acid from *Salvia miltiorrhiza* exhibits potent anti-HIV action. Punicalagin, chebulagic acid, and punicalin are hydrolysable tannins from *Terminalia chebula* that exhibit anti-HIV action. Numerous lignans have antiviral activities, while naphthoquinones such as plumbagin, 1,4-naphthoquinone, juglone, and vitamin K3 all exhibit HIV inhibitory activity [77, 79].

Several natural materials have been employed as primary compounds because of their explicit efficacy and the rising amount of molecules showing anti-HIV activity that have been identified from plants. New therapies using these natural compounds are required because HIV-1 resistance to the ARV medications has been rising, and because agents that are less expensive and hazardous than the ones now utilized are necessary. The primary unmet need is for the development of anti-HIV drugs with a new mechanism of action, acceptable toxicity, and a reduced resistance profile that may be used to create therapies that specifically target viral replication. With this context in mind, the World Health Organization has advocated for the study of HIV/AIDS treatment using traditional or "ethno" medicine. In light of this, it is important to assess the efficacy and cost-effectiveness of traditional medicine [24, 70]. The above findings provide evidence that numerous herbs, many of which are often used to treat various ailments, are effective against HIV. These reports are priceless since they serve as indicators for decision-making at different levels and the discovery of new lead compounds.

### *11.8.1 ALKALOIDS*

Alkaloids are a class of naturally occurring poisonous amines that are primarily generated by plants as a defensive mechanism to ward off herbivores. Alkaloids primarily cause their harmful effects by interfering with the body's central nervous system, digestive system, reproductive system, and immunological system. Within the category of grain legumes, only lupins are known to have significant levels of alkaloids, while faba beans, peas, and oil seeds do not contain any. Major alkaloids found in *Lupinus albus* include lupanine, albine, and 13-hydroxylupanine, while in *Lupinus luteus*, lupanine and sparteine were found to be in the majority. Recent harvests of low-alkaloid lupin cultivars, popularly known as sweet lupins, had an average alkaloid concentration below 0.288 $kg^{-1}$. Bioactive chemicals, including nicotine, physostigmine, and serotonin, were discovered in *Mucuna* seeds. Several cases of alkaloids have shown efficacy against HIV. Polycitone A, an aromatic alkaloid extracted from the marine ascidian *Polycitor* sp., is one of the natural compounds having noteworthy effect on reverse transcriptase (RT). Both RNA- and DNA-directed DNA polymerases are sensitive to polycitone A's strong inhibitory action [38]. *P. somniferum*, a member of the *Papaveraceae* family, is a source of papaverine, an alkaloid that may block HIV replication. The quinolone buchapine was first isolated from the plant *Evodia roxburghiana* [39]. It has been proven to prevent the cytopathogenic effects of HIV-1. Nitidine is derived from the roots of the plant *Toddalia asiatica*, which belongs to the Rutaceae family. *O*-demethylbuchenavianine, an alkaloid related to piperidine flavones found in *Buchenavia capitata* of the Combretaceae family, indicates inhibition of HIV activity. Harmine, which originates from the *S. setchuensis*, has been demonstrated to suppress HIV replication in H9 cells [27]. *L. floridana* is a source for 1-methoxy cathinone, which has been shown to be effective against HIV. Isolated from *Tripterygium wilfordii* and *Tripterygium hypoglaucum*, the sesquiterpene pyridine alkaloids such as hypoglaunine B, troponin B, and troponin A have been demonstrated to exhibit anti-HIV activities [18].

### 11.8.2 COUMARINS

The first coumarins were identified by Vogel in 1820 from the plant *Dipteryx odorata* Willd. (Fabaceae), also known as "coumaroun" locally. This polyphenolic component belongs to a group of colorless and crystalline oxygenated heterocyclic compounds. Derivatives of either the furan or pyran nucleus with an additional oxygen atom make up oxygenated heterocyclic compounds. In contrast to the rarity of furan derivatives in plants, pyran derivatives are more often observed due to their widespread use in the construction of a wide range of chemicals. Derivatives of pyran are ketones, often in the form of -pyron or -pyron. Condensation of pyron derivatives with benzene in plants results in the secondary metabolites coumarin (benzopyrone) and chromone (benzopyrone). Calanolides, a coumarin found in many species of the tropical tree genus *Calophyllum* (Clusiaceae), are an example of a nonnucleoside specific reverse transcriptase inhibitor of the virus. The *Calophyllum lanigerum* may be used to extract calanolide A, calanolide B, and its derivative 7,8-dihydrocalanolide B, all of which inhibit the cytopathogenic effects of HIV-1 on host cells. The HIV-1 replication inhibitors cordatolide A and B have structural similarities with calanolides. *Calophyllum cordato-oblongum* is the source of these chemicals. The pyrocoumarin derivative suksdorfin [61, 78], which is found in the fruits of the Apiaceae plants *A. morii* and *L. suksdorfii*, has been shown to suppress the replication of the virus in a T-cell line.

### 11.8.3 FLAVONOIDS

An essential category of natural products, flavonoids are polyphenolic secondary metabolites of plants that may be found in a broad variety of foods and drinks. Cancer, Alzheimer's disease, atherosclerosis, and other disorders benefit from their plethora of biochemical and antioxidant effects. Flavonoids have been linked to a wide range of health benefits and are used in nutraceuticals, pharmaceuticals, medicines, and cosmetics. They are able to regulate major cellular enzyme processes while also possessing antioxidative, anti-inflammatory, antimutagenic, and anticarcinogenic capabilities. Several enzymes, including xanthine oxidase, cyclooxygenase, lipoxygenase, and phosphoinositide 3-kinase, have been shown to be very sensitive to their inhibition. Several polyphenols, including flavonoids, have shown promising anti-HIV action. They have been shown to exhibit antiviral activity in several cell cultures and possess antioxidant characteristics [52]. Baicalin, an anti-HIV flavonoid derived from *Scutellaria baicalensis*, suppresses HIV replication in peripheral blood mononuclear cell in a dose-dependent way. Prenylated flavonoids produced from the extract of *Monotes africanus*, such as 6,8-diprenyl-aromadendrin and 6,8-diprenylkaempferol, exhibit anti-HIV activity in an XTT-based, whole-cell screen [40]. Ethanolic extract of *Acer okamotoanum* from the Aceraceae family yields flavonoid gallate ester and quercetin 3-O-(2-galloyl)-a-L-arbinopyranose, both of which suppress HIV-1 integrase activity [30]. Methanolic extracts of the leaves and twigs of *Rhus succedanea*, a member of the Anacardiaceae family, yield the polymerase inhibitors hinokiflavone, robustaflavone, and biflavonoids. Wikstrol B, a biflavonoid, may be extracted from the roots of *Wikstroemia indica*, a member of the Thymelaeaceae family [26]. It has been shown to have anti-HIV action. Hops (*H. lupulus*) contain a compound called xanthohumol, a prenylchalcone that has been shown to suppress HIV-1.

### 11.8.4 LIGNANS

Lignans have a 2,3-dibenzylbutane structure and are phenolic dimers. The synthesis of lignin in the plant cell wall requires the presence of these chemicals, which are known to occur as minor ingredients in many plants. Glycosidic forms of the chemicals predominate. Lignans are a class of chemicals that are often connected with fiber and may be found in a wide variety of plant meals and beverages. Secoisolariciresinol diglucoside, the form of dietary lignans present in flaxseed, has the greatest concentration. Sesamin, matairesinol, pinoresinol, and lariciresinol are some other lignans found in food. A group of gut bacteria called the *Bacillus coagulans* complex may transform plant lignans into the compounds enterolignans, enterodiol, and enterolactone. Multiple lignans have been shown to inhibit virus replication [14] Chloroform extract of *Phyllanthus myrtifolius*/*Phyllanthus urinaria* of the Euphorbiaceae family yields phyllamyricin B and its lactone retrojusticidin B, both of which suppress HIV-RTase activity. *Anogeissus acuminata* extracts containing anolignan B, anolignan A, and dibenzylbutadiene lignans have been demonstrated to inhibit HIV-1 RTase

[54]. Gomisin, which is extracted from the interior of the *Kadsura* plant, is one of the most effective inhibitors of HIV replication.

### 11.8.5 QUINONES

The biological pigments known as quinones are present in a wide variety of species, including bacteria, fungi, higher plants, and even certain mammals. There are several different types of quinones found in nature, including benzoquinones, naphthoquinones, anthraquinones, and polycyclic quinones. Naphthoquinones include, for instance, the vitamin K compound phylloquinone. Coma and medullary center paralysis have been linked to quinones. Hematuria and albuminuria might develop. Quinines have been shown to produce skin irritation and redness in experimental animals after prolonged contact. Naphthoquinones such as plumbagin, 1,4-naphthoquinone, juglone, and vitamin K3 have been shown to have HIV-inhibiting properties [41]. Conocurvone is a trimeric naphthoquinone isolated from the *Conospermum incurvum* plant in the Proteaceae family [17]. It has potent anti-HIV action.

### 11.8.6 TERPENES

Terpenes are a class of hydrocarbons having five carbon atoms and eight hydrogen atoms ($C_5H_8$); they are widespread in nature and thought to have descended from isoprene. The oxygenated derivatives of these hydrocarbons are called terpenoids and are sometimes referred to by this term. The essential oils of many plants, especially evergreens and citrus trees, include a class of volatile unsaturated hydrocarbons known as terpenes. Some triterpenoids have shown ARV efficacy via a variety of methods. Inhibition of HIV replication was seen in H9 lymphocyte cells after treatment with betulinic acid, platanic acid, and oleanolic acid, all of which were isolated from *Syzygium claviflorum* leaves [41]. The Sapindaceae family tree, *Xanthoceras sorbifolium*, yields oleanolic acid, which has been shown to inhibit HIV-1 replication in these cells. Maslinic acid isolated from the *G. japonicum* has shown strong inhibitory effect against HIV-1 protease. Celasdin B, isolated from an ethanolic extract of the plant species *Celastrus hindsii* of the family Celastraceae, has been shown to inhibit HIV replication in H9 cells. The ethyl acetate extract of

*Garcinia speciosa*'s stems and bark yields the protostanes garcisaterpenes A and C, which have been shown to inhibit HIV-1 reverse transcriptase activity. Suberosol produced from ethanolic extract of leaves and stems of *Polyalthia suberosa*, Annonaceae family, has been proven to suppress HIV replication in H9 cells. Another chemical that inhibits HIV replication in these cells is lancilactone C, a triterpene lactone that can be isolated from the roots and stems of *Kadsura lancilimba* [54]. Methanolic extract of the plant genus *Croton tiglium* (Euphorbiaceae) yields the phorbol diester 12-*O*-tetradecanoylphorbol-13-acetate, which can block the cytopathogenic effects of HIV-1. *Homalanthus nutans*, a member of the Euphorbiaceae family, is harvested for its prostratin, a phorbol ester with anti-HIV effects.

### 11.8.7 PHENOLICS

Phenolic molecules, the most common kind of secondary metabolite in plants, are present in almost every plant species native to Algeria. Flavonoids, phenolic acids, tannins, stilbenes, and lignans are all types of phenolic chemicals, but they all have a similar chemical structure consisting of an aromatic ring with one or more hydroxyl substituents. *Centaurea* spp. (*Cheirolophus*, *Rhaponticoides*, and *Volutaria*) native to Algeria have high levels of phenolic chemicals. There are a total of 65 distinct flavonoid structures identified in this research, making them the most numerous of all the phenolic compounds. Simple phenols and phenolic acids are also present in certain species. Prolonged administration of polyphenol-rich fruit juices is thought to be promising for HIV-positive persons due to increased phytohemagglutinin-induced lymphocytes proliferation. Multiple viral systems have shown the virucidal effects of tannins and related phenolic compounds. Abd-Elazem et al. [1] found that lithospermic acid, which was derived from *S. miltiorrhiza*, had potent anti-HIV activity in H9 cells. Hydrolyzable tannins found in *T. chebula*, such as punicalagin, chebulagic acid, and punicalin, have anti-HIV action [30]. Repandusinic acid, which is derived from the Euphorbiaceae plant *Phyllanthus niruri*, has been demonstrated to inhibit HIV-1 RTase. *Arnebia euchroma* (Boraginaceae) aqueous acetone extract yields monopotassium and monosodium salts of isomeric caffeic acid tetramer, which has been demonstrated to suppress HIV replication. The pericarp of the *Camellia japonica* tree is where you will find the anti-HIV compound known as camelliatannin H. *T. chebula*, a member of the Combretaceae family, is the source of the HIV integrase inhibitors galloyl glucose and gallic acid. Extracted from the pericarps of *Mallotus japonicus*, mallotojaponin is a dimeric phloroglucinol derivative that blocks HIV-1 reverse transcriptase function. Curcuminoids, derived from the *Curcuma longa* rhizome, have been demonstrated to block HIV-1 and HIV-2 protease [56]. *Pothomorphe peltata*, a member of the Piperaceae family, is the source of peltatol A, a prenylated catechol dimer with anti-HIV action.

### *11.8.8 SAPONINS*

Natural saponin chemicals are found in almost every cell of legume plants. The complex and chemically varied group of chemicals known as saponins gets its name from its propensity to produce stable, soap-like foams in aqueous solutions. Saponins are compounds that are made up of a carbohydrate moiety coupled to a steroid or triterpenoid. Due to their wide range of both harmful and perhaps useful effects, saponins have recently garnered a lot of attention. Saponins are components that have been shown to provide a variety of health benefits, including lowering cholesterol and protecting the body's immune system against cancer. The rhizome of *Cimicifuga racemosa* (black cohosh) yields actein, a tetracyclic triterpenoid saponin with potent anti-HIV action [60].

### *11.8.9 XANTHONES*

The chemical formula for xanthone is $O[C_6H_4]_2CO$, and it is classified as an organic compound. It is constantly white in color. As a larvicide and ovicide for codling moth eggs, xanthone has been in use since its introduction in 1939. Urea levels in the blood may be measured using a compound called xanthydrol, which is made from xanthone. It also has photocatalytic properties. *Swertia franchetiana* is the source of swertifrancheside, a flavonone–xanthone glucoside that has been found to block HIV-1 RT [67]. *Maclura tinctoria*, a member of the Moraceae family, is the source of macluraxanthone B, a prenylated xanthone with anti-HIV action [23].

## 11.9 SUMMARY

Despite the relative lack of focus on maternal variables, there is enough data to draw the conclusion that maternal HIV infection has a negative impact on newborn outcomes in the early years. The focus has largely shifted from the numerous causes of these negative effects to feeding practices and ARV exposure. However, studies have indicated that these negative effects continue to exist even while breastfeeding and ARV usage have improved results. Even while it is unclear whether the virus itself or the stimulated maternal environment is more to blame, evidence indicating the degree of this influence is influenced by the severity of maternal sickness, further supports the idea that the mechanism is at least partially related to *in utero* exposure. For the purpose of developing an effective maternal and/or infant HIV-1 vaccine to aid in the creation of an HIV-free generation, larger and better controlled studies that examine maternal neutralizing antibodies with defined fine-epitope specificity and their function in preventing or reducing MTCT risk in the context of ART may provide crucial information. Different types of plant-based products have been found effective in the control of HIV infection from mother to baby, although a lot of studies need to be conducted in this regard.

## KEYWORDS

- **fetus**
- **HIV**
- **infant**
- **infection**
- **mechanism**
- **transmission**

## REFERENCES

1. Abd-Elazem, I. S., Chen, H. S., Bates, R. B., & Huang, R. C. (2002). Isolation of two highly potent and non-toxic inhibitors of human immunodeficiency virus type 1 (HIV-1) integrase from *Salvia miltiorrhiza*. *Antiviral Research*, *55*, 91–106.
2. Auvert, B., Sobngwi-Tambekou, J., Cutler, E., Nieuwoudt, M., Lissouba, P., Puren, A., & Taljaard, D. (2009). Effect of male circumcision on the prevalence

of high-risk human papillomavirus in young men: Results of a randomized controlled trial conducted in Orange Farm, South Africa. *The Journal of infectious diseases*, *199*(1), 14–19.

3. Auvert, B., Taljaard, D., Lagarde, E., Sobngwi-Tambekou, J., Sitta, R., & Puren, A. (2005). Randomized, controlled intervention trial of male circumcision for reduction of HIV infection risk: The ANRS 1265 trial. *PLoS Medicine*, *2*(11), e298.
4. Backé, E., Unger, M., Jimenez, E., Siegel, G., Schäfer, A., & Vogel, M. (1993). Fetal organs infected by HIV-1. *AIDS*, *7*(6), 896–897.
5. Bailey, R. C., Moses, S., Parker, C. B., Agot, K., Maclean, I., Krieger, J. N., Williams, C. F., Campbell, R. T., & Ndinya-Achola, J. O. (2007). Male circumcision for HIV prevention in young men in Kisumu, Kenya: A randomized controlled trial. *Lancet*, *369*(9562), 643–656.
6. Bakas, C., Zarou, D. M., & de Caprariis, P. J. (1996). First-trimester spontaneous abortions and the incidence of human immunodeficiency virus seropositivity. *Journal of Reproductive Medicine*, *41*(1), 15–18.
7. Behets, F. M., Matendo, R., Vaz, L. M. E., Kilese, N., Nanlele, D., Kokolomami, J., Okitolando, E. W., & Van Rie, A. (2006). Preventing vertical transmission of HIV in Kinshasa, Democratic Republic of the Congo: A baseline survey of 18 antenatal clinics. *Bulletin of the World Health Organization*, *84*(12), 969–975.
8. Bergström, S., Sonnerborg, A., Osman, N. B., & Libombo, A. (1995). HIV infection and maternal outcome of pregnancy in Mozambican women: A case control study. *Genitourinary Medicine*, *71*(5), 323–324.
9. Bertolli, J., St Louis, M. E., Simonds, R. J., Nieburg, P., Kamenga, M., Brown, C., Tarande, M., Quinn, T., & Ou, C. Y. (1996). Estimating the timing of mother-to-child transmission of human immunodeficiency virus in a breast-feeding population in Kinshasa, Zaire. *Journal of Infectious Diseases*, *174*(4), 722–726.
10. Braddick, M. R., Kreiss, J. K., Embree, J. B., Datta, P., Ndinya-Achola, J. O., Pamba, H., Maitha, G., Roberts, P. L., Quinn, T. C., & Holmes, K. K. (1990). Impact of maternal HIV infection on obstetrical and early neonatal outcome. *AIDS (London, England)*, *4*(10), 1001–1005.
11. Braddick, M. R., Kreiss, J. K., Embree, J. B., Datta, P., Ndinya-Achola, J. O., Pamba, H., Maitha, G., Roberts, P. L., Quinn, T. C., & Holmes, K. K. (1990). Impact of maternal HIV infection on obstetrical and early pregnancy outcome. *AIDS*, *4*(10), 1001–1005.
12. Bulterys, M., Chao, A., Dushimimana, A., & Saah, A. (1996). Fatal complications after Caesarian section in HIV-infected women. *AIDS*, *10*(8), 923–924.
13. Burns, D. N., Landesman, S., Minkoff, H., Wright, D. J., Waters, D., Mitchell, R. M., Rubinstein, A., Willoughby, A., & Goedert, J. J. (1998). The influence of pregnancy on human immunodeficiency virus type 1 infection: Antepartum and postpartum changes in human immunodeficiency virus type 1 viral load. *American Journal of Obstetrics and Gynecology*, *178*(2), 355–359.
14. Byabamazina, C. R., Asiimwe, O. G., & Malamba, S. (1995). HIV/Syphilis serology as an indicator of past pregnancy outcomes among antenatal attendees in Kampala (abstract TuC108). In: *IXth International Conference on AIDS and STD in Africa*, Kampala.
15. Charlton, J. L. (1998). Antiviral activity of lignans. *Journal of Natural Products*, *61*, 1447–1451.

16. Cherie, N., & Mebratu, A. (2018). *Adverse Birth Outcomes and Associated Factors among Delivered Mothers in Dessie Referral Hospital* (pp. 1–6). North-East, Ethiopia.
17. Connor, E. M., Sperling, R. S., Gelber, R., Kiselev, P., Scott, G., O'Sullivan, M. J., VanDyke, R., Bey, M., Shearer, W., & Jacobson, R. L. (1994). Reduction of maternal-infant transmission of human immunodeficiency virus type 1 with zidovudine treatment. Pediatric AIDS clinical trials group protocol 076 study group. *New England Journal of Medicine*, *331*(18), 1173–1180.
18. Decosterd, L. A., Parsons, I. C., Gustafson, K. R., Cardellina, J. H., Mcmahon, J. B., Cragg, G. M., Murata, Y., Pannell, L. K., & Steiner, J. R. (1993). HIV inhibitory natural products. 11. Structure, absolute stereochemistry, and synthesis of conocurvone, a potent, novel HIV-inhibitory naphthoquinone trimer from a *Conospermum* sp. *Journal of the American Chemical Society, 115*, 6673–6679.
19. Duan, H., Takaishi, Y., Imakura, Y., Jia, Y., Li, D., Cosentino, L. M., & Lee, K. H. (2000). Sesquiterpene alkaloids from *Tripterygium hypoglaucum* and *Tripterygium wilfordii*: A new class of potent Anti-HIV agents. *Journal of Natural Products, 63*, 357–361.
20. Evans, C., Jones, C. E., & Prendergast, A. J. (2016). HIV-exposed, uninfected infants: New global challenges in the era of paediatric HIV elimination. *Lancet. Infectious Diseases*, *16*(6), e92–e107.
21. Fentie, E. A., Yeshita, H. Y., & Bokie, M. M. (2022). Low birth weight and associated factors among HIV positive and negative mothers delivered in northwest Amhara region referral hospitals, Ethiopia, 2020 a comparative cross-sectional study. *PLoS One,* (2), *17*(2), e0263812.
22. Gray, G., McIntyre, J. A., & Pettifor, J. (1995). Difference in growth and illness between breastfed and formula fed infants born to HIV positive women in Soweto (abstract ThB280). In: *IXth International Conference on AIDS and STD in Africa*, Kampala.
23. Gray, R. H., Kigozi, G., Serwadda, D., Makumbi, F., Watya, S., Nalugoda, F., Kiwanuka, N., Moulton, L. H., Chaudhary, M. A., Chen, M. Z., Sewankambo, N. K., Wabwire-Mangen, F., Bacon, M. C., Williams, C. F., Opendi, P., Reynolds, S. J., Laeyendecker, O., Quinn, T. C., & Wawer, M. J. (2007). Male circumcision for HIV prevention in men in Rakai, Uganda: A randomized trial. *Lancet*, *369*(9562), 657–666.
24. Groweiss, A., Cardellina, J. H., & Boyd, M. R. (2000). HIV-Inhibitory prenylated *Xanthones* and flavones from *Maclura tinctoria*. *Journal of Natural Products, 63*, 1537–1539.
25. Hedimbi, M., & Chinsembu, K. C. (2012). Ethnomedicinal study of plants used to manage HIV/AIDS-related disease conditions in the Ohangwena region, Namibia. *International Journal of Medicinal Plants Research, 1*, 4–11.
26. Hocke, C., Morlat, P., Chene, G., Dequae, L., & Dabis, F. (1995). Prospective cohort study of the effect of pregnancy on the progression of human immunodeficiency virus infection. *Obstetrics & Gynecology*, *86*(6), 886–891.
27. Hu, K., Kobayashi, H., Dong, A., Iwasaki, S., & Yao, X. (2000). Antifungal, antimitotic and anti-HIV-1 agents from the roots of *Wikstroemia indica*. *Planta Medica, 66*, 564–567.

28. Ishida, J., Wang, H. K., Oyama, M., Cosentino, M. L., Hu, C. Q., & Lee, K. H. (2001). Anti-AIDS agents. 46.1 anti-HIV activity of harman, an anti-HIV principle from *Symplocos setchuensis*, and its derivatives. *Journal of Natural Products*, *64*, 958–960.
29. Jensen, L. P., O'Sullivan, M. J., Gomez-del-Rio, M., Setzer, E. S., Gaskin, C., & Penso, C. (1984). Acquired immune deficiency syndrome in pregnancy. *American Journal of Obstetrics and Gynecology*, *148*(8), 1145–1146.
30. Kemp, M. W. (2014). Preterm birth, intrauterine infection, and fetal inflammation. *Frontiers in Immunology*, *5*, 574.
31. Kim, H. J., Woo, E. R., Shin, C. G., & Park, H. (1998). A new flavonol glycoside gallate ester from *Acer okamotoanum* and its inhibitory activity against human immunodeficiency virus-1 (HIV-1) integrase. *Journal of Natural Products, 61*, 145–148.
32. Kloos, H., Assefa, Y., Adugna, A., Mulatu, M. S., & Mariam, D. H. (2007). Utilization of antiretroviral treatment in Ethiopia between February and December 2006: Spatial, temporal, and demographic patterns. *International Journal of Health Geographics*, *6*, 45.
33. Klugman, K. P., Patel, J., Sischy, A., & McIntyre, J. A. (1991). Serological markers of sexually transmitted diseases associated with HIV-1 infection in pregnant black women. *South African Medical Journal*, *80*(5), 243–244.
34. Kuhn, L., Kasonde, P., Sinkala, M., Kankasa, C., Semrau, K., Scott, N., Tsai, W. Y., Vermund, S. H., Aldrovandi, G. M., & Thea, D. M. (2005). Does severity of HIV disease in HIV-infected mothers affect mortality and morbidity among their uninfected infants? *Clinical Infectious Diseases: An Official Publication of the Infectious Diseases Society of America*, *41*(11), 1654–1661.
35. Kuhn, L., Meddows-Taylor, S., Gray, G., & Tiemessen, C. (2002). Human immunodeficiency virus (HIV)-specific cellular immune responses in newborns exposed to HIV in utero. *Clinical infectious diseases*, *34*(2), 267–276.
36. Lee, A. C., Katz, J., Blencowe, H., Cousens, S., Kozuki, N., Vogel, J. P., & Black, R. E. (2013). National and regional estimates of term and preterm babies born small for gestational age in 138 low-income and middle-income countries in 2010. *The Lancet Global Health*, *1*(1), e26–e36.
37. Leroy, V., De Clercq, A., Ladner, J., Bogaerts, J., Van de Perre, P., & Dabis, F. (1995). Should screening of genital infections be part of antenatal care in areas of high HIV prevalence?: A prospective cohort study from Kigali, Rwanda, 1992–1993. The Pregnancy and HIV (EGE) Group. *Genitourinary Medicine*, *71*(4), 207–211.
38. López, M., Palacio, M., Goncé, A., Hernàndez, S., Barranco, F. J., García, L., Loncà, M., Coll, J. O., Gratacós, E., & Figueras, F. (2015). Risk of intrauterine growth restriction among HIV-infected pregnant women: A cohort study. *European Journal of Clinical Microbiology and Infectious Diseases*, *34*(2), 223–230.
39. Loya, S., Rudi, A., Kashman, Y., & Hizi, A. (1999). Polycitone-A: A novel and potent general inhibitor of retroviral reverse transcriptases and cellular DNA polymerases. *Biochemical Journal*, *344*, 85–92.
40. McCormick, J. L., Mckee, T. C., Cardellina, J. H., & Boyd, M. R. (1996). HIV inhibitory natural products: Quinoline alkaloids from *Euodia roxburghiana*. *Journal of Natural Products, 59*, 469–471.

41. Meragelman, K. M., Mckee, T. C., & Boyd, M. R. (2001). Anti-HIV prenylated flavonoids from *Monotes africanus*. *Journal of Natural Products, 64*, 546–548.
42. Min, B. S., Miyashiro, H., & Hattori, M. (2002). Inhibitory effects of quinones on RNase H activity associated with HIV-1 reverse transcriptase. *Phytotherapy Research, 16*(Suppl. 1), S57–S62.
43. Minkoff, H. (1995). Pregnancy and HIV infection. In: *HIV Infection in Women* (pp. 173–188). Raven Press.
44. Minkoff, H., Nanda, D., Menez, R., & Fikrig, S. (1987). Pregnancies resulting in infants with acquired immune deficiency syndrome or AIDS related complex. *Obstetrics and Gynecology, 69*(3 Pt 1), 285–287.
45. Miotti, P. G., Chiphangwi, J. D., & Dallabetta, G. A. (1992). The situation in Africa. *Bailliere's Clinical Obstetrics and Gynaecology, 6*(1), 165–186.
46. Mofenson, L. M. (1997). Interaction between the timing of perinatal human immunodeficiency virus infection and the design of preventive and therapeutic interventions. *Acta Paediatrica,. 421*(Supp. L), 1–9.
47. Naniche, D., Bardají, A., Lahuerta, M., Berenguera, A., Mandomando, I., Sanz, S., Aponte, J. J., Sigauque, B., Alonso, P. L., & Menéndez, C. (2009). Impact of maternal human immunodeficiency virus infection on birth outcomes and infant survival in rural Mozambique. *American Journal of Tropical Medicine and Hygiene, 80*(5), 870–876.
48. Naniche, D., Varior-Krishnan, G. A. Y. A. T. H. R. I., Cervoni, F., Wild, T. F., Rossi, B., Rabourdin-Combe, C. A., & Gerlier, D. (1993). Human membrane cofactor protein (CD46) acts as a cellular receptor for measles virus. *Journal of virology, 67*(10), 6025–6032.
49. Newell, M. L., Coovadia, H., Cortina-Borja, M., Rollins, N., Gaillard, P., & Dabis, F. (2004). Mortality of infected and uninfected infants born to HIV-infected mothers in Africa: A pooled analysis. *The Lancet, 364*(9441), 1236–1243.
50. Newell, M. L. (1998). Mechanisms and timing of mother-to-child transmission of HIV-1. *Aids, 12*(8), 831–837.
51. Newell, M. L., Gray, G., & Bryson, Y. J. (1997). Prevention of mother-to child transmission of HIV-1 transmission. *AIDS, 11*(Suppl. A), S165–S172.
52. Novitsky, V., Bussmann, H., Logan, A., Moyo, S., van Widenfelt, E., Okui, L., Mmalane, M., Baca, J., Buck, L., Phillips, E., Tim, D., McLane, M. F., Lei, Q., Wang, R., Makhema, J., Lockman, S., DeGruttola, V., & Essex, M. (2013). Phylogenetic relatedness of circulating HIV-1C variants in Mochudi, Botswana. *PLoS One, 8*(12), e80589.
53. Orhan, D. D., Ozcelik, B., Ozgen, S., & Ergun, F. (2010). Antibacterial, antifungal, and antiviral activities of some flavonoids. *Microbiological Research, 165*, 496–504.
54. Read, J. (1998). Mode of delivery and vertical transmission of HIV-1: A meta-analysis from fifteen prospective cohort studies (abstract 23603). In: *12th World AIDS Conference*, Geneva, June 28. The International Perinatal HIV Group.
55. Rimando, A. M., Pezzuto, J. M., Farnsworth, N. R., Santisuk, T., Reutrakul, V., & Kawanishi, K. (1994). New lignans from *Anogeissus acuminata* with HIV-1 reverse transcriptase inhibitory activity. *Journal of Natural Products, 57*, 896–904.
56. Rollins, N. C., Coovadia, H. M., Bland, R. M., Coutsoudis, A., Bennish, M. L., Patel, D., & Newell, M. L. (2007). Pregnancy outcomes in HIV-infected and uninfected

women in rural and urban South Africa. *Journal of Acquired Immune Deficiency Syndromes*, *44*(3), 321–328.

57. Roth, G. N., Chandra, A., & Nair, M. G. (1998). Novel bioactivities of *Curcuma longa* constituents. *Journal of Natural Products, 61*, 542–545.
58. Ryder, R. W., & Temmerman, M. (1991). The effects of HIV-1 infection during pregnancy and the perinatal period on maternal and child health in Africa. *AIDS*, *5*(Suppl. 1), S75–S85.
59. Ryder, R. W., Nsuami, M., Nsa, W., Kamenga, M., Badi, N., Utshudi, M., & Heyward, W. L. (1994). Mortality in HIV-1 seropositive women, their spouses and their newly born children during 36 months of follow up in Kinshasa, Zaire. *AIDS*, *8*(5), 667–672.
60. Ryder, R. W., Nsa, W., Hassig, S. E., Behets, F., Rayfield, M., Ekungola, B., & Curran, J. W. (1989). Perinatal transmission of the human immunodeficiency virus type 1 to infants of seropositive women in Zaire. *New England Journal of Medicine*, *320*(25), 1637–1642.
61. Sakurai, N., Wu, J. H., Sashida, Y., Mimaki, Y., Nikaido, T., & Koike, K. (2004). Anti-AIDS agents, *part* 57: Actein, an anti-HIV principle from the rhizome of *Cimicifuga racemosa* (black cohosh), and the anti-HIV activity of related saponins. *Bioorganic & Medicinal Chemistry Letters*, *14*, 1329–1332.
62. Sayal, S. K., Banerjee, S., Das, A., Gupta, C. M., Doiphade, V. V., Gogte, R. B., & Uppal, S. S. (1998). Role of ayurvedic drugs in treatment of HIV infection. *Medical Journal, Armed Forces India*, *54*(4), 374.
63. Shearer, W. T., Langston, C., Lewis, D. E., Pham, E. L., Hammill, H. H., Kozinetz, C. A., Kline, M. W., Hanson, I. C., & Popek, E. J. (1997). Early spontaneous abortion and fetal thymic abnormalities in maternal-to-fetal HIV infection. *Acta Paediatrica*, *421*, 60–64.
64. Soto-Ramirez, L. E., Renjifo, B., McLane, M. F., McLane, M. F., Marlink, R., O'Hara, C., Sutthent, R., Wasi, C., Vithayasai, P., Vithayasai, V., Apichartpiyakul, C., Auewarakul, P., Peña Cruz, V., Chui, D. S., Osathanondh, R., Mayer, K., Lee, T. H., & Essex, M. (1996). HIV-1 Langerhans' cell tropism associated with heterosexual transmission of HIV. *Science*, *271*(5253), 1291–1293.
65. Temmerman, M. (1994). Human immunodeficiency virus and women. *Journal of Obstetrics and Gynaecology*, *14*(suppl. 2), s70–s74.
66. Temmerman, M., Plummer, F. A., Mirza, N. B., Ndinya-Achola, J. O., Wamola, I. A., Nagelkerke, N., Brunham, R. C., & Piot, P. (1990). Infection with HIV as a risk factor for adverse obstetrical outcome. *AIDS*, *4*(11), 1087–1093.
67. Tomilola, O. R., Bolanle, O. E., & Olufunmilayo, O. M. (2023). Unintended pregnancies among HIV-positive women in sub-Saharan Africa: A scoping review protocol. *Systematic Reviews*, *12*(1), 12.
68. UNAIDS. (2015). HIV/AIDS fact sheet 2015. http://www.unaids.org/sites/default/files/media_asset/20150901_FactSheet_2015_en.pdf; (accessed on 03 March 2024).
69. Wang, J. N., Hou, C. Y., Liu, Y. L., Lin, L. Z., Gil, R. R., & Cordell, G. A. (1994). Swertifrancheside, an HIV-reverse transcriptase inhibitor and the first flavone-xanthone dimer, from *Swertia franchetiana*. *Journal of Natural Products, 57(2), 211–217.*
70. Wang, J. (2009). The effect of combination of traditional Chinese medicine (TCM) and highly active antiretroviral therapy (HAART) on immune reconstitution of HIV/AIDS patients. Clinicaltrials.gov

71. Weisser, M., Rudin, C., Battegay, M., Pfluger, D., Kully, C., & Egger, M. (1998). The Swiss HIV cohort study (SHCS), and the Swiss collaborative HIV and pregnancy study (SCHPS). Does pregnancy influence the course of HIV infection? Evidence from two large Swiss cohort studies? *Journal of Acquired Immune Deficiency Syndromes and Human Retrovirology*, *17*(5), 404–410.
72. World Health Organization (WHO). (2002). *WHO Traditional Medicine Strategy 2002–2005* (p. 61). World Health Organization.
73. World Health Organization. (2010). Guidelines on HIV and infant feeding 2010: Principles and recommendations for infant feeding in the context of HIV and a summary of evidence. http://www.who.int/maternal_child_adolescent/documents/9789241599535/en/; (accessed on 03 March 2024).
74. World Health Organization, UNAIDS, United Nations Population Fund, & United Nations Children's Fund, author. (2010). *HIV and infant feeding guidelines: Principles and Recommendations for Infant Feeding in the Context of HIV and a Summary of Evidence*. WHO; UNAIDS; UNFPA. United Nations Children's Fund.
75. World Health Organization. (2012). Born to soon: The global action report on preterm birth [Internet]. http://www.who.int/pmnch/media/news/2012/201204_borntoosoon-report.pdf; (accessed on 03 March 2024).
76. Wuhib, T., Legesse, T., Morrison, L., Dempsey, H. F., Mereke, N., & Ghebreyesus, T. A. (2006). Global Fund-PEPFAR HIV/AIDS partnership in Ethiopia for maximum impact (Abstract TUPE0875). In: *Abstracts of the XVI International Aids Conference, Toronto*.
77. Xu, H. X., Wan, M., Dong, H., But, P. P., & Foo, L. Y. (2000). Inhibitory activity of flavonoids and tannins against HIV-1 protease. *Biological and Pharmaceutical Bulletin*, *23*(9), 1072–1076.
78. Xu, H. X., & Lee, S. F. (2001). Activity of plant flavonoids against antibiotic-resistant bacteria. *Phytotherapy Research: An International Journal Devoted to Pharmacological and Toxicological Evaluation of Natural Product Derivatives*, *15*(1), 39–43.
79. Xu, H. X., Zeng, F. Q., Wan, M., & Sim, K. Y. (1996). Anti-HIV triterpene acids from Geum japonicum. *Journal of Natural Products*, *59*(7), 643–645.
80. Yu, D., Suzuki, M., Xie, L., Morris-Natschke, S. L., & Lee, K. H. (2003). Recent progress in the development of coumarin derivatives as potent anti-HIV agents. *Medicinal Research Reviews*, *23*, 322–345.
81. Zaba, B., Calvert, C., Marston, M., Isingo, R., Nakiyingi-Miiro, J., Lutalo, T., Crampin, A., Robertson, L., Herbst, K., Newell, M. L., Todd, J., Byass, P., Boerma, T., & Ronsmans, C. (2013). Effect of HIV infection on pregnancy-related mortality in sub-Saharan Africa: Secondary analyses of pooled community-based data from the network for analyzing longitudinal population-based HIV/AIDS data on Africa (alpha). *Lancet*, *381*(9879), 1763–1771.

# CHAPTER 12

# Dry Vagina: Challenges, Causes, Issues, and Remedies

ANAMIKA CHAUHAN* and MEGH R. GOYAL

*Corresponding author

## ABSTRACT

Dry vagina is referred to as vaginal dryness or vaginal atrophy. It is a multifaceted condition that affects a significant proportion of women across various age groups. This chapter comprehensively explores the challenges posed by vaginal dryness, its underlying causes, and the wide array of remedies available for its management. Vaginal dryness can result in discomfort, pain, and adversely impact a woman's quality of life. This chapter begins by delving into the physiological and hormonal changes that contribute to vaginal dryness, particularly during menopause but also at other life stages. Additionally, we investigate the psychosocial aspects of this condition, such as its impact on sexual satisfaction, relationships, and emotional well-being. This chapter examines the efficacy, safety, and potential side effects associated with each treatment approach. The chapter also highlights the importance of open communication between patients and healthcare providers in diagnosing and addressing vaginal dryness. Additionally, the chapter underscores the significance of holistic approaches that consider both physical and emotional factors in managing this condition. Ultimately, this chapter aims to provide valuable insights into the challenges posed by vaginal dryness, its root causes, the broader issues it can engender, and the diverse range of remedies available, facilitating informed decision-making for individuals and healthcare practitioners alike.

Holistic Approaches for Women's Sustainable Health, Volume 1: Foundations, Innovations, Challenges, and Management. Megh R. Goyal, Anamika Chauhan, and Junaid Ahmad Malik (Eds)


DOI: 10.1201/9781779641632-15

## 12.1 INTRODUCTION

### 12.1.1 BRIEF INTRODUCTION ON VAGINAL DRYNESS

Vaginal dryness, medically termed as atrophic vaginitis, is a prevalent condition affecting a significant proportion of women, particularly during and postmenopause. This condition arises when the vaginal tissues are deficient in moisture. One primary etiological factor is hormonal alterations, especially a reduction in estrogen levels. Estrogen plays a crucial role in maintaining vaginal health, and its diminishment can lead to the thinning, drying, and inflammation of the vaginal walls [39].

Various other elements contribute to vaginal dryness which includes certain drugs such as antihistamines and antidepressants, medical treatments such as chemotherapy, autoimmune disorders, smoking, and insufficient sexual arousal [27]. Additionally, psychological factors such as stress and anxiety can also influence vaginal lubrication [23]. Symptomatically, vaginal dryness can manifest as itching, burning, discomfort during intercourse, light bleeding postintercourse, and a decrease in vaginal lubrication. These symptoms can substantially affect a woman's life, encompassing her sexual health and general well-being [7, 20].

Addressing vaginal dryness involves various remedies, contingent on the underlying cause. Hormone therapy, particularly estrogen therapy, is frequently employed for menopausal vaginal dryness. Over-the-counter lubricants and moisturizers also offer symptomatic relief. Lifestyle modifications, such as smoking cessation and stress management, can be beneficial. Furthermore, engaging in regular sexual activity or vaginal stimulation can enhance blood flow to the vagina, aiding in maintaining its health [26, 43].

### 12.1.2 IMPORTANCE OF THE ISSUE OF VAGINAL DRYNESS

Addressing the issue of vaginal dryness is critical due to its profound impact on various aspects of a woman's life. This condition, while often associated with menopause, can affect women of any age and has significant physical, emotional, and relational consequences. Physically, vaginal dryness can cause discomfort, itching, and soreness, especially during intercourse. This can result in diminished sexual desire and a consequent strain on intimate relationships. Women experiencing vaginal dryness often report decreased sexual satisfaction, which can affect their overall quality of life [20]. Emotionally, the symptoms of vaginal dryness can lead to feelings of inadequacy, anxiety, and decreased self-esteem.

According to the North American Menopause Society [39], many women feel embarrassed or hesitant to discuss these symptoms with their healthcare providers, which can delay diagnosis and treatment. From a relational perspective, the discomfort and pain associated with vaginal dryness can lead to avoidance of sexual activity, which can strain intimate relationships [17]. A study by the National Institute on Aging [31] noted that communication between partners often diminishes when sexual health issues are not addressed, potentially leading to misunderstandings and emotional distance.

Moreover, untreated vaginal dryness can lead to more severe health issues such as increased susceptibility to vaginal infections and urinary problems. According to Mayo Clinic [27], maintaining vaginal health is crucial for preventing these complications. Therefore, addressing vaginal dryness is not just about alleviating physical symptoms; it is also about improving a woman's overall quality of life, emotional well-being, and the health of her intimate relationships. Healthcare providers play a vital role in this process by offering effective treatments and creating an environment where women feel comfortable discussing such issues.

This review chapter focuses on: (1) the efficacy, safety, and potential side effects associated with each treatment approach; (2) the importance of open communication between patients and healthcare providers in diagnosing and addressing vaginal dryness, emphasizing the need for personalized treatment plans; (3) underscores the significance of holistic approaches that consider both physical and emotional factors in managing this condition; (4) valuable insights into the challenges posed by vaginal dryness, its root causes, the broader issues it can engender; and (5) the diverse range of remedies available, facilitating informed decision-making for individuals and healthcare practitioners alike.

## 12.2 VAGINAL DRYNESS: UNDERSTANDING THE CHALLENGES

Vaginal dryness, a significant health issue affecting a broad spectrum of women, is often underreported and undertreated. This condition, characterized by the drying and thinning of the vaginal walls, primarily results from a decrease in estrogen levels. While commonly associated with menopause, it can affect women of all ages due to various factors such as hormonal imbalances, certain medications, and health conditions [39]. The challenge in addressing vaginal dryness lies not only in its physical symptoms but also in the psychological and relational impacts it can have. Physically, women may experience discomfort, itching, pain during intercourse, and increased susceptibility to infections [23]. These symptoms can lead to a decreased quality of life, which indicates a significant impact on sexual function and satisfaction [20]. Psychologically, vaginal dryness can lead to feelings of embarrassment, anxiety, and a decrease in self-esteem.

Many women are hesitant to discuss these symptoms with healthcare providers, contributing to a delay in diagnosis and treatment [27]. This reluctance is often due to social stigmas and a lack of awareness about the condition. From a relational standpoint, the discomfort and pain associated with vaginal dryness can lead to avoidance of sexual activity, thereby affecting intimate relationships. According to a study by WebMD [43], communication between partners about sexual health is crucial, yet often challenging in the context of vaginal dryness. Effective treatment of vaginal dryness requires a multifaceted approach, including hormonal therapies, over-the-counter lubricants and moisturizers, and lifestyle changes. Patient education and open communication with healthcare providers are key to successfully managing this condition [39]. The importance of addressing vaginal dryness extends beyond physical comfort, encompassing emotional well-being and the health of intimate relationships. Increased awareness and open dialogue about this condition are essential for improving the lives of many women who suffer in silence.

## *12.2.1 DEFINITIONS AND TERMINOLOGIES*

### *12.2.1.1 ATROPHIC VAGINITIS*

It combines "atrophy" (thinning of tissue) and "vaginitis" (inflammation of the vagina). It describes the condition where the vaginal walls become thinner, less elastic, and more prone to inflammation, primarily due to reduced estrogen levels [32].

### *12.2.1.2 DYSPAREUNIA*

Dyspareunia refers to painful sexual intercourse, a frequent complaint among women suffering from vaginal dryness. The lack of adequate lubrication and decreased elasticity of the vaginal tissue contribute to this discomfort [4].

#### *12.2.1.3 ESTROGEN*

It plays a pivotal role in female reproductive health. Estrogen maintains the structure and function of the vaginal wall, and its decrease, especially during menopause, leads to symptoms such as dryness, itching, and discomfort [35].

#### *12.2.1.4 HORMONE REPLACEMENT THERAPY*

A treatment modality is used to alleviate menopausal symptoms, including vaginal dryness, by replacing diminished estrogen levels [36].

#### *12.2.1.5 MENOPAUSE*

It is a life stage when a woman's menstrual periods permanently stop, typically occurring in the late 40s to early 50s. Menopause is associated with a natural decline in estrogen levels, often resulting in vaginal dryness [34].

#### *12.2.1.6 NATURAL VAGINAL LUBRICATION*

Natural vaginal lubrication, produced by glands in the vagina, decreases with lower estrogen levels. This reduction in lubrication can lead to dryness and discomfort during sexual activity [22].

#### *12.2.1.7 NONHORMONAL THERAPIES*

Nonhormonal therapies encompass over-the-counter lubricants and moisturizers that offer symptomatic relief for vaginal dryness without hormone replacement [33].

#### *12.2.1.8 VAGINAL ATROPHY*

Vaginal atrophy pertains to the thinning, drying, and inflammation of the vaginal walls due to decreased estrogen levels [40].

### 12.2.2 PREVALENCE ACROSS DIFFERENT AGE GROUPS

#### 12.2.2.1 MENOPAUSE AND POSTMENOPAUSE

The prevalence of vaginal dryness increases significantly during and after menopause. A study by The North American Menopause Society (NAMS, 2013) [40] found that up to 60–70% of postmenopausal women experience some degree of vaginal dryness. This condition is primarily attributed to the significant drop in estrogen levels that occurs during menopause [38].

#### 12.2.2.2 PERIMENOPAUSE

This transitional phase leading up to menopause often begins in the 40s. Changes in estrogen levels during this stage can start to cause irregular menstrual cycles and symptoms such as hot flashes and vaginal dryness. According to Avis et al. (2009) [2] in menopause, approximately 40% of perimenopausal women report symptoms of vaginal dryness.

#### 12.2.2.3 REPRODUCTIVE AGE

In younger women of reproductive age, vaginal dryness is less common but not rare. Factors such as hormonal birth control, breastfeeding, and certain medications can contribute to reduced estrogen levels, leading to dryness. A study by Leiblum et al. [25] reported that hormonal fluctuations during the menstrual cycle can also affect vaginal lubrication.

#### 12.2.2.4 SENIOR WOMEN

The prevalence continues to rise with age, as vaginal tissue naturally atrophies over time. A study by Dennerstein et al. [10] indicated that postmenopausal women in their 60s and 70s report higher rates of vaginal dryness, with estimates ranging from 70% to 80%.

### 12.2.3 IMPACT ON WOMEN'S QUALITY OF LIFE

Vaginal dryness can have a substantial impact on a woman's quality of life. This condition, characterized by symptoms such as itching, burning, soreness, and pain during sexual intercourse, not only causes physical discomfort but also has significant emotional and relational consequences [16]. The discomfort and pain associated with vaginal dryness can lead to a decreased interest in sexual activity and a diminished quality of sexual experiences, potentially straining intimate relationships [37]. Additionally, the emotional toll should not be underestimated, as women experiencing vaginal dryness may develop feelings of self-consciousness, lowered self-esteem, and even anxiety or depression [29]. Overall, the combination of physical discomfort, decreased sexual satisfaction, and emotional distress can profoundly affect a woman's general well-being and quality of life (Table 12.1) [2].

**TABLE 12.1** Common Symptoms and Manifestations

| Symptom | Description | Reference |
| --- | --- | --- |
| Decreased sexual desire | A reduction in libido, often because of discomfort or pain associated with vaginal dryness. | [24] |
| Dryness | A lack of natural vaginal lubrication, leading to a feeling of dryness inside the vagina. | [40] |
| Itching and burning | Uncomfortable sensations in the vaginal area, including itching and burning, often related to the irritation caused by dryness. | [32] |
| Light bleeding postintercourse | Occasional light bleeding or spotting following sexual activity, attributed to the fragility of the dry vaginal tissue. | [10] |
| Pain during intercourse (Dyspareunia) | Experiencing pain or discomfort during sexual intercourse due to reduced lubrication and elasticity of the vaginal tissue. | [4] |
| Urinary symptoms | Increased frequency of urination, urinary incontinence, or urinary tract infections, as changes in the vagina can affect the urinary tract. | [33] |

## 12.3 CAUSES AND CONTRIBUTING FACTORS

### *12.3.1 HORMONAL CHANGES DURING MENOPAUSE*

During menopause, women experience a significant decline in estrogen levels. Estrogen is a key hormone accountable for upholding the health and elasticity of vaginal tissue, as well as lubrication. As estrogen levels drop, the vaginal walls become thinner, less elastic, and more prone to dryness and irritation [34].

### 12.3.2 CHANGES IN VAGINAL TISSUE

The decrease in estrogen during menopause also leads to changes in vaginal tissue. These changes include reduced blood flow and diminished production of natural lubricants. As a result, the vaginal tissue becomes more fragile, less acidic, and more susceptible to infections and inflammation, contributing to discomfort and dryness [36].

### 12.3.3 OTHER LIFE STAGES AND MEDICAL CONDITIONS

#### 12.3.3.1 BREASTFEEDING

Breastfeeding can prolong the period of low estrogen levels postpartum [1]. The body prioritizes lactation over reproduction during breastfeeding, leading to lower estrogen levels and, consequently, vaginal dryness [3].

#### 12.3.3.2 MEDICATIONS

Certain medications, including hormonal birth control, antidepressants, antihistamines, and some blood pressure drugs, can affect vaginal lubrication. These medications can alter hormone levels or affect bodily functions that contribute to moisture production in the vagina [35].

#### 12.3.3.3 POSTPARTUM

After childbirth, women often experience hormonal fluctuations, with a significant drop in estrogen, like menopause. This decrease can lead to vaginal dryness, as the body temporarily reduces its production of estrogen during the postpartum period [25].

### 12.3.4 CANCER TREATMENTS

Treatments for cancer, such as chemotherapy and radiation therapy, especially when directed at the pelvic area, can significantly affect the ovaries and reduce estrogen production. The decrease in estrogen levels can result in vaginal dryness. Additionally, hormonal therapies for breast cancer can also contribute to this condition [9].

## 12.4 PSYCHOLOGICAL AND EMOTIONAL FACTORS

### *12.4.1 STRESS*

Stress can significantly impact the body's hormonal balance, including the production of estrogen, which is crucial for vaginal lubrication. Chronic stress can lead to an imbalance in the body's stress hormones, like cortisol, which in turn can affect sexual health and lead to symptoms like vaginal dryness [44].

### *12.4.2 ANXIETY*

Anxiety, much like stress, can disturb the steady operational process of the body's endocrine system, affecting hormonal levels and sexual function. Anxiety can also lead to psychological barriers that impact sexual arousal and lubrication, further contributing to vaginal dryness [5].

### *12.4.3 RELATIONSHIP DYNAMICS*

The quality of a woman's intimate relationships can significantly impact her sexual health. Relationship issues, such as poor communication, lack of emotional connection, or unresolved conflicts, can lead to reduced sexual arousal and subsequently to vaginal dryness [6].

## 12.5 PSYCHOSOCIAL IMPACT

### *12.5.1 EFFECT ON SEXUAL SATISFACTION*

Vaginal dryness can significantly reduce sexual satisfaction due to discomfort and pain during intercourse. This reduction in sexual pleasure can also lead to decreased sexual desire and frequency [21].

### 12.5.2 RELATIONSHIP ISSUES AND COMMUNICATION

The discomfort associated with vaginal dryness can lead to avoidance of sexual intimacy, potentially causing relationship strain. Additionally, there can be a lack of communication about this issue between partners due to embarrassment or misunderstanding [30].

### 12.5.3 EMOTIONAL WELL-BEING

Women experiencing vaginal dryness may suffer from reduced self-esteem and body image issues. This can result in feelings of inadequacy, anxiety, and depression, impacting general emotional well-being [11].

### 12.5.4 SOCIAL STIGMA AND MISCONCEPTIONS

Vaginal dryness is often surrounded by social stigma and misconceptions, which can discourage individuals from seeking help or discussing the issue openly. Many women feel isolated or believe that vaginal dryness is an inevitable and unmanageable part of aging [41].

## 12.6 TREATMENT OPTIONS

### 12.6.1 LIFESTYLE MODIFICATIONS

Vaginal dryness, a condition often associated with a decline in estrogen levels, can be effectively managed through various lifestyle modifications. Regular sexual activity is beneficial as it promotes blood flow and natural lubrication in the vagina, a fact underscored by Leiblum and Koochaki [24] in their study on the impact of vaginal dryness. The use of over-the-counter vaginal moisturizers and lubricants is another key approach, as highlighted by Edwards and Panay [13], offering immediate relief by supplementing the body's natural lubrication and reducing discomfort during intercourse.

Additionally, maintaining adequate hydration and a balanced diet rich in phytoestrogens, found in foods like soy products and flaxseeds, may help manage symptoms. This dietary approach is supported by Gandhi et al. [16], who emphasized its role in supporting overall health, including vaginal tissue health. Stress management techniques like yoga, meditation, or counseling are beneficial in regulating the body's hormonal balance, thus potentially alleviating symptoms of vaginal dryness, as suggested by Green et al. [18]. Finally, avoiding irritants such as scented soaps, douches, and certain laundry detergents is crucial, as these can further irritate the vaginal tissue, a point made by Farage et al. [14] in their comprehensive study on skin aging.

### 12.6.2 HORMONE THERAPY

Hormone therapy is a central component in the treatment of vaginal dryness, particularly for symptoms stemming from menopausal changes. Estrogen-based treatments are commonly prescribed for this purpose. These treatments can be systemic, like oral estrogen, or local, like vaginal creams, rings, or tablets, which specifically target the vaginal area with minimal systemic absorption. A key study by NAMS [41] highlights the effectiveness of these estrogen-based therapies in alleviating the symptoms of vaginal dryness by replenishing estrogen levels, thereby restoring the normal function and structure of vaginal tissue.

For those who cannot or prefer not to use hormonal treatments, nonhormonal alternatives are available. These include vaginal moisturizers and lubricants, which can provide symptomatic relief. Another nonhormonal option is ospemifene, a selective estrogen receptor modulator, which is effective in treating vaginal dryness and discomfort during intercourse. A study by Bachmann et al. [5] emphasizes the utility of ospemifene as a viable nonhormonal alternative for postmenopausal women.

### 12.6.3 INNOVATIVE APPROACHES

Innovative approaches to treating vaginal dryness, particularly those outside the realm of conventional hormone therapy, are gaining attention. These include regenerative medicine techniques for vaginal rejuvenation and the use of herbs and herbal medicines, including Ayurvedic treatments.

#### 12.6.3.1 REGENERATIVE MEDICINE AND VAGINAL REJUVENATION

##### 12.6.3.1.1 Laser Therapy

Laser therapy, specifically $CO_2$ laser therapy, is a notable regenerative medicine technique used for vaginal rejuvenation. This approach involves the use of laser energy to stimulate collagen production in the vaginal tissues, thereby improving elasticity and moisture levels. A study by Salvatore et al. [34] in the *Journal of Sexual Medicine* demonstrated the efficacy of this therapy in improving the symptoms of vaginal atrophy.

#### 12.6.3.1.2 Platelet-Rich Plasma

Another regenerative method is the use of platelet-rich plasma (PRP) injections. PRP involves injecting a concentration of a patient's platelets to accelerate the healing of injured tissues. According to a research article by Hersant et al. [19] in *Aesthetic Surgery Journal*, PRP has been found beneficial in enhancing vaginal tissue regeneration and improving symptoms of dryness.

### 12.6.3.2 HERBS AND HERBAL MEDICINES, AND AYURVEDIC MEDICINES

#### 12.6.3.2.1 Ayurvedic Remedies

Ayurvedic medicine uses a variety of herbs and treatments for managing menopausal symptoms. Commonly used herbs include Ashwagandha and Shatavari. A study by Modi et al. [28] points out the beneficial effects of these herbs in balancing hormones and improving overall women's health.

#### 12.6.3.2.2 Phytoestrogens

Herbal treatments often focus on plants with phytoestrogens, which are plant-derived compounds that mimic estrogen. Herbs such as red clover, soy, and flaxseed are commonly used. A review by Bedell et al. [8] highlights the potential of phytoestrogens in alleviating menopausal symptoms, including vaginal dryness.

### 12.6.3.3 EFFICACY, SAFETY, AND POTENTIAL SIDE EFFECTS OF TREATMENTS

The treatment of vaginal dryness encompasses various options, each with its own efficacy, safety profile, and potential side effects. Hormonal therapy, particularly estrogen-based treatments, is highly effective in alleviating symptoms of vaginal dryness, improving lubrication, and reducing discomfort during intercourse. The North American Menopause Society [40] highlights their effectiveness but also notes potential side effects like breast tenderness, nausea, and an increased risk of thrombotic events in certain women. Nonhormonal alternatives such as vaginal moisturizers and lubricants are effective for temporary relief, especially during sexual activity, and are considered safe for most women, including those who cannot use hormonal therapies [12].

Innovative treatments like laser therapy and PRP injections in regenerative medicine show promise. Salvatore et al. [34] documented the benefits of laser therapy in improving vaginal health, though concerns about long-term safety remain. Herbal and Ayurvedic medicines, with phytoestrogens and other plant-based compounds, offer alternative relief, but their efficacy and safety vary, and more rigorous studies are needed for conclusive evidence [8, 28].

## 12.7 HOLISTIC APPROACHES TO MANAGEMENT

### *12.7.1 THE IMPORTANCE OF PATIENT–PROVIDER COMMUNICATION*

A holistic approach to managing vaginal dryness underscores the importance of effective patient–provider communication. Open and empathetic dialogue is essential for accurately diagnosing the condition, understanding its impact on the patient's life, and devising a treatment plan that aligns with the patient's needs and preferences. This communication is not only about medical history and symptoms but also involves discussing sensitive topics such as sexual health and personal relationships, which are often impacted by vaginal dryness. Flynn et al. [15] emphasized the significant role of communication in patient care, particularly in sensitive areas like sexual health. Their study highlights that patients who have open lines of communication with their healthcare providers report a better understanding of their condition and treatment options. This understanding is critical for patient adherence to treatment and overall satisfaction with care. Moreover, effective communication fosters a therapeutic relationship built on trust and mutual understanding, which is particularly important in conditions like vaginal dryness that can have significant physical, emotional, and psychosocial implications. The ability of healthcare providers to engage in empathetic and nonjudgmental communication can greatly enhance the quality of care and patient outcomes.

### *12.7.2 PERSONALIZED TREATMENT PLANS*

Personalized treatment plans are a cornerstone in the holistic management of vaginal dryness, addressing the unique needs and circumstances of each individual. This personalized approach is crucial because the causes and experiences of vaginal dryness can vary greatly among women. Factors such as age, underlying health conditions, menopausal status, lifestyle, and individual symptoms must be considered when crafting a treatment plan. According to Kingsberg and Simon [21], personalized treatment plans for vaginal dryness should consider not only the physical symptoms but also the emotional and psychosocial impacts [42]. This includes considering how symptoms affect sexual function, intimacy, and quality of life. Personalized care may involve a combination of therapies such as hormonal or nonhormonal treatments, lifestyle adjustments, and even counseling or sex therapy, depending on the patient's specific symptoms, preferences, and overall health. Furthermore, Nappi and Kokot-Kierepa [30] highlighted the importance of understanding patient preferences and experiences in managing menopausal symptoms, including vaginal dryness. They emphasize that personalized care leads to better patient satisfaction and treatment adherence, ultimately improving outcomes.

### *12.7.3 INTEGRATING PHYSICAL AND EMOTIONAL CARE*

Integrating physical and emotional care is crucial in the holistic management of vaginal dryness, a condition that impacts not only physical health but also carries significant emotional and psychosocial implications. This integrated approach acknowledges that the symptoms of vaginal dryness, such as discomfort during intercourse, can lead to emotional distress, reduced self-esteem, and strain in intimate relationships.

The importance of addressing both physical and emotional aspects is highlighted by Nappi and Kokot-Kierepa [30], who emphasized that vaginal dryness can significantly impact a woman's quality of life, sexual function, and emotional well-being. Their research suggests that treatment should focus not only on alleviating physical symptoms but also on addressing related emotional and psychological issues, including anxiety, depression, and relationship challenges. According to Dennerstein et al. [10], the psychological impact of vaginal dryness is often underappreciated. They argue for a more comprehensive approach to treatment, which includes counseling and support, alongside medical interventions. This approach helps women cope with the emotional aspects of the condition, improves communication with partners, and leads to better overall treatment outcomes.

### *12.7.4 ADDRESSING UNDERLYING CAUSES*

Addressing the underlying causes of vaginal dryness is crucial for its effective management. Vaginal dryness can stem from a range of factors, including hormonal changes and lifestyle influences. Understanding these root causes is essential for developing an effective treatment plan. Hormonal changes, especially the decline in estrogen levels during menopause, are a primary cause of vaginal dryness, as highlighted by NAMS [39]. This hormonal imbalance leads to thinning and drying of the vaginal tissues, making it imperative for treatment plans to focus on hormonal regulation, whether through hormone replacement therapy or alternatives that mitigate these changes. In addition to hormonal factors, certain medications and health conditions can contribute to vaginal dryness. For instance, antidepressants, antihistamines, and some cancer treatments can adversely affect vaginal lubrication, as noted by Robinson et al. [33].

Moreover, lifestyle factors such as smoking and inadequate hydration can exacerbate the condition, underlining the need for lifestyle modifications as part of a comprehensive treatment strategy. Furthermore, psychological factors such as stress and anxiety can impact hormonal balance and exacerbate symptoms of vaginal dryness, as discussed by Dennerstein et al. [10]. Addressing these psychological components through stress management techniques or counselling can be beneficial in managing the condition holistically.

## 12.8 SUMMARY

In conclusion, vaginal dryness is a multifaceted condition with physical, emotional, and psychosocial dimensions. Its management requires a comprehensive approach that addresses not only the symptoms but also the underlying causes. Hormonal changes, particularly during menopause, are a primary factor, but other elements such as medications, lifestyle choices, and psychological factors also play significant roles. The importance of patient–provider communication cannot be overstated. It is the foundation for understanding individual patient needs and developing personalized treatment plans. These plans may include hormonal therapies, nonhormonal alternatives such as lubricants and moisturizers, or innovative approaches such as regenerative medicine techniques. Moreover, the integration of physical and emotional care is vital, as the condition can significantly impact sexual health, emotional well-being, and intimate relationships. Additionally, addressing the underlying causes, be they hormonal imbalances, side effects of medication, lifestyle factors, or psychological issues, is crucial for effective and long-lasting treatment. This holistic approach, which encompasses lifestyle modifications, stress management, and counselling, alongside medical treatments, ensures a more comprehensive and satisfying management of vaginal dryness. Ultimately, the goal is to improve the quality of life for women experiencing this condition, empowering them with knowledge and treatment options to manage their symptoms effectively. As research continues to evolve, it is hoped that awareness around vaginal dryness will increase, encouraging more women to seek the care and support they need.

## KEYWORDS

- **hormonal changes**
- **menopause**
- **psychosocial impact**
- **quality of life**
- **sexual discomfort**
- **treatment options**
- **vaginal dryness**
- **women's health**

## REFERENCES


1. Avery, M. D., & Duckett, L. (2013). Maternal and infant outcomes in the postpartum period. *Journal of Midwifery & Women's Health, 58*(6), 645–653.
2. Avis, N. E., Colvin, A., Bromberger, J. T., Hess, R., Matthews, K. A., Ory, M., & Schocken, M. (2009). Change in health-related quality of life over the menopausal transition in a multiethnic cohort of middle-aged women: Study of Women's Health Across the Nation (SWAN). *Menopause, 16*(5), 860–869.
3. Avis, N. E., Crawford, S. L., & Green, R. (2018). Vasomotor symptoms across the menopause transition: Differences among women. *Obstetrics and Gynecology Clinics, 45*(4), 629–640.
4. Bachmann, G., Bancroft, J., Braunstein, G., Burger, H., Davis, S., Dennerstein, L., & Leiblum, S. (2006). Female androgen insufficiency: The Princeton consensus statement on definition, classification, and assessment. *Fertility and Sterility, 85*(4), 1137–1146.
5. Bachmann, G., Bouchard, C., Hoppe, D., Ranganath, R., Altomare, C., Vieweg, A., & Grainger, D. (2010). Efficacy and safety of low-dose regimens of conjugated estrogens cream administered vaginally. *Menopause, 17*(4), 709–719.
6. Bancroft, J., Loftus, J., & Long, J. S. (2003). Distress about sex: A national survey of women in heterosexual relationships. *Archives of Sexual Behavior, 32*(3), 193–208.
7. Basson, R., Leiblum, S., Brotto, L., Derogatis, L., Fourcroy, J., Fugl-Meyer, K., & Schultz, W. (2003). Definitions of women's sexual dysfunction: Advocating expansion and revision. *Journal of Psychosomatic Obstetrics & Gynecology, 24*(4), 221–229.
8. Bedell, S., Nachtigall, M., & Naftolin, F. (2014). The pros and cons of plant estrogens for menopause. *Journal of the American Association of Nurse Practitioners, 26*(4), 214–221.
9. Carter, J., Lacchetti, C., Andersen, B. L., Barton, D. L., Bolte, S., Damast, S., & Wollins, D. S. (2018). Interventions to address sexual problems in people with cancer: American Society of Clinical Oncology Clinical Practice Guideline Adaptation of Cancer Care Ontario Guideline. *Journal of Clinical Oncology, 36*(5), 492–511.
10. Dennerstein, L., Dudley, E. C., & Burger, H. (2009). Are changes in sexual functioning during midlife due to aging or menopause? *Fertility and Sterility, 82*(3), 456–460.
11. Dennerstein, L., Dudley, E. C., & Burger, H. (2009). Psychological and sexual well-being in women with vulvovaginal atrophy. *Climacteric, 12*(4), 355–366.
12. Dennerstein, L., Koochaki, P., Barton, I., & Graziottin, A. (2006). Hypoactive sexual desire disorder in menopausal women: A survey of Western European women. *Journal of Sexual Medicine, 3*(2), 212–222.
13. Edwards, D., & Panay, N. (2016). Treating vulvovaginal atrophy/genitourinary syndrome of menopause: How important is vaginal lubricant and moisturizer composition? *Climacteric, 19*(2), 151–161.
14. Farage, M. A., Miller, K. W., & Maibach, H. I. (2013). Degenerative changes in aging skin. In: *Textbook of Aging Skin* (pp. 25–36). Springer-Verlag: Berlin Heidelberg.
15. Flynn, K. E., Reese, J. B., Jeffery, D. D., Abernethy, A. P., Lin, L., Shelby, R. A., & Weinfurt, K. P. (2018). Patient experiences with communication about sex during and after cancer treatment. *Psycho-Oncology, 27*(1), 19–27.

16. Gandhi, J., Chen, A., Dagur, G., Suh, Y., Smith, N., Cali, B., & Khan, S. A. (2017). Genitourinary syndrome of menopause: An overview of clinical manifestations, pathophysiology, etiology, evaluation, and management. *American Journal of Obstetrics and Gynecology, 217*(6), 704–711.
17. Goldstein, I., & Alexander, J. L. (2005). Practical aspects of diagnosis and management. *Urologic Clinics of North America, 32*(4), 469–476.
18. Green, S. M., Habib, F. W., & Smith, M. A. (2018). The impact of mindfulness meditation in promoting a culture of safety on an acute psychiatric ward. *Perspectives in Psychiatric Care, 54*(3), 358–365.
19. Hersant, B., SidAhmed-Mezi, M., Belkacemi, Y., & Rodriguez, A. (2016). Efficacy of autologous platelet-rich plasma use for orthopedic indications: A meta-analysis. *Aesthetic Surgery Journal, 36*(3), 113–123.
20. Jenkins, A., & O'Doherty, K. C. (2021). The clean vagina, the healthy vagina, and the dirty vagina: Exploring women's portrayals of the vagina in relation to vaginal cleansing product use. *Feminism & Psychology, 31*(2), 192–211.
21. Kingsberg, S. A., & Simon, J. A. (2018). The impact of vaginal atrophy on sexual health and quality of life in postmenopausal women. *Journal of Women's Health, 27*(3), 297–304.
22. Leeman, L. M., & Rogers, R. G. (2012). Sex after childbirth: Postpartum sexual function. *Obstetrics & Gynecology,* 119(3), 647–655.
23. Leiblum, S. R. (Edn.). (2006). *Principles and Practice of Sex Therapy*. Guilford Press.
24. Leiblum, S. R., & Koochaki, P. E. (2008). A review of the prevalence and impact of vaginal dryness in postmenopausal women. *Journal of Sexual Medicine, 5*(4), 1057–1064.
25. Leiblum, S. R., Koochaki, P. E., Rodenberg, C. A., Barton, I. P., & Rosen, R. C. (2006). Hypoactive sexual desire disorder in postmenopausal women: US results from the women's international study of health and sexuality (WISHeS). *Journal of Sexual Medicine*, 3(1), 212–222.
26. Louis, J. M., Bryant, A., Ramos, D., Stuebe, A., & Blackwell, S. C. (2019). Interpregnancy care. *American Journal of Obstetrics and Gynecology, 220*(1), B2–B18.
27. Mayo Clinic. (2021). *Vaginal Dryness: Symptoms and Causes*. https://www.mayoclinic.org; (accessed on 31 May 2024).
28. Modi, M., Deo, V., & Kadam, V. (2010). Ayurveda for the management of menopausal symptoms. *International Journal of Pharmaceutical Sciences and Research, 1*(6), 1–14.
29. Nappi, R. E., & Kokot-Kierepa, M. (2012). Vaginal Health: Insights, views & attitudes (VIVA)—Results from an international survey. *Climacteric, 15*(1), 36–44.
30. Nappi, R. E., & Lachowsky, M. (2010). Menopause and sexuality: Prevalence of symptoms and impact on quality of life. *Maturitas, 66*(4), 398–405.
31. National Institute on Aging (NIA). (2021). *Sex and Menopause: Treatment for Symptoms.* https://www.nia.nih.gov/health/vaginal-dryness (accessed on 31 May 2024).
32. Portman, D. J., & Gass, M. L. S. (2014). Genitourinary syndrome of menopause: New terminology for vulvovaginal atrophy from the International Society for the Study of

Women's Sexual Health and The North American Menopause Society. *Menopause, 21*(10), 1063–1068.
33. Robinson, D., Cardozo, L., Milsom, I., Pons, M. E., Kirby, M., Koelbl, H., & Vella, M. (2014). Estrogens and overactive bladder. *Neurourology and Urodynamics*, *33*(7), 1086–1091.
34. Salvatore, S., Nappi, R. E., Parma, M., Chionna, R., Lagona, F., Zerbinati, N., & Candiani, M. (2015). Sexual function after fractional microablative $CO_2$ laser in women with vulvovaginal atrophy. *Journal of Sexual Medicine*, *12*(3), 745–752.
35. Santoro, N., Epperson, C. N., & Mathews, S. B. (2015). Menopausal symptoms and their management. *Endocrinology and Metabolism Clinics*, 44(3), 497–515.
36. Shifren, J. L., & Schiff, I. (2010). Role of hormone therapy in the management of menopause. *Obstetrics & Gynecology*, *115*(4), 839–855.
37. Simon, J. A., Kokot-Kierepa, M., Goldstein, J., & Nappi, R. E. (2013). Vaginal health in the United States - results from the vaginal health: Insights, views & attitudes survey. *Menopause, 20*(10), 1043–1048.
38. Sturdee, D. W., & Panay, N. (2010). Recommendations for the management of postmenopausal vaginal atrophy. *Climacteric, 13*(6), 509–522.
39. The North American Menopause Society. (2013). The 2012 hormone therapy position statement. *Menopause, 20*(3), 330–356.
40. The North American Menopause Society. (2017). The 2017 hormone therapy position statement. *Menopause*, *24*(7), 728–753.
41. The North American Menopause Society. (2020). The 2020 hormone therapy position statement. *Menopause, 27*(9), 976–992.
42. Thomas, H. N., & Thurston, R. C. (2016). A biopsychosocial approach to women's sexual function and dysfunction at midlife: A narrative review. *Maturitas*, *87*, 49–60.
43. WebMD. (2023). *Understanding Vaginal Dryness Treatment*. https://www.webmd.com; (accessed on 31 May 2024).
44. West, S. L., D'Aloisio, A. A., Agans, R. P., Kalsbeek, W. D., & Borisov, N. N. (2008). Prevalence of low sexual desire and hypoactive sexual desire disorder in a nationally representative sample of US women. *Archives of Internal Medicine*, *168*(13), 1441–1449.

# CHAPTER 13

# Impact of Pesticides on Neurological and General Health of Women

KHURSHEED AHMAD WANI, UFAQ SUMERA, and
JUNAID AHMAD MALIK*

*Corresponding author

## ABSTRACT

Neurological health impacts have diverse reasons, and among them, pesticide exposure is considered to be one of the main reasons. Women and children are considered vulnerable to the pesticide poisoning at very low doses. The treatment for the same is very limited, and there is a hope that botanicals may prove very useful in the treatment of diseases caused by pesticides. This chapter will review the different types of neurological and general health impacts to women due to pesticides and the role of botanicals in treating these diseases.

## 13.1 INTRODUCTION

For the most part, pests like weeds, insects, and fungus (plant diseases) may be managed with the use of pesticides. Pesticides are often categorized as herbicides, fumigants, insecticides, or fungicides depending on their intended purpose or target organism. Organophosphates (OPs), organochlorines (OCs), carbamates (CBAs), and pyrethroids (PYRs) are common chemical categories for insecticides. Many pesticides, or combinations of pesticides, are often introduced to individuals in a

Holistic Approaches for Women's Sustainable Health, Volume 1: Foundations, Innovations, Challenges, and Management. Megh R. Goyal, Anamika Chauhan, and Junaid Ahmad Malik (Eds)


DOI: 10.1201/9781779641632-16

sequential or simultaneous fashion. It is challenging to determine the effects of individual agents due to the high degree of correlation between these exposures, especially within functional or chemical groups [8].

Poverty, lack of knowledge, and education all contribute to the high rates of pesticide poisoning and suicide in developing nations. An estimated 300,000 people are poisoned by pesticides each year, with over 250,000 losing their lives as a result. There have been several reports of cases of pesticide poisoning from various nations, including India. India is fourth in the world for pesticide usage and second in Asia for pesticide production, mostly due to the country's reliance on traditional agricultural practices. In contrast to developing nations that impose a greater acute risk of poisoning, India mostly uses insecticides rather than other types of pesticides (such as herbicides, weedicides, etc.). The majority of the reported cases of poisoning leading to suicide in various parts of India are likely to be associated with OP pesticides, including monocrotophos and others. According to Zhang et al., there has been new evidence linking pesticide exposure on the job to impaired neurobehavioral function and increased mental illness in Chinese agricultural laborers [32]. There are many types of pesticides, such as insecticides, weedicides, fungicides, rodenticides, and fumigants, which are chemical or chemical mixtures that are often used to deter insects, weeds, fungus, and rodents. There are many types of insecticides, including PYRs, OCs, CBAs, and OPs, all of which disrupt the insects' neurological systems and kill them. Overuse of pesticides increases the likelihood of exposure, which may occur either accidentally or as a result of working with the chemicals in production, application, harvesting, crop handling, or public health purposes. The widespread and careless use of pesticides in many contexts, including homes, farms, veterinary clinics, and workplaces and parks, makes human exposure to these chemicals very likely. It is not uncommon for people who are suicidal to knowingly consume the pesticide [3].

A significant form of exposure is the contamination of food by crops consistently treated with pesticides. This is because these pesticides accumulate in the tissue, milk, and food products of animals. While this is going on, it is concerning because exposed peoples biological tissues and food contain large amounts of OP and PYR residues and their metabolites, which might have negative health impacts. Dewan et al. [8] showed that newborns' birth weight, crown heel length, head circumference, mid-arm circumference, and ponderal index are affected by high amounts of OPs in the mother's blood, cord blood, and breast milk from the placenta. Pregnant mothers and preschoolers have had PYR metabolites found in their urine. Dosage, exposure route, duration, and metabolic rate are potential factors in pesticide toxicity. It may take some time for the long-term effects of conditions, including infertility, birth abnormalities, endocrine disruption, neurological diseases, and cancer, to become apparent. When working with pesticides, whether spraying, mixing, or loading, farm workers may experience both short-term and long-term exposure. As a result of not knowing the harmful effects of pesticides and not wearing protective gear while applying them, the exposure pattern became very high [12].

Women may be more exposed to pesticides via other agricultural duties, even when they do not apply the pesticides themselves. Working in their own fields or for a floriculture or horticulture company involves tasks such as weeding, harvesting, planting, or packaging. Indirect exposure to pesticides may occur in households where women are expected to do domestic duties, in addition to direct exposure that occurs during field labor. Additional sources of exposure include pesticide storage, disposal of empty pesticide containers, prevention of malaria, spray drift, and the duty for cleaning contaminated equipment and clothes.

According to these interactions, women face more risks in the home and in agriculture. The lack of knowledge, information, or training, and safety equipment that comes with being poor makes their already limited resources even more inadequate. In addition, many women operate in fields that employ pesticides, and they do so without adequate safety gear. Pesticides that are both highly hazardous and long-lasting are used in agriculture due to market liberalization, privatization of agricultural inputs, and the lack of effective enforcement of pesticide regulations throughout much of Africa. These pesticides, which are inexpensive and widely utilized in African agriculture—a sector in which women play a significant role—continue to be accessible illegally via parallel open markets [18].

Another biological difference between the sexes is that women are more easily damaged by pesticides. Hormonal changes after menopause, pregnancy, or breastfeeding, as well as increased amounts of adipose tissue, make women more vulnerable to pesticide dangers, which may cause acute to chronic illnesses. Babies whose moms were exposed to the substance when they were pregnant or nursing may also suffer from developmental delays and other health problems. According to Bai et al., neurotoxins are manufactured or otherwise foreign chemicals that harm the CNS, peripheral nerves, and sensory organs in a variety of ways, including structural, biochemical, and functional damage. Thus, sensory, motor, and cognition problems may be caused by exposure to neurotoxins. Pesticides are among the neurotoxic compounds that induce neurocognitive impairments in agricultural workers more often than any other. According to Muñoz-Quezada et al. [19], pesticide exposure in the workplace without proper protective gear is recognized as a problem in public health. According to Muñoz-Quezada et al. [19], the demand from the food business and the rise in insect resistance have caused pesticide sales and applications to surge globally. This results in a greater risk of exposure for workers, who are already at increased risk due to factors such as low levels of education, inadequate training, low-risk perception, inadequate personal protective equipment uses, unsafe working conditions, lack of supervision, and inherent biological susceptibility. Occupational diseases related to acute or chronic pesticide poisoning have been reported in the literature. Exposure to pesticides at low levels over time may create chronic neurological consequences, even if large concentrations are necessary to cause acute poisoning or death. Pesticides such as PYRs, CBAs, OCs, and OPs are widely used. Most of these pesticides have an effect on how ion channels in neurons work or how synapses communicate with one another [22].

There has been enough evidence that pesticides, particularly OPs and OCs, have negative impacts on neurodevelopment and neurocognitive function since the latter decade of the 20th century. OC insecticides are now illegal on a global scale because of their extreme toxicity and environmental persistence. Despite their decreased persistence, OP and CBA insecticides are nonetheless highly or moderately dangerous and are subject to stricter regulations for their sale and usage. Furthermore, their usage has been somewhat reduced owing to the stringent regulations imposed by industrialized nations on imported agri-food items concerning pesticide residues.

However, in the middle of the 20th century, scientists altered the natural chrysanthemum pyrethrins insecticides utilized by many European, African, and Asian nations to produce synthetic PYR pesticides. As an ostensibly less harmful and less persistent alternative to CBAs and OPs, they have recently emerged. The majority of their current sales come from domestic usage, where they are most often employed to combat pests such as pediculosis in people and mites in domestic animals, as well as widespread use in agriculture. Epidemiological studies have linked environmental exposure to these pesticides to worse neurocognitive function, and new research has shown negative neurological effects in animals [23].

Because of their supposedly low toxicity to humans, PYR insecticides such as deltamethrin, permethrin, and cypermethrin are often marketed and suggested for use around the house. But new research shows that they are not completely safe for humans to consume; in fact, they are neurotoxic compounds with a laundry list of negative effects: These three pesticides have different effects on the body: permethrin on fertility, the immune system, enzymatic activity, cardiovascular health, and hepatic metabolism; deltamethrin on inflammation, nephrotoxicity, and hepatotoxicity; and alpha-cypermethrin on diabetes and lipids [27].

PYRs may be categorized into several levels based on the danger classifications proposed by the World Health Organization [31]: Group II (yellow label) is moderately dangerous, Group III (blue label) is significantly harmful, and Group IV (red label) is severely hazardous. PYRs work in the neurological system by interacting with sodium channels and causing neuronal cells to undergo extended depolarization. Acute intoxication symptoms help differentiate between two classes of PYRs: (1) Type I, which alters the opening and shutting of sodium channels in neuronal membranes, and (2) Type II, which does not. It produces systemic tremors, violent conduct, hypersensitivity, and motor ataxia; (2) Type II, which impacts the chloride, sodium, and GABA channels, leading to salivation and motor dysfunction.

## 13.2 PATHWAYS

Pathways of women's exposure to pesticides are as follows.

### *13.2.1 OCCUPATIONAL EXPOSURE*

Little is known about the pesticide exposure that women face on the job, and studies that do exist mostly focus on male farmers and agricultural laborers. The gender division of labor and the societal construction of pesticide application as men's job contribute to the belief that only males are occupationally exposed to pesticides, which is why women's exposure to these chemicals does not get the attention it needs. In other parts of sub-Saharan Africa, however, women do the same thing when it comes to applying pesticides. Research conducted in four randomly chosen parishes in the Tororo area of Eastern Uganda found that 80% of families led by women used pesticides on their crops. One research found that 38% of the women who grew coffee trees in the two districts that make up Uganda's Mt. Elgon area used pesticides [21]. Another place where women are discovered applying pesticides is in the Brong Ahafo area of Ghana, where 18% of the population consists of women. The fact that 45.6% of the women surveyed in Kwa-Zulu-Natal, South Africa, admitted to directly handling pesticides on their subsistence farms provides another pertinent example. All 68 women who were interviewed for this study lived in the Ashanti area of Ghana and worked as pesticide applicators for their vegetable crops. Zseleczky et al. [33] state that in the Brong Ahafo area of Ghana, pesticide application is typically seen as a male-dominated activity. However, it is worth noting that some women have admitted to applying pesticides to their own tomatoes. Similarly, 94% of the women in that part of Ghana were engaged in high-exposure occupations, such as pesticide mixing for use on vegetable fields (Figure 13.1).

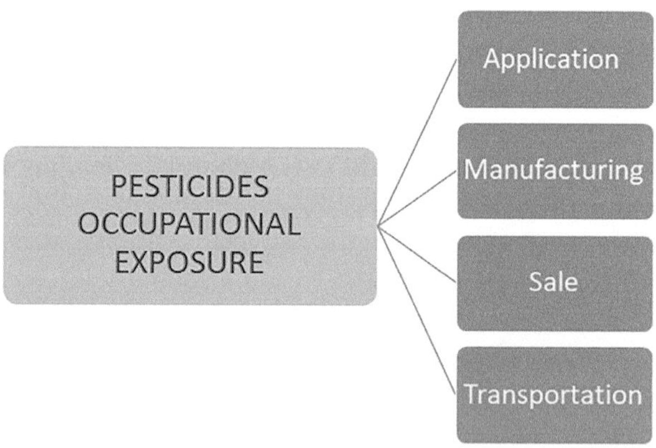


**FIGURE 13.1** Pesticides occupational exposure.

Unfortunately, the tools and insecticides used by women who participate in direct applications are often tainted. In Uganda, for instance, women often use traditional application techniques, such as physically sweeping with a grass-bristled broom and a plastic basin, which might lead to worker contamination. Potentially dangerous chemicals may also pose the most threats to these ladies. To illustrate the point, this farm makes use of pesticides such as the moderately dangerous endosulfan and the obsolete or unclassified profenofos, which are believed to be neurotoxins and cholinesterase inhibitors, respectively. Pesticide residues on soil, foliage, or crops may expose women more than men, even when they do not handle the pesticides themselves. Women were seen weeding in the field during the peak spraying season on smallholder farms in Ghana, Mali, and Uganda. This means that they are at significantly increased risk of exposure to the high residues carried as aerosols. Similarly, women in horticulture farms in Kenya and flower farms in Ethiopia were hired for short-term and supposedly dangerous jobs such as planting, weeding, thinning, disease checking, harvesting, packaging, or transportation. Due to the informal nature of many women's jobs in these fields, they are much less likely to have access to formal education and training opportunities than their male counterparts. Because of both biological and societal reasons, women may have negative health effects as a result of the widespread use of pesticides in the floriculture and horticulture industries. More knowledge-based and gender-oriented research and interventions are needed, since all of the results shown in this study show that even women who do not apply pesticides directly may be exposed *via* other agricultural duties [20].

### 13.2.2 NONOCCUPATIONAL EXPOSURE

Women face additional risks at home, where they may wash pesticide-contaminated clothes and equipment, in addition to the risks they face on the job as pesticide applicators or farm laborers. When women or members of their households wear dirty clothes while working in the field, they often bring them home to wash. Due to the fact that women often bring pesticide residue on their clothes home, this might add to their exposure. The potential for exposure via household pesticides is another significant route to investigate. Reusing empty pesticide containers for home use raises serious concerns about the exposure of women. Some Tanzanian women have found creative ways to recycle old pesticide containers, turning them into containers for oil, water, milk, wheat, salt, and even kerosene. Water was collected and stored by women in South Africa using repurposed vessels. The kids were caught consuming water from the empty bottles. Women sometimes reuse the big barrels that were used for mixing pesticides after tomato picking for water storage in their houses. Worries about the exposure of women to pesticides used in the home are also widespread, but there is a dearth of data on the subject. Pesticides are sprayed on grain after harvest in Ghana, according to studies, so it looks fresh and appealing to buyers. Women are disproportionately responsible for applying pesticides to areas around their houses. There is a danger to those handling the grain, merchants, and consumers if pesticide residues infect food sources. Pesticide residues in the house are especially worrisome for children, whose immune systems are still developing. Children spend a lot of time at home, are more prone to hand-to-mouth behavior, absorb chemicals at a greater rate, and have a reduced capacity to metabolize and expel chemicals [10].

Most women might be exposed to malaria via DDT, even though its usage has decreased in several African nations owing to resistance. Since women often spend the majority of their time in and around the house taking care of domestic duties, they are at increased risk of being exposed to indoor spraying. Breast milk from women in malaria-endemic regions has been shown to have higher quantities of DDT residues and its metabolites. Another way that women might be exposed to pesticides is *via* spray drifts, which can happen on farms where women labor in the fields or even reach their homes. Because of the heavy burdens they bear at home and in the fields, women are disproportionately vulnerable to the contamination of their food, water, and clothes that might occur when spray drift reaches their homes. Researchers in South Africa's Western Cape found that farmwomen had asthma and other allergy problems, which they linked in part to a drift that made its way to their homes [30].

## 13.3 HEALTH IMPACTS OF PESTICIDE EXPOSURE

Although it is difficult to show direct correlations, exposure to pesticides, whether at work or elsewhere, has been linked to many health issues in women. Garcia [11] states that although the dangers of pesticides are the same for both sexes, women are more vulnerable due to inherent biological distinctions between the sexes. Due to hormonal changes that occur during menopause, pregnancy, and lactation, as well as a higher average amount of adipose tissue in women, women are more susceptible to the harmful effects of pesticide absorption from polluted environments than men.

Evidence suggests that women who were not applicators of pesticides had comparable or worse health issues than males, contradicting the idea that the health implications of pesticides are greatest for those who handle them directly. Women in Zimbabwean commercial farms had an abnormally high rate of cholinesterase and central nervous system problems; women in Kenyan flower farms had an abnormally high rate of cardiovascular disease and gastrointestinal disease, respectively, due to exposure to OPs and CBAs, in contrast to men, who were all pesticide applicators. As a result of their employment or entry into sprayed fields, these women come into constant contact with pesticide residues. Along with a lack of access to safety gear, they lacked proper training on the dangers of pesticides [7].

Studies examining the negative effects of pesticides on the health of women in sub-Saharan Africa are few, especially when compared to the proportion of women working in agriculture in this region. According to research conducted in rural South Africa, Heeren et al. [12] found that OPs and CBAs were a cause of birth malformations in women who were active in farming, who reused empty pesticide containers as water storage, and who dipped cattle to avoid ticks. Exposure to OCs has been associated with an increased risk of cancer, diabetes, hypertension, and reproductive dysfunction in female horticulture workers in Tanzania. Several pesticides from the World Health Organization classes II and Ib were found to be present in South African workplaces, including methamidophos, monocrotophos, methyl carbamate, deltamethrin, cypermethrin, dimethoate, lambda-cyhalothrin, paraquat, and glyphosate, according to another study. Women who are pregnant or who spend a lot of time in greenhouses are more likely to have complications during their pregnancies, such as miscarriages, early births, and spontaneous abortions. Pregnant women who were exposed to pesticides had a higher risk of having infants with abnormalities. Because many pesticides are endocrine disrupters, hormone-related malignancies disproportionately affect women. It is common for women to develop hormone-related malignancies, including tumors of the thyroid, endometrium, ovary, bone, and breast. While doing research outside of Africa, we came across other instances of women suffering from chronic ailments. Spouses of pesticide applicators have a higher risk of cancer, according to reports, which is associated with women's exposure to OPs. Additionally, it is said that OP exposure during pregnancy is associated with placental and fetal problems, as well as preterm births, miscarriages, and disruptions of the endocrine system. It is very uncommon for OPs (such as chlorpyrifos), PYRs, and herbicides (such as 2,4-D) to be present during pregnancy, which may lead to problems and negative effects on the developing kid and the fetus, including miscarriages and stillbirths. More instances of elevated thyroid hormone levels in women residing in highly polluted areas have been reported, and increased pesticide levels in the urine of wives of pesticide applicators who were present in a field during the application of 2,4-D have been reported (Figure 13.2) [4].

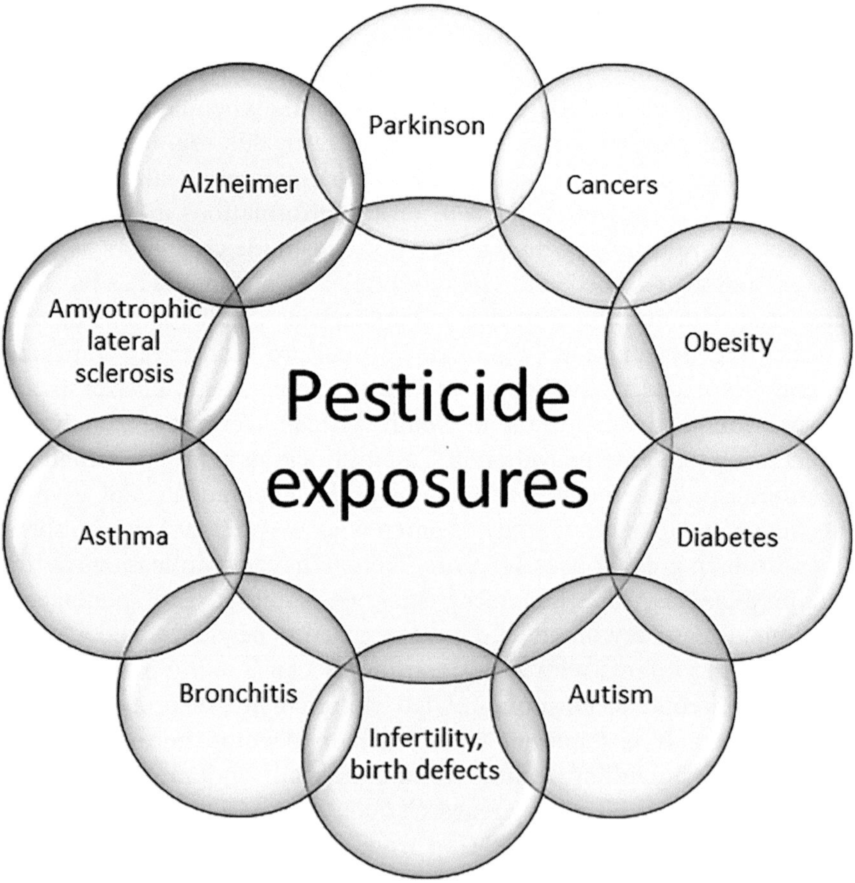


**FIGURE 13.2** Health impacts of pesticide exposure.

## 13.4 IMPACT ON REPRODUCTIVE HEALTH

During the third trimester of pregnancy, 75% of French women did not smoke, 44% were nulliparous, 43% had finished high school, and the average age of pregnant women was 29 in 2003 (as reported in a nationwide perinatal survey). Although they only made up a tiny fraction of Brittany's pregnant women, the PELAGIE research found that, compared to the rest of the country, the women who participated had higher levels of education and smoked less [26]. The research did find recognized risk variables for birth weight and head circumference outcomes, despite the enrolment bias that implies the mothers included in the study were likely healthy (Figure 13.3).

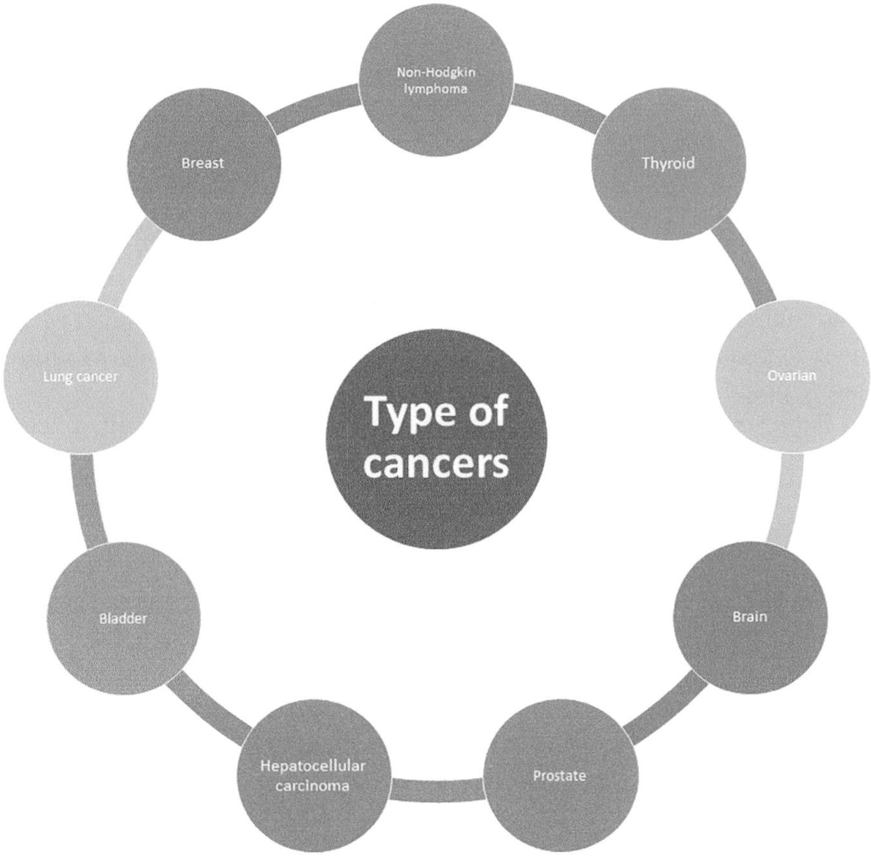


**FIGURE 13.3** Reproductive health effects on women due to pesticides.

The incidence of HPE (holoprosencephaly) was found to be two times higher in cases where mothers reported using personal insect repellents both before and throughout pregnancy. There is a lack of data on environmental exposures and HPE, despite the growing body of evidence implicating pesticides in the complicated etiologies of birth abnormalities. However, such studies have examined characteristics such as the mother's work and her state or country of residency during pregnancy. Although exposure rates were modest overall, they were much lower for mothers, and neither paternal nor maternal occupational exposures to pesticides were linked to HPE in this research. In contrast, we did discover that those who reported living next to a field had a higher risk of HPE. In addition, while the exposure rates were low and the confidence interval was broad, there were weak relationships between HPE and household herbicide exposures during pregnancy [5]. The neurotoxicity of pesticides, their propensity to be more harmful to the developing brain, and their links to other birth abnormalities are some of the reasons why pesticides might be teratogens in HPE. Thus, anencephaly, which may include microcephaly but is pathophysiologically and clinically distinct from HPE, is one of many severe congenital brain abnormalities connected to prenatal exposure to pesticides. Orofacial clefts, which are connected to pesticide exposure in the mother, often occur with HPE and have been shown to be associated with sonic hedgehog signaling in animal models. This research adds to the existing evidence linking pesticides to serious fetal abnormalities by suggesting that pesticide exposure during pregnancy increases the likelihood of HPE [9].

Exposure to pesticides and acaricides used on pets, as well as pest management agents used around the home, was associated with an increased risk of HPE. We saw no changes in risk when we limited the study to instances where the mother personally applied these chemicals. It is interesting to note that exposures to pesticides for pets were related to an elevated risk for HPE. It is suggested that the risks do not only come from the mother applying the products herself, but also from other household members using them, which could lead to higher levels of pesticide residue in dust and other home environment components. This raises important questions regarding the origins of pesticide exposures. Evidence suggests that pesticides used in homes might cause higher-than-recommended levels of residues to linger in the air and on surfaces for up to two weeks after a single application.

Future research should look at pesticide use in food, since this was not addressed in this one, and might be a major exposure factor. Studies evaluating pesticide biomarkers in serum during pregnancy would be ideal for identifying parent chemicals and determining the magnitude of exposures to determine dose-dependent associations with risk for HPE. This would complement epidemiological and animal studies that investigate exposures to specific pesticides and co-ingredients. It would be wise for future HPE research to look at potential links to pesticide mixture exposures, since they have been linked to an increased risk of aberrant development, such as neural tube abnormalities, compared to isolated exposures [29].

Furthermore, results should be carefully evaluated due to the fact that exposure evaluation depended on retrospective reporting, which may be influenced by both reporting bias and recollection bias. This is especially true for serious birth abnormalities as HPE. It was believed that the recollection bias would be equally skewed across the cases and controls, leading to findings that were biased toward the null; hence, WBS controls were used to try to control for the latter [6]. It was difficult to utilize questionnaire data to evaluate certain windows using a retrospective approach, while women were more likely to report exposures throughout all windows of pregnancy, according to the findings. The length of time between the administration of the proband and survey completion was greater in the HPE cohort, which is one variation between the characteristics of the cases and controls. Because of this disparity, it is possible that the two groups' propensity for accurate recollection of events occurring during pregnancy is differently hindered. In order to reduce the impact of this disparity, all multiple regression models included the duration from delivery to survey as a covariate. In spite of these caveats, HPE and other congenital malformations continue to pose serious health and public health problems, including high rates of fetal death and morbidity. Prospective studies of preconception and early pregnancy outcomes are challenging and expensive since birth abnormalities are rare and complex. This is only a preliminary examination of possible correlations; more investigation into topics like exposure biomarkers and prospective designs is required [7].

## 13.5 NEUROBEHAVIORAL, NEUROMOTOR, AND NEUROCOGNITIVE EFFECTS

Outcomes associated with PYR exposure were not found in four trials, which means that there was no evidence of impacts or connections with neurobehavioral, neuromotor, or neurocognitive outcomes. Some studies have limitations, such as a small sample size [16], the lack of a control group in one of the manuscripts [32], and the possibility of memory bias in another study that relied solely on patients' own reports of their pesticide use in the past [28]. In a study conducted by Ismail et al. [14], neurobehavioral performance, sociodemographic variables, neurological symptoms, and exposure to PYRs were investigated. The researchers used cholinesterase levels to measure OP exposure. A number of executive and motor speed/coordination tasks, including the symbol digit test delay, tapping (TAP) with a nonpreferred hand, and TAP with alternate hands, showed that an applicator performed poorly. Problems with memory and motor speed/coordination were linked to khat eating.

Huang et al. [13] examined the effects of PYR exposure on conventional nerve conduction in Chinese applicators, although they only found a correlation with a reduction in ulnar nerve conduction after brief exposure. Kori et al. [15] discovered that among agricultural workers in India who are chronically exposed to high and medium levels of pesticides, the majority of workers who keep pesticides (PYRs and others) at home had signs of stress ($p < 0.01$) and anxiety ($p < 0.05$). The majority of these workers employed PYRs as pesticides; 7% of farmers used a very risky PYR, and 34% used a moderately dangerous one. When comparing agricultural workers with high and medium chronic pesticide exposure, the negative health consequences were more pronounced in the former group (19.7% high depression, 10.3% medium anxiety, and 41.6% high sleep problems, compared to 32.7% and 36.2% medium, respectively). Importantly, this research just used bivariate chi-square tests to determine whether there was a correlation between exposure and symptoms.

Most farmers used PYRs (71.1% full-time and 73.3% part-time), although full-time workers also used OPs, according to another study involving male and female agricultural workers [17]. The percentage of full-time employees with an abnormal neuromotor diagnostic was 5.22%, whereas the percentage of part-time employees was 8.63%. Out of 139 part-time farmers, three exhibited impairment in the cerebellum. Thus, neuromotor symptoms were identical among full-time and part-time farmers due to equivalent exposure to PYR insecticides. The lack of a control group that was not exposed to pesticides was a major flaw in this study. However, PYR exposure was shown in just one study with South African women using urine concentrations of particular metabolites. This study used the Q16 questionnaire to assess neurological symptoms. Farm women were more likely to have all Q16 symptoms than city women, according to this paper. There was a positive correlation between three PYR metabolites (*cis*-DCCA, *trans*-DCCA, and DBCA) and three Q16 symptoms (reading difficulties, note-taking difficulties, and buttoning issues); however, these associations might be due to chance since numerous comparisons were conducted. Odds ratio = 8.93; 95% CI = 1.71–46.5 were the highest connection for a PYR metabolite between buttoning issues and DBCA.

van Wendel et al. [25] concluded with a comparison of neurobehavioral and neurotonic functioning results with urine metabolites of PYRs from three communities in Costa Rica. The children of agricultural workers living near or working in large- and small-scale banana plantations were included in the study. Processing speed scores were shown to be worse in those with higher amounts of 3-PBA, particularly in females. Research on the link between PYR pesticide exposure and neurological effects is limited, but what little there is confirms the dangers that workers face on the job and children whose parents work in agriculture face health risks as well. In 66% of the studies included in this meta-analysis, people working in agriculture or their children exposed to PYR pesticides showed signs of impaired neurobehavioral, neuromotor, or neurocognitive function, most commonly related to issues with processing speed and attention. Motor coordination-related neurobehavioral function is impacted by other sleep-related neurological changes and peripheral nervous system responses. Neurobehavioral abnormalities and other health issues are more likely to occur when other harmful pesticides, such as herbicides and OPs, are exposed at the same time [5].

Additional research has looked into the neurobehavioral effects of PYR exposure in children and the general population [26]. It has also compared the levels of PYR metabolites in schoolchildren with similar studies, revealing that the risk is also rising in the nonoccupational population [19]. Research on this pesticide should be intensified, according to the papers included in this review. It has been promoted by the agrochemical industry as a safer alternative to traditional methods of controlling and eliminating insect pests in both urban and rural settings.

Additionally, PYR sales have been on the rise recently, with the product being positioned as a safer alternative to pesticides like OPs, which pose a greater threat to human health. Neurobehavioral and neurodevelopmental disorders may be caused by low-dose OP exposure over time, as has been shown in several studies for over 20 years. The quality of life of both children and adults is affected, and they contribute to environmental pollution [1]. Evidence suggests that they are also carcinogenic, genotoxic, and associated with immunological and reproductive changes.

There is evidence that PYR exposure on the job poses a danger to the neurobehavioral health of agricultural workers, and the majority of the research in this area is of moderate or high quality (83%). In addition to studying the effects of other dangerous pesticides like OPs, further research is needed to assess the long-term exposure to PYRs using biomarkers and the neurological outcomes using validated neurobehavioral and neuromotor tests. To address the issue of neurotoxic relationships, the real-life risk simulation method could be used as an auxiliary tool to decrease the number of animal studies and the high expense of human population-based longitudinal studies. This would speed up the delivery of evidence, which in turn would enable authorities to take swift action and implement policies to control pesticide use [24]. The sale of PYRs and other pesticides should be regulated more strictly, workers should be trained on their safe use, and potential risks to human health should be monitored. This is based on the assumption that PYR use is increasing rapidly, outpacing the scientific evidence regarding its effects on human health and the environment.

It is recommended that future epidemiological studies evaluating neuro outcomes include brain functioning metrics such as EEG recordings or functional magnetic resonance imaging. With these tools, in addition to the traditional neurobehavioral and neurocognitive assessments, we can learn more about the effects of long-term PYR exposure on human brain activity. Research on the impact of OP exposure on the structure of the brain and the cognitive functioning of children and adolescents has previously made use of several of these neuroimaging techniques. Lastly, we think it would be a good idea to explore how microRNAs are changed as a result of pesticide exposure in the workplace and Parkinson's disease, as well as other neurological disorders and cancers [2] (Table 13.1).

**TABLE 13.1** Herbs for Treatment of Diseases Caused by Pesticides

| S. No. | Name of Plant | Diseases That Can Be Treated |
|---|---|---|
| | **General health disorders** | |
| a | *Emblica officinalis*, *Ephedra sinica*, *Ephedra trifurca*, *Ephedra nevadensis*, *Eucalyptus* spp., *Foeniculum vulgare*, *Ginkgo biloba*, *Gnaphalium* spp., *Lippia dulcis*, *Lobelia inflate*, *Mentha pulegium*, *Origanum* spp., *Talauma mexicana*, *Thea sinensis*, *Theobroma cacao*, *Tussilago farfara*, *Verbascum thapsus* | Asthma |
| b | *Echinacea purpurea*, *Andrographic paniculata*, *Allium sativum*, *Panax quinquefolius* | Bronchitis |
| c | *Punica granatum*, *Matricaria chamomilla*, *Vitex agnus-castus*, *Withania somnifera*, *Trifolium pratense*, *Camellia sinensis*, *Phoenix Dactylifera*, *Cinnamomum cassia* and *Cinnamomum verum*, *Foeniculum Vulgare*, *Glycyrrhiza glabra* | Infertility |
| e | *Ginkgo biloba* and *Withania somnifera* | Hyperactivity disorder |
| f | *Chamomillae anthodium*, *Calendulae flos*, *Hamamelis virginiana* L., *Hamamelidis folium*, *Aloe barbadensis* Mill., *Althaea officinalis* L., *Avenae fructus*, *Avenae stramentum*, *Symphyti radix*, *Millefolii herba*, *Plantago lanceolata* L., *Salvia officinalis* L., *Hyperici herba*, *Oenotherae oleum*, *Juglandis folium*, *Trigonellae foenugraeci semen* | Rashes, blisters, skin irritations |
| g | *Foeniculum vulgare*, *Ruta graveolens*, *Emblica officinalis*, *Terminalia chebula*, *Peganum harmala*, *Zingiber officinalis*, *Ferula assa-foetida*, *Rheum ribes*, and *Terminalia bellerica* | Blindness |
| h | *Zingiber officinale* Roscoe, *Elettaria cardamomum* Maton, *Matricaria chamomilla*, *Mentha piperita* L. | Nausea |
| i | *Zingiber officinale* Roscoe, *Curcuma longa*, *Prunus dulcis*, *Crocus sativus* | Dizziness |
| j | *Berberis aristata*, *Potentilla tormentilla*, *Ceratonia siliqua*, *Malus domestica*, *Creosote bush*, *Psidium guajava* L., *Atropa belladonna*, *Phaseolis vulgaris* | Diarrhea |
| k | *Momordica charantia*, *Trigonella foenum*, *Gymnema sylvestre*, *Hoodia gordonii*, *Opuntia* spp., *Artemisia dracunculus* L., *Allium sativum*, *Ginkgo biloba*, *Aloe vera* | Diabetes |
| l | *Rhizoma coptidis*, *Panax ginseng* C. A. Mey, *Radix Lithospermi*, *Ephedra sinica* Stapf., *Rheum palmatum* L., *Astragalus membranaceus* (Fisch.), *Carthamus tinctorius* L. (Hong Hua), *Ganoderma lucidum* | Obesity |
| | **Cancers** | |
| a | *Prunella vulgaris*, *Sophora flavescens*, *Scutellaria baicalensis*, *Salvia miltiorrhiza*, and *Hedyotis diffusa* | NonHodgkin lymphoma |
| b | *Ginseng biloba*, *Allium sativum*, *Curcuma longa*, *Curcuma longa*, *Echinacea*, *Arctium lappa*, *Nigella sativa* | Breast cancer |
| c | *Polyalthia longifolia*, *Cymbopogon citratus*, *Litchi chinensis*, *Maytenus royleanus*, *Sutherlandia frutescens*, *Acanthopanax trifoliatus*, *Azadirachta indica*, *Ipomoea batatus* | Prostate cancer |

**TABLE 13.1** *(Continued)*

| S. No. | Name of Plant | Diseases That Can Be Treated |
|---|---|---|
| d | *Rasagenthi lehyam*, *Berberis vulgaris* L., *Catharanthus roseus*, *Handroanthus impetiginosa*, *Taxus baccata* var., *Cannabis sativa*, *Taxus brevifolia*, *Podophyllum peltatum*, *Nothapodytes foetida* | Lung cancer |
| e | *Solanum nigrum* L., *Curcuma longa* | Bladder cancer |
| f | *Curcuma aromatic*, *Vitis vinifera*, *Arachis hypogaea*, *Berries*, *Silybum marianum* | Hepatocellular carcinoma |
| g | *Rhizoma coptidis*, *Folium isatidis*, *Acidum citricum*, *Radix stellariae*, *Trifolium fragiferum* | Stomach cancer |
| h | *Coptis chinensis*, *Berberis wilsonae* Hemsl. et Wils, *Pseudolarix amabilis*, *Lithospermum erythrorhizon* | Thyroid cancer |
| i | *Phyllanthus emblica*, *Vaccinium myrtillus*, *Zingiber officinale* Roscoe, *Taxus brevifolia*, *Withania somnifera*, *Curcuma longa* | Ovarian cancer |
| j | *Curcuma longa* L., *Zingiber officinale* Roscoe, *Allium sativum* L., *Trigonella foenum-graecum* L., *Sesamum indicum*, *Linum usitatissimum* L. | Colorectal cancer |
| | **Neurological disorders** | |
| a | *Ginkgo biloba*, *Withania somnifera*, *Curcuma longa*, *Bacopa monnieri*, *Convolvulus pluricaulis*, *Evolvulus alsinoides* | Alzheimer's disease |
| b | *Ginkgo biloba*, *Withania somnifera*, *Manasamitrav vataka*, *Galphimia glauca* | Anxiety |
| c | *Humulus lupulus* L., *Piper methysticum* G. Forst, *Lavandula angustifolia* Mill., *Melissa officinalis* L., *Passiflora incarnata* L., *Mentha aquatica* L. and *Mentha spicata* L., *Crocus sativus* L., *Valeriana officinalis* L. | Depression and stress |
| d | *Centella asiatica*, *Ampelopsis grossedentata*, green tea, *Picrorhi zarhizoma*, *Cornus officinalis*, *Radix astragali*, *Liliaceae allium* | Amyotrophic lateral sclerosis |
| e | *Withania somnifera*, *Curcuma longa*, *Convolvulus pluricaulis*, *Centella asiatica*, *Celastrus paniculatus*, *Nardostachys jatamansi*, *Coriandrum sativum*, *Ficus carica* | Dementia |
| f | *Veratrum viride*, *Stachys officinalis*, *Caulophyllum thalictroides*, *Piper methysticum*, *Viscum* sp., *Artemisia vulgaris*, *Chimaphila umbellata*, *Scutellaria laterifolia* and *Scutellaria baicalensis*, *Valeriana officinalis* | Epilepsy and seizures |
| g | *Ginkgo biloba*, *Zingiber officinale*, *Curcuma longa*, *Hypericum perforatum*, *Valeriana officinalis*, *Vaccinium macrocarpon*, *Nigella sativa*, *Piper methysticum*, *Crocus sativus*, *Panax ginseng*, *Boswellia papyrifera*, *Vitis vinifera*, *Gastrodia elata*, *Camellia sinensis*, *Oenothera biennis* | Multiple sclerosis |
| h | *Mucuna pruriens*, *Ginkgo biloba* L., *Carthamus tinctorius* L., *Tinospora cordifolia* | Parkinson's disease |
| I | *Zingiber officinale*, *Astragalus membranaceus*, *Ginkgo biloba*, *Centella asiatica*, *Acorus calamus*, *Paeonia lactiflora*, *Lobelia inflata*, and *Actaea racemosa* | Autism |
| J | *Piper methysticum*, *Matricaria chamomilla*, *Passiflora incarnata*, *Valeriana officinalis*, *Lavandula anugustifolia*, *Ganoderma lucidum*, *Hypericum perforation* (St. Johns Wort), *Coriandrum sativum* | Insomnia |

## 13.6 SUMMARY

Eleven plants were researched for their beneficial effects on female fertility out of the many plants that were useful in treating different types of female reproductive diseases. Many reproductive disorders, including polycystic ovary syndrome, endometriosis, polypeptide disorder, hypothalamic dysfunction, hyperprolactinemia, polyphenol-induced disease, menopausal symptoms, osteoporosis, and cancers of the reproductive system (cervical, ovarian, uterine/endometrial, vaginal, and vulvar cancers) are effectively prevented or treated with these plants. By conducting thorough examinations into the bioactivity of different chemicals isolated from these plants' extracts, new and effective medications may be produced after further pharmacological, phytochemical, and toxicological studies.

## KEYWORDS

- **women**
- **neurological disorders**
- **health**
- **pesticides**
- **botanicals**

## REFERENCES

1. Alavanja, M. C., & Bonner, M. R. (2012). Occupational pesticide exposures and cancer risk: A review. *The Journal of Toxicology and Environmental Health: Part B, Critical Reviews*, *15*, 238–263.
2. Aloizou, A. M., Siokas, V., Sapouni, E. M., Sita, N., Liampas, I., & Brotis, A. G. (2020). Parkinson's disease and pesticides: Are microRNAs the missing link? *Science of the Total Environment*, *744*, 140591.
3. Alshalati, M. (2021). *Limited Knowledge and Unsafe Practices in usage of Pesticides and the Associated Toxicity Symptoms among Farmers in Tullo and Finchawa Rural Kebeles, Hawassa City, Sidama Regional State, Southern Ethiopia. Emerging Contaminants*. IntechOpen: London, UK.
4. Anakwue, R. (2019). Cardiotoxicity of pesticides: Are Africans at risk? *Cardiovascular Toxicology*, *19*, 95–104.

5. Belay, T., & Negash, T. (2020). Perceptions of flower farm workers on the health effects of chemicals exposures around Bahir Dar town, Ethiopia. *Asian Research Journal of Agriculture, 12*(1), 36–46.
6. Berkowitz, G. S., Wetmur, J. G., Birman-Deych, E., Obel, J., Lapinski, R. H., Godbold, J. H., Holzman, I. R., Wolff, M. S. (2004). In utero pesticide exposure, maternal paraoxonase activity, and head circumference. *Environmental Health Perspectives, 112*, 388–391.
7. Costa, C., Teodoro, M., Rugolo, C. A., Alibrando, C., Giambò, F., & Briguglio, G. (2020). MicroRNAs alteration as early biomarkers for cancer and neurodegenerative diseases: New challenges in pesticides exposure. *Toxicology Reports, 7*, 759–767.
8. Dewan, P., Jain, V., Gupta, P., & Banerjee, B. D. (2012). Organochlorine pesticide residues in maternal blood, cord blood, placenta, and breast milk and their relation to birth size. *Chemosphere, 90*(5), 1704–1710.
9. Fiedler, N., Rohitrattana, J., Siriwong, W., Suttiwan, P., Ohman Strickland, P., & Ryan, P. B. (2015). Neurobehavioral effects of exposure to organophosphates and pyrethroid pesticides among Thai children. *Neurotoxicology, 48*, 90–99.
10. Food and Agriculture Organization (FAO). (1999). *Guidelines for the Management of Small Quantities of Unwanted and Obsolete Pesticides*. Food and Agriculture Organization.
11. Garcia, A. (2003). Pesticide exposure and women's health. *American Journal of Industrial Medicine, 44*, 584–594.
12. Heeren, G., Tyler, J., & Mandeya, A. (2003). Agricultural chemical exposures and birth defects in the Eastern Cape Province, South Africa. *Environmental Health, 2*(11), 1–8.
13. Huang, X., Zhang, C., Hu, R., Li, Y., Yin, Y., & Chen, Z. (2016). Association between occupational exposures to pesticides with heterogeneous chemical structures and farmer health in China. *Scientific Reports, 6*, 25190.
14. Ismail, A. A., Almalki, M., Agag, A., Solan, Y. M., & Bani, I. A. (2018). Pesticide application and khat chewing as predictors of the neurological health outcomes among pesticide applicators in a vector control unit, Saudi Arabia. *International Journal of Occupational and Environmental Medicine, 9*, 32–44.
15. Kori, R. K., Singh, M. K., Jain, A. K., & Yadav, R. S. (2018). Neurochemical and behavioral dysfunctions in pesticide exposed farm workers: A clinical outcome. *Indian Journal of Clinical Biochemistry, 33*, 372–381.
16. Lu, C., Essig, C., Root, C., Rohlman, D. S., McDonald, T., & Sulzbacher, S. (2009). Assessing the association between pesticide exposure and cognitive development in rural Costa Rican children living in organic and conventional coffee farms. *International Journal of Adolescent Medicine and Health, 21*, 609–621.
17. Lu, J. L. (2009). Comparison of pesticide exposure and physical examination, neurological assessment, and laboratory findings between full-time and part-time vegetable farmers in the Philippines. *Environmental Health and Preventive Medicine, 14*, 345–352.
18. Motsoeneng, P. M., & Dalvie, M. A. (2015). Relationship between urinary pesticide residue levels and neurotoxic symptoms among women on farms in the Western Cape, South Africa. *International Journal of Environmental Research and Public Health, 12*, 6281–6299.

19. Muñoz-Quezada, M. T., Lucero, B. A., Iglesias, V., Muñoz, M. P., Cornejo, C., & Achu, E. (2016). Chronic exposure to organophosphate (OP) pesticides and neuropsychological functioning in farm workers: A review. *International Journal of Occupational and Environmental Health, 22*, 68–79.
20. Naidoo, S., London, L., & Rother, H. (2010). Pesticide safety training and practices in South African women working in small-scale agriculture. *Occupational and Environmental Medicine, 67*, 823–828.
21. Ochago, R. (2018). Gender and pest management: Constraints to integrated pest management uptake among smallholder coffee farmers in Uganda. *Cogent Food & Agriculture, 4*(1), 1540093.
22. Ross, S. M., McManus, I. C., Harrison, V., & Mason, O. (2013). Neurobehavioral problems following low-level exposure to organophosphate pesticides: A systematic and meta-analytic review. *Critical Reviews in Toxicology, 43*(1), 21–44.
23. Shafer, T. J., Meyer, D. A., & Crofton, K. M. (2005). Developmental neurotoxicity of pyrethroid insecticides: Critical review and future research needs. *Environmental Health Perspectives, 113*(2), 123–136.
24. Tsatsakis, A., Goumenou, M., Liesivuori, J., Dekant, W., & Hernández, A. F. (2019). Toxicology for real-life risk simulation—Editorial preface to this special issue. *Toxicology Letters, 309*, 33–34.
25. van Wendel de Joode, B., Mora, A. M., Lindh, C. H., Hernández-Bonilla, D., Córdoba, L., Wesseling, C., et al. (2016). Pesticide exposure and neurodevelopment in children aged 6–9 years from Talamanca, Costa Rica. *Cortex, 85*, 137–150.
26. Viel, J. F., Rouget, F., Warembourg, C., Monfort, C., Limon, G., & Cordier, S. (2017). Behavioural disorders in 6-year-old children and pyrethroid insecticide exposure: The PELAGIE mother-child cohort. *Occupational and Environmental Medicine, 74*, 275–281.
27. Voorhees, J., Rohlman, D., Lein, P., & Pieper, A. (2017). Neurotoxicity in preclinical models of occupational exposure to organophosphorus compounds. *Frontiers in Neuroscience, 10*, 590.
28. Weisskopf, M., Moisan, F., Tzourio, C., Rathouz, P., & Elbaz, A. (2013). Pesticide exposure and depression among agricultural workers in France. *American Journal of Epidemiology, 178*, 1051–1058.
29. Weselak, M., Arbuckle, T. E., & Foster, W. (2007). Pesticide exposures and developmental outcomes: The epidemiological evidence. *Journal of Toxicology and Environmental Health B, 10*(1–2), 41–80.
30. Whitworth, K., Bornman, R., Archer, J., Kudumu, M., Travlos, G., & Wilson, R. (2014). Predictors of plasma DDT and DDE concentrations among women exposed to indoor residual spraying for malaria control in the South African Study of Women and Babies (SOWB). *Environmental Health Perspectives, 122*(6), 545–552.
31. World Health Organization. (2009). *Health Implications from Monocrotophos Use: A Review of the Evidence in India*. World Health Organization: Geneva.
32. Zhang, C., Sun, Y., Hu, R., Huang, J., Huang, X., & Li, Y. (2018). A comparison of the effects of agricultural pesticide uses on peripheral nerve conduction in China. *Scientific Reports, 8*, 9621.

33. Zseleczky, L., Elisa, M., & Haleegoah, C. (2014). Embodied livelihoods and tomato farmers' gendered experience of pesticides in Tuobodom, Ghana. *Gender, Technology and Development, 18*(2), 249–274.

CHAPTER 14

# Management Techniques for Female Health

FAISAL SUALEH HAYYAT,* V. GOPINATH,
SHOWKEEN BILAL AHMAD GUL, MOHAMMAD MUZAMIL SHAH,
SAQIB BASHIR, TASLEEMA JAN, UROOJ NISSAR, SEEHAM JALEEL, and
SYED ABEERA ANDRABI

*Corresponding author

## ABSTRACT

This chapter explores various strategies and approaches to promote and maintain women's health across different life stages. The chapter begins with an overview of the importance of prioritizing women's health and the unique healthcare needs specific to females. It delves into the physiological and hormonal changes that occur during puberty, menstruation, pregnancy, and menopause, highlighting the impact of these changes on women's health and well-being. The chapter discusses preventive measures and health promotion initiatives tailored to address common female health issues such as reproductive health, breast health, pelvic floor disorders, and gynecological conditions. It provides insights into screening methods, diagnostic tools, and evidence-based interventions in managing female-specific health concerns. Furthermore, the chapter explores the role of lifestyle modifications, dietary practices, physical activity, and stress management techniques in promoting optimal female health outcomes. It also examines the importance of holistic and integrative approaches to women's health care, encompassing psychological support, emotional vigor, and

Holistic Approaches for Women's Sustainable Health, Volume 1: Foundations, Innovations, Challenges, and Management. Megh R. Goyal, Anamika Chauhan, and Junaid Ahmad Malik (Eds)


DOI: 10.1201/9781779641632-17

social elements of health. The chapter emphasizes empowering women to participate actively in decision-making processes regarding their health and to advocate for comprehensive and patient-centered care. By addressing the multifaceted aspects of female health management, this chapter aims to equip healthcare professionals, researchers, and policymakers with valuable insights and practical strategies to enhance the quality of care and support for women across diverse populations and settings.

## 14.1 INTRODUCTION

The realm of women's health encompasses a myriad of complex physiological, psychological, and social factors that influence well-being throughout the lifespan. From puberty to menopause and beyond, women experience unique health challenges that demand specialized care and attention [8]. Understanding these intricacies is essential for devising effective management techniques tailored to meet different necessities of women across different stages of life. This chapter serves as a comprehensive exploration of management techniques for female health, encompassing various aspects such as reproductive health, hormonal balance, mental well-being, and lifestyle interventions [25]. By synthesizing the latest research findings, clinical insights, and practical recommendations, this chapter aims to provide healthcare professionals, policymakers, and individuals with the knowledge and tools necessary to optimize women's health outcomes. Throughout this chapter, we will delve into the physiological mechanisms underlying female health, examining the intricate interplay of hormones, genetics, and environmental factors. We will explore evidence-based strategies for managing common reproductive health issues, including menstrual disorders, contraception, fertility optimization, and menopausal symptoms.

Furthermore, this chapter will address the importance of mental health in women's overall well-being, highlighting the prevalence of conditions such as anxiety, depression, and eating disorders, and discussing therapeutic approaches and support systems. Additionally, we will discuss the impact of lifestyle factors such as diet, exercise, sleep, and stress management on female health outcomes, offering practical recommendations for promoting holistic wellness. By fostering a deeper understanding of the multifaceted nature of women's health and providing actionable insights into effective management strategies, this chapter aims to empower females to take an active role in their healthiness. Through collaborative efforts between healthcare providers, researchers, policymakers, and individuals, we can strive toward a future where every woman has access to comprehensive, compassionate, and evidence-based care that honors her unique needs and enhances her quality of life.

## 14.2 IMPORTANCE OF WOMEN'S HEALTH

Women's health plays a pivotal role in the overall well-being of societies worldwide. Understanding the significance of women's health involves recognizing the unique physiological, psychological, and social factors that influence women's lives.

### *14.2.1 ECONOMIC IMPACT*

Investing in women's health has far-reaching economic benefits, including increased productivity, reduced healthcare costs, and improved socio-economic outcomes for individuals and communities. By prioritizing women's health, societies can foster greater gender equality and promote sustainable development [21].

### *14.2.2 PHYSIOLOGICAL FACTORS*

Women have distinct biological and anatomical characteristics that require specialized health care. From reproductive health, including menstruation, pregnancy, and menopause, to conditions like polycystic ovary syndrome (PCOS) and endometriosis, addressing these physiological aspects is essential for maintaining women's health and preventing complications [16].

### 14.2.3 PREVENTIVE CARE

Emphasizing preventive care and early intervention is key to maintaining women's health. Regular screenings for cervical and breast cancer, vaccinations against human papillomavirus (HPV), and education on healthy lifestyle behaviors can help prevent diseases and improve health outcomes [13].

### 14.2.4 PSYCHOLOGICAL FACTORS

Women may encounter specific mental health challenges, including hopelessness, anxiety, and eating disorders, which can have profound effects on their overall well-being. Recognizing and addressing these psychological factors are crucial for promoting mental wellness and improving quality of life [2].

### 14.2.5 REPRODUCTIVE RIGHTS

Ensuring women's reproductive rights, including access to contraception, family planning services, and safe abortion care, is essential for empowering women to make informed decisions about their bodies and reproductive health [14].

### 14.2.6 SOCIAL FACTORS

Social determinants, such as socioeconomic status, access to education, healthcare resources, and cultural beliefs, significantly impact women's health outcomes. Disparities in these areas can exacerbate health inequalities and limit access to essential services, underscoring the importance of addressing social factors in promoting women's health equity [9].

Recognizing the importance of women's health involves acknowledging the multifaceted nature of women's lives and addressing physiological, psychological, and social factors. By investing in women's health and promoting equitable access to healthcare services, societies can foster healthier, more resilient communities and empower women to lead fulfilling lives.

## 14.3 PHYSIOLOGICAL CHANGES ACROSS LIFE STAGES

Women experience a continuum of physiological changes throughout their lives, each stage marked by distinct transitions and adaptations to support reproductive function and overall health.

### *14.3.1 PUBERTY*

Puberty heralds the onset of sexual maturation and reproductive capability in girls, typically occurring between the ages of 8 and 14 years. This developmental phase is orchestrated by the hypothalamic–pituitary–gonadal axis, leading to hormonal changes and physical transformations [1].

#### *14.3.1.1 HORMONAL CHANGES*

Puberty is initiated by the activation of the hypothalamus, which secretes gonadotropin-releasing hormone, stimulating the pituitary gland to release follicle-stimulating hormone (FSH) and luteinizing hormone (LH). These hormones trigger the production of estrogen and progesterone by the ovaries, leading to the development of secondary sexual characteristics.

#### *14.3.1.2 PHYSICAL TRANSFORMATIONS*

Estrogen promotes breast development, widening of the hips, growth of pubic and underarm hair, and the onset of menstruation (menarche). Meanwhile, testosterone, though present in smaller amounts, contributes to the development of muscle mass and facial hair in boys.

### *14.3.2 MENSTRUATION*

Menstruation, or the menstrual cycle, is a complex physiological process regulated by hormonal fluctuations and involving the shedding of the uterine lining in the absence of pregnancy [17]. This cyclical event typically lasts around 28 days and is divided into several phases.

#### *14.3.2.1 FOLLICULAR PHASE*

Initiated by the rise in FSH, this phase involves the development of ovarian follicles and the thickening of the uterine lining (endometrium) in preparation for potential implantation.

#### *14.3.2.2 OVULATION*

Triggered by a surge in LH, ovulation marks the release of a mature egg from the ovary, ready for fertilization.

#### *14.3.2.3 LUTEAL PHASE*

Following ovulation, the ruptured follicle transforms into the corpus luteum, which produces progesterone to support the uterine lining and prepare for implantation. If fertilization does not occur, hormone levels decline, leading to menstruation and the shedding of the endometrium.

### ***14.3.3 PREGNANCY***

Pregnancy encompasses a series of profound physiological changes designed to support fetal growth and development within the maternal environment [27]. These changes are orchestrated by hormonal signals and adaptations in various organ systems:

#### *14.3.3.1 HORMONAL SHIFTS*

Pregnancy is characterized by elevated levels of estrogen and progesterone, which promote uterine growth, maintain the endometrium, and suppress ovulation to prevent further menstruation.

#### *14.3.3.2 CARDIOVASCULAR CHANGES*

Increased blood volume, cardiac output, and heart rate accommodate the metabolic demands of pregnancy and ensure an adequate oxygen and nutrient supply to the fetus.

#### *14.3.3.3 RESPIRATORY ADAPTATIONS*

Hormonal influences and mechanical changes, such as diaphragm elevation and increased tidal volume, enhance respiratory function to meet the oxygen needs of both mother and fetus.

### ***14.3.4 MENOPAUSE***

Menopause signifies the cessation of menstruation and the end of reproductive function, typically occurring between the ages of 45 and 55 [10]. This natural transition is characterized by hormonal fluctuations, physiological changes, and potentially associated symptoms.

#### *14.3.4.1 HORMONAL DECLINE*

As women age, ovarian function declines, leading to decreased production of estrogen and progesterone. This hormonal imbalance can result in symptoms such as hot flashes, night sweats, vaginal dryness, and mood disturbances.

#### *14.3.4.2 BONE HEALTH*

The maintenance of bone density relies heavily on estrogen, and its decline during menopause elevates the risk of osteoporosis and bone fractures. Adequate calcium intake, weight-bearing exercise, and hormone replacement therapy may help mitigate these risks [6].

Understanding the intricate physiological changes across different life stages is essential for providing tailored healthcare interventions and support to women. By addressing the unique needs and challenges associated with each phase, healthcare providers can empower women to navigate these transitions with confidence and optimize their overall health and well-being.

## 14.4 PREVENTIVE MEASURES AND HEALTH PROMOTION

Promoting women's health and well-being involves implementing preventive measures and health promotion strategies tailored to address the unique needs and challenges across various domains of female health.

### *14.4.1 REPRODUCTIVE HEALTH*

Maintaining reproductive health is essential for women's overall well-being and fertility. Key preventive measures and health promotion strategies are given below.

#### *14.4.1.1 CONTRACEPTION*

Offering a variety of contraceptive options empowers women to make informed choices about family planning and effectively prevent unintended pregnancies. Options include hormonal contraceptives (e.g., birth control pills, patches, injections), barrier methods (e.g., condoms, diaphragms), intrauterine devices, and permanent sterilization (e.g., tubal ligation).

#### *14.4.1.2 SEXUAL HEALTH EDUCATION*

Comprehensive sexual health education empowers women with knowledge about reproductive anatomy, contraception, sexually transmitted infections (STIs), and healthy relationships. Education should emphasize the importance of consent, communication, and practicing safe sex to prevent STIs and unintended pregnancies.

#### *14.4.1.3 REGULAR SCREENING*

Routine screenings for cervical cancer, breast cancer, and sexually transmitted infections are crucial for early detection and intervention. Pap smears, mammograms, and STI testing enable healthcare providers to identify abnormalities and provide timely treatment and support.

##### *14.4.1.4 PRECONCEPTION COUNSELING*

Counseling women of reproductive age about preconception health and planning can optimize pregnancy outcomes and reduce the risk of complications. Topics may include optimizing nutrition, managing chronic conditions, avoiding teratogens, and achieving a healthy lifestyle before conception [5].

### ***14.4.2 BREAST HEALTH***

Maintaining breast health is paramount for early detection and prevention of breast cancer and further breast-related disorders. Preventive measures and health promotion strategies are given below.

#### *14.4.2.1 BREAST SELF-EXAMINATION*

Encouraging women to perform regular breast self-examination (BSE) enables them to become familiar with the normal texture and appearance of their breasts and detect any changes or abnormalities. Educating women about the proper technique for performing BSE and the signs of breast cancer can facilitate early detection and prompt medical evaluation.

#### *14.4.2.2 CLINICAL BREAST EXAMINATION*

Healthcare providers should conduct regular clinical breast examinations (CBEs) as part of preventive care visits. CBE allows for a thorough assessment of breast tissue, identification of lumps or masses, and referral for further diagnostic evaluation if necessary.

#### *14.4.2.3 MAMMOGRAPHY SCREENING*

Recommending regular mammograms for women aged 40 and older, or earlier for those with a family history or other risk factors, is crucial for spotting breast cancer at an early stage, when treatment outcomes are most favorable. Mammography screening can identify suspicious lesions or abnormalities that may require additional imaging or biopsy for diagnosis.

#### *14.4.2.4 BREASTFEEDING SUPPORT*

Promoting breastfeeding initiation and providing support for breastfeeding mothers can contribute to improved maternal and infant health outcomes. Breastfeeding offers numerous benefits, including reduced risk of breast cancer, ovarian cancer, and osteoporosis for mothers, as well as enhanced immunity and optimal nutrition for infants [12].

### ***14.4.3 PELVIC FLOOR DISORDERS***

Pelvic floor disorders such as urinary incontinence, pelvic organ prolapse, and fecal incontinence can markedly affect the quality of life for women. Preventive measures and health promotion strategies are given below.

#### *14.4.3.1 PELVIC FLOOR EXERCISES*

Encouraging women to perform pelvic floor exercises, such as Kegel exercises, can strengthen the muscles supporting the pelvic organs and improve bladder and bowel control. Physical therapists specializing in pelvic floor rehabilitation can provide guidance on proper technique and personalized exercise programs.

#### *14.4.3.2 HEALTHY LIFESTYLE HABITS*

Maintaining a healthy weight, avoiding smoking, and practicing good bowel and bladder habits can help prevent pelvic floor disorders. Excess weight and smoking are risk factors for pelvic floor dysfunction, while maintaining a healthy diet and staying hydrated can support overall pelvic health.

#### *14.4.3.3 PRENATAL AND POSTPARTUM CARE*

Providing comprehensive prenatal and postpartum care is essential for preventing and managing pelvic floor disorders related to pregnancy and childbearing. Educating women about pelvic floor health, addressing concerns related to labor and delivery, and offering postpartum rehabilitation services can support pelvic floor function and recovery.

#### *14.4.3.4 TREATMENT OPTIONS*

For women experiencing pelvic floor disorders, a range of treatment options are available, including physical therapy, medication, behavioral interventions, and surgical procedures. Individualized treatment plans should consider the severity of symptoms, impact on quality of life, and patient preferences [7].

### ***14.4.4 GYNECOLOGICAL CONDITIONS***

Gynecological conditions encompass a diverse range of disorders affecting the female reproductive system, including menstrual disorders, ovarian cysts, endometriosis, and uterine fibroids. Preventive measures and health promotion strategies are given below.

#### *14.4.4.1 REGULAR GYNECOLOGICAL EXAMINATION*

Encouraging women to schedule routine gynecological examinations enables healthcare providers to assess reproductive health, screen for gynecological conditions and provide preventive care. Examinations may include pelvic exams, Pap smears, and discussions about contraception, sexual health, and menstrual irregularities.

#### *14.4.4.2 EDUCATION AND AWARENESS*

Providing education and raising awareness about common gynecological conditions can empower women to recognize symptoms, seek timely medical attention, and advocate for their health needs. Providing information about symptoms, risk factors, treatment options, and available resources can empower women to make informed decisions about their health care.

#### *14.4.4.3 LIFESTYLE MODIFICATIONS*

Incorporating healthy lifestyle habits, such as maintaining a balanced diet, engaging in regular physical activity, managing stress, and ensuring adequate sleep, can promote gynecological health and lower the risk of various conditions. For example, maintaining a healthy weight may help prevent PCOS and improve fertility outcomes.

#### *14.4.4.4 MANAGEMENT OF MENSTRUAL DISORDERS*

For women undergoing menstrual complaints, for example uneven periods, heavy bleeding, or painful menstruation, various management options are available, including hormonal therapy, nonsteroidal antiinflammatory drugs, and surgical interventions. Treatment plans should be tailored to address underlying causes and alleviate symptoms while preserving fertility and quality of life [11].

By implementing preventive measures and health promotion strategies tailored to address reproductive health, breast health, pelvic floor disorders, and gynecological conditions, healthcare providers can empower women to prioritize their health, detect potential issues early, and access appropriate care and support.

## 14.5 SCREENING AND DIAGNOSTIC METHODS

Screening and diagnostic methods are essential tools in the early detection, diagnosis, and management of various health conditions affecting women. From cervical cancer to breast abnormalities, these methods play a crucial role in promoting early intervention and improving health outcomes.

### *14.5.1 CERVICAL CANCER SCREENING*

Cervical cancer screening aims to recognize precancerous variations or early stage cancer in the cervix, typically using the Pap smear (Papanicolaou test) or HPV testing.

#### *14.5.1.1 PAP SMEAR*

During a Pap smear, cells from the cervix are collected and examined under a microscope for abnormalities such as dysplasia or cervical intraepithelial neoplasia. Regular Pap smears are recommended for women aged 21–65, with frequency determined by age and risk factors.

#### *14.5.1.2 HPV TESTING*

HPV testing detects high-risk strains of the HPV, which are associated with an increased risk of cervical cancer. HPV testing may be performed alone or in conjunction with a Pap smear as part of cervical cancer screening algorithms [3].

### ***14.5.2 BREAST CANCER SCREENING***

Breast cancer screening aims to detect breast abnormalities, including tumors and calcifications, using various imaging modalities.

#### *14.5.2.1 MAMMOGRAPHY*

Mammography is the primary screening tool for breast cancer, involving low-dose X-rays to capture images of the breast tissue. Regular mammograms are recommended for women aged 40 and older, with frequency determined by age, risk factors, and individual preferences.

#### *14.5.2.2 BREAST ULTRASOUND*

Breast ultrasound may be used as a supplemental imaging modality for women with dense breast tissue or those at increased risk of breast cancer. Ultrasound can provide additional information about suspicious findings detected on mammography or clinical examination.

#### *14.5.2.3 BREAST MRI*

Breast magnetic resonance imaging (MRI) is reserved for women at high risk for breast cancer including those with a strong family history or genetic predisposition. MRI is more sensitive than mammography for detecting breast lesions but may yield more false-positive results [20].

### 14.5.3 COLORECTAL CANCER SCREENING

Colorectal cancer screening aims to detect precancerous polyps or early stage cancer in the colon or rectum, typically using colonoscopy, fecal occult blood testing (FOBT), or stool DNA testing.

#### 14.5.3.1 COLONOSCOPY

Colonoscopy involves inserting a flexible tube equipped with a camera into the colon to examine the intestinal lining and identify any abnormalities such as polyps or tumors. Colonoscopy is considered the gold standard for colorectal cancer screening and allows for the simultaneous removal of precancerous lesions.

#### 14.5.3.2 FECAL OCCULT BLOOD TESTING

FOBT identifies blood in the stool, which may specify the existence of colorectal cancer or precancerous polyps. Both guaiac-based and immunochemical FOBTs are available and may be performed at home or in a clinical setting.

#### 14.5.3.3 STOOL DNA TESTING

Stool DNA testing analyzes stool samples for genetic alterations associated with colorectal cancer. This noninvasive screening method may be used as an alternative to colonoscopy for individuals at average risk of colorectal cancer [26].

### 14.5.4 DIAGNOSTIC IMAGING

Diagnostic imaging modalities, such as ultrasound, computed tomography, and MRI, play a crucial role in diagnosing various gynecological conditions, including ovarian cysts, uterine fibroids, and pelvic inflammatory disease.

#### *14.5.4.1 TRANSVAGINAL ULTRASOUND*

Transvaginal ultrasound allows for detailed imaging of the pelvic organs, including the uterus, ovaries, and fallopian tubes. This imaging modality is commonly used to evaluate pelvic pain, abnormal bleeding, and infertility.

#### *14.5.4.2 PELVIC MRI*

Pelvic MRI provides high-resolution images of the pelvic anatomy and is particularly useful for assessing complex gynecological conditions such as endometriosis, adenomyosis, and pelvic masses.

#### *14.5.4.3 HYSTEROSALPINGOGRAPHY*

Hysterosalpingography is a specialized X-ray procedure used to evaluate the uterine cavity and fallopian tubes. This imaging test may be performed to assess infertility, identify uterine abnormalities, or confirm tubal patency [24].

By utilizing appropriate screening and diagnostic methods tailored to individual risk factors and health concerns, healthcare providers can detect health conditions early, facilitate timely intervention, and improve outcomes for women across the lifespan.

## 14.6 LIFESTYLE MODIFICATIONS AND HEALTH BEHAVIORS

Lifestyle modifications and health behaviors play a critical role in promoting women's health and preventing chronic diseases. By adopting healthy habits and making positive changes to their lifestyle, women can enhance their overall well-being and reduce the risk of various health conditions.

### *14.6.1 NUTRITION*

#### *14.6.1.1 BALANCED DIET*

Promoting a balanced diet that includes fruits, vegetables, whole grains, lean proteins, and healthy fats encourages women to consume essential nutrients and promotes overall health. Emphasizing portion control, mindful eating, and moderation of processed foods and sugary beverages can help maintain a healthy weight and prevent chronic diseases such as obesity, diabetes, and cardiovascular disease.

#### *14.6.1.2 HYDRATION*

Promoting adequate hydration by encouraging women to drink plenty of water throughout the day supports proper bodily functions, including digestion, circulation, and temperature regulation. Limiting intake of caffeinated and alcoholic beverages, which can contribute to dehydration, is also important for maintaining hydration levels [19].

### ***14.6.2 PHYSICAL ACTIVITY***

#### *14.6.2.1 REGULAR EXERCISE*

Encouraging women to engage in regular physical activity, such as aerobic exercise, strength training, and flexibility exercises, enhances cardiovascular fitness, supports muscles and bones, and recovers mood and mental well-being. Advising at least 150 min of moderate-intensity aerobic activity or 75 min of vigorous-intensity aerobic activity per week, complemented by muscle-strengthening activities on 2 or more days per week, adheres to current physical activity guidelines.

#### *14.6.2.2 ACTIVE LIFESTYLE*

Encouraging women to incorporate physical activity into their daily routine, such as walking or biking to work, taking the stairs instead of the elevator, and participating in recreational activities with family and friends, promotes an active lifestyle and reduces sedentary behavior [29].

### ***14.6.3 STRESS MANAGEMENT***

#### *14.6.3.1 MINDFULNESS PRACTICES*

Introducing mindfulness practices, such as meditation, deep breathing exercises, and yoga, can help women reduce stress, improve emotional resilience, and enhance overall well-being. Encouraging regular practice of mindfulness techniques can promote relaxation, increase self-awareness, and cultivate a sense of inner calm.

#### *14.6.3.2 HEALTHY COPING MECHANISMS*

Encouraging women to develop healthy coping mechanisms for managing stress, such as engaging in hobbies, spending time in nature, seeking social support, and maintaining a positive outlook, promotes adaptive responses to challenging situations and reduces the risk of stress-related health problems [15].

### ***14.6.4 SLEEP HYGIENE***

#### *14.6.4.1 ESTABLISHING ROUTINE*

Promoting good sleep hygiene by encouraging women to begin a steady sleep schedule, generate a relaxing bedtime routine, and make a relaxed sleep environment supports healthy sleep habits and improves sleep quality. Emphasizing the importance of prioritizing sleep and setting aside sufficient time for rest and relaxation is essential for overall well-being.

#### *14.6.4.2 LIMITING STIMULANTS*

Advising women to limit consumption of stimulants, such as caffeine and electronic devices, particularly before bedtime, can reduce sleep disturbances and promote restful sleep. Educating women about the effects of stimulants on sleep patterns and offering alternatives, such as herbal tea or reading, can support healthy sleep habits [18].

### ***14.6.5 SUBSTANCE USE AND ABUSE***

#### *14.6.5.1 TOBACCO CESSATION*

Offering tobacco cessation support and resources to women who smoke or use tobacco products can reduce the risk of tobacco-related diseases such as lung cancer, heart disease, and respiratory disorders. Providing counseling, nicotine replacement therapy, and behavioral interventions can assist women in quitting smoking and maintaining long-term abstinence.

#### *14.6.5.2 ALCOHOL MODERATION*

Promoting moderation and responsible drinking behavior among women who consume alcohol can reduce the risk of alcohol-related harm, including liver disease, cardiovascular problems, and accidents. Advising women to adhere to recommended guidelines for alcohol consumption and avoid excessive drinking can support overall health and well-being.

By promoting lifestyle modifications and health behaviors, healthcare providers can empower women to take control of their health and make positive changes that contribute to long-term well-being and disease prevention.

## 14.7 HOLISTIC APPROACHES TO WOMEN'S HEALTH

Holistic approaches to women's health acknowledge the interconnectedness of the mind, body, and spirit. They strive to enhance overall well-being by addressing the physical, emotional, social, and spiritual dimensions of health.

### *14.7.1 MIND-BODY PRACTICES*

#### *14.7.1.1 MINDFULNESS MEDITATION*

Incorporating mindfulness meditation practices into women's health care can promote relaxation, reduce stress, and enhance emotional resilience. Mindfulness-based interventions, such as mindfulness-based stress reduction and mindfulness-based cognitive therapy, offer evidence-based strategies for managing anxiety, depression, and chronic pain.

#### *14.7.1.2 YOGA AND TAI CHI*

Encouraging women to engage in yoga and tai chi practices can improve flexibility, strength, and balance, while also promoting mental clarity and emotional well-being. These mind–body practices integrate physical postures, breathing techniques, and meditation to support holistic health and vitality [4].

### 14.7.2 NUTRITIONAL MEDICINE

#### 14.7.2.1 FUNCTIONAL NUTRITION

Applying principles of functional nutrition to women's health care involves assessing individual nutritional needs, identifying potential nutrient imbalances or deficiencies, and recommending personalized dietary interventions. Integrating functional medicine approaches, such as elimination diets, nutritional supplementation, and gut health optimization, can support digestive health, hormonal balance, and immune function.

#### 14.7.2.2 HERBAL MEDICINE

Incorporating herbal medicine into women's health care involves using plant-based remedies, such as botanical extracts, teas, and tinctures, to address various health concerns. Herbal preparations may offer therapeutic benefits for menstrual irregularities, menopausal symptoms, and reproductive health conditions, with careful consideration of safety, efficacy, and potential interactions with medications [28].

### 14.7.3 ENERGY-BASED THERAPIES

#### 14.7.3.1 ACUPUNCTURE

Integrating acupuncture into women's health care involves using fine needles to stimulate specific acupoints and restore balance to the body's energy flow (qi). Acupuncture may be used to address a wide range of women's health concerns, including menstrual disorders, fertility issues, and menopausal symptoms, with growing evidence supporting its effectiveness.

#### *14.7.3.2 REIKI AND ENERGY HEALING*

Offering reiki and energy healing therapies as complementary modalities for women's health care can promote relaxation, reduce pain, and enhance overall well-being. These energy-based practices involve the gentle manipulation of subtle energy fields to support physical, emotional, and spiritual healing.

### *14.7.4 MIND-BODY-SPIRIT INTEGRATION*

#### *14.7.4.1 HOLISTIC HEALTH COACHING*

Providing holistic health coaching services to women empowers them to take an active role in their health journey and make informed choices that align with their values and goals. Holistic health coaches collaborate with clients to address lifestyle factors, set realistic goals, and implement sustainable behavior changes that support holistic well-being.

#### *14.7.4.2 SPIRITUAL CARE AND COUNSELING*

Recognizing the importance of spirituality in women's health, offering spiritual care and counseling services can provide emotional support, foster resilience, and promote a sense of purpose and meaning. Spiritual care may involve exploring beliefs, values, and existential concerns, as well as facilitating connections to community resources and support networks.

### *14.7.5 COMMUNITY AND SOCIAL SUPPORT*

#### *14.7.5.1 GROUP-BASED INTERVENTIONS*

Implementing group-based interventions, such as support groups, wellness workshops, and community health programs, can foster social connections, reduce isolation, and promote collective empowerment among women. Group settings offer opportunities for sharing experiences, exchanging information, and providing mutual encouragement and support.

#### *14.7.5.2 CULTURAL COMPETENCE*

Recognizing the diverse cultural backgrounds and perspectives of women, integrating cultural competence into women's health care involves respecting individual beliefs, values, and traditions. Culturally sensitive approaches ensure that women receive care that is respectful, inclusive, and responsive to their unique needs and preferences.

By embracing holistic approaches to women's health, healthcare providers can support women in achieving optimal health and well-being across the lifespan, addressing the physical, emotional, social, and spiritual dimensions of health in a comprehensive and integrated manner.

## 14.8 EMPOWERMENT AND PATIENT-CENTERED CARE

Empowerment and patient-centered care are foundational principles in women's health that prioritize collaboration, autonomy, and respect for individual values and preferences. By empowering women to actively participate in their healthcare decisions and providing personalized, compassionate care, healthcare providers can promote positive health outcomes and enhance patient experience [23].

### *14.8.1 SHARED DECISION-MAKING*

#### *14.8.1.1 INFORMED CONSENT*

Providing women with clear, understandable information about their health conditions, treatment options, and potential risks and benefits empowers them to make informed decisions that align with their values and preferences. Informed consent empowers women to actively participate in their care and promotes transparency and trust in the patient–provider relationship.

#### *14.8.1.2 SHARED DECISION-MAKING*

Engaging women in shared decision-making processes involves collaborative discussions between healthcare providers and patients to explore treatment options, discuss risks and benefits, and arrive at mutually agreed-upon care plans. Shared decision-making honors women's autonomy, values diversity, and fosters a sense of partnership and empowerment in healthcare decision-making.

### *14.8.2 HEALTH EDUCATION AND ADVOCACY*

#### *14.8.2.1 HEALTH LITERACY*

Providing health education resources and materials in accessible formats empowers women to understand their health conditions, navigate the healthcare system, and advocate for their needs. Health literacy initiatives may include written materials, multimedia resources, and interactive workshops designed to promote understanding and self-advocacy.

#### *14.8.2.2 COMMUNITY ENGAGEMENT*

Engaging women in community-based health promotion activities, advocacy campaigns, and peer support networks fosters empowerment, social connection, and collective action. Community engagement initiatives empower women to address systemic barriers to health equity, advocate for policy change, and promote community-wide health initiatives.

### *14.8.3 CULTURALLY RESPONSIVE CARE*

#### *14.8.3.1 CULTURAL COMPETENCE*

Recognizing and respecting the diverse cultural backgrounds, beliefs, and values of women is essential for providing culturally responsive care. Culturally competent healthcare providers strive to understand and accommodate cultural differences, language preferences, and health beliefs to ensure that care is respectful, inclusive, and effective.

##### *14.8.3.2 TRAUMA-INFORMED CARE*

Implementing a trauma-informed approach to care involves understanding and addressing the profound impact of past trauma on women's health and well-being. It requires creating a supportive and safe environment that facilitates healing and promotes resilience. Trauma-informed care emphasizes empowerment, choice, and collaboration while minimizing retraumatization and fostering trust in the therapeutic relationship.

#### *14.8.4 ADVOCACY AND POLICY CHANGE*

##### *14.8.4.1 WOMEN'S HEALTH ADVOCACY*

Advocating for women's health rights, access to care, and reproductive autonomy at the individual, community, and policy levels promotes empowerment and social justice. Women's health advocacy efforts may involve grassroots organizing, coalition building, and legislative advocacy to address systemic inequities and promote policies that support women's health and well-being.

##### *14.8.4.2 POLICY CHANGE*

Engaging in policy change initiatives to address social determinants of health, such as poverty, discrimination, and access to health care, can create supportive environments that empower women to lead healthy lives. Policy change efforts may focus on issues such as paid family leave, affordable childcare, reproductive rights, and healthcare coverage for essential services [22].

By embracing empowerment and patient-centered care principles in women's health, healthcare providers can foster collaborative partnerships with women, promote informed decision-making, and advocate for policies and systems that advance health equity and improve outcomes for all women.

### 14.9 CONCLUSION AND FUTURE DIRECTIONS

Women's health encompasses a broad spectrum of physiological, psychological, and social factors that influence well-being across the lifespan. From reproductive health and breast health to pelvic floor disorders and gynecological conditions, addressing the unique needs and challenges of women requires a multifaceted approach that integrates evidence-based interventions, holistic care principles, and patient-centered practices. Through preventive measures, screening and diagnostic methods, lifestyle modifications, and empowerment initiatives, healthcare providers can empower women to take control of their health, make informed decisions, and access the resources and support they need to thrive. By embracing a holistic view of health and wellness that encompasses mind, body, and spirit, healthcare providers can promote resilience, enhance quality of life, and foster a sense of empowerment and self-efficacy in women.

Looking ahead, the future of women's health holds tremendous promise for innovation, collaboration, and progress. As advancements in technology, research, and healthcare delivery continue to evolve, there are several key areas where future efforts can focus to further improve women's health outcomes.

### 14.9.1 HEALTH EQUITY

Addressing disparities in women's health outcomes, particularly among marginalized and underserved populations, is paramount for achieving health equity. Future efforts should prioritize culturally responsive care, community engagement, and advocacy for policies and programs that promote health equity and social justice.

### 14.9.2 PRECISION MEDICINE

Embracing personalized medicine approaches that consider individual differences in genetics, lifestyle factors, and social determinants of health can optimize preventive care, screening strategies, and treatment interventions tailored to women's unique needs and preferences.

### 14.9.3 INTEGRATIVE HEALTH MODELS

Integrating complementary and alternative medicine modalities, such as acupuncture, herbal medicine, and mind–body practices, into mainstream health care can expand treatment options, improve patient satisfaction, and enhance holistic approaches to women's health and wellness.

### *14.9.4 DIGITAL HEALTH SOLUTIONS*

Utilizing digital health technologies, such as telemedicine, mobile apps, and wearable devices, can improve access to care, enable remote monitoring, and empower women to take an active role in managing their health and making informed decisions.

### *14.9.5 RESEARCH AND INNOVATION*

Investing in research and innovation in women's health, including basic science, clinical trials, and translational research, can drive discovery, inform evidence-based practice, and address critical gaps in knowledge and understanding of women's health conditions and treatment outcomes.

In closing, by embracing a comprehensive, patient-centered approach to women's health that prioritizes empowerment, equity, and innovation, we can collectively work toward a future where all women have the opportunity to achieve optimal health and well-being.

## 14.10 SUMMARY

This chapter on "Management Techniques for Female Health" delves into a comprehensive examination of the multifaceted aspects of women's health management. It underscores the intricate interplay between biological, psychological, and social factors that shape women's health outcomes and experiences throughout their lives. Throughout the chapter, the importance of adopting a proactive approach to women's health is emphasized, starting with education and awareness. Women need access to accurate, culturally sensitive information about their bodies, reproductive health, and the importance of preventive care. By empowering women with knowledge, healthcare providers can enable them to make informed decisions about their health and advocate for their well-being. A central focus of the chapter is on preventive measures and health promotion strategies tailored to women's unique needs. From routine screenings for cervical and breast cancer to counseling on reproductive health and contraception, preventive care is paramount in identifying potential health issues early and facilitating timely intervention. Additionally, promoting healthy lifestyle behaviors, such as balanced nutrition, regular physical activity, stress management, and adequate sleep, plays a crucial role in preventing chronic diseases and promoting overall well-being. The chapter also explores the diverse array of diagnostic methods and treatment interventions available for addressing common women's health concerns. From advanced imaging techniques for gynecological conditions to minimally invasive surgical procedures for pelvic floor disorders, healthcare providers have an array of tools at their disposal for diagnosing and managing women's health conditions effectively. Moreover, the integration of evidence-based interventions, such as hormonal therapies, behavioral interventions, and complementary therapies, underscores the importance of tailoring treatment plans to individual needs and preferences. An underlying theme woven throughout the discussion is the significance of patient-centered care and empowerment in women's health management. Recognizing women as active participants in their healthcare journey, healthcare providers strive to cultivate collaborative partnerships that honor women's autonomy, preferences, and values. By engaging in shared decision-making, providing compassionate support, and fostering open communication, healthcare providers can create a supportive environment where women feel empowered to take ownership of their health and well-being. Looking ahead, the chapter highlights the need for continued research, innovation, and advocacy in women's health. As advancements in technology, precision medicine, and integrative health models continue to evolve, there are abundant opportunities to further enhance women's health outcomes and address disparities in care. By embracing a holistic, patient-centered approach to women's health management that prioritizes empowerment, equity, and innovation, healthcare providers can work toward a future where all women have the opportunity to thrive.

## KEYWORDS

- **holistic approaches**
- **patient empowerment**
- **patient-centered care**
- **preventive care**
- **screening methods**
- **women's health**

## REFERENCES

1. Abreu, A. P., & Kaiser, U. B. (2016). Pubertal development and regulation. *Lancet Diabetes Endocrinology, 4*(3), 254–264. doi:10.1016/s2213-8587(15)00418-0
2. Alegría, M., NeMoyer, A., Falgàs Bagué, I., Wang, Y., & Alvarez, K. (2018). Social determinants of mental health: Where we are and where we need to go. *Current Psychiatry Reports, 20*(11), 95. doi:10.1007/s11920-018-0969-9
3. Basoya, S., & Anjankar, A. (2022). Cervical cancer: Early detection and prevention in reproductive age group. *Cureus, 14*(11), e31312. doi:10.7759/cureus.31312
4. Boyd, J. E., Lanius, R. A., & McKinnon, M. C. (2018). Mindfulness-based treatments for posttraumatic stress disorder: A review of the treatment literature and neurobiological evidence. *Journal of Psychiatry & Neuroscience, 43*(1), 7–25. doi:10.1503/jpn.170021
5. Britton, L. E., Alspaugh, A., Greene, M. Z., & McLemore, M. R. (2020). CE: An evidence-based update on contraception. *The American Journal of Nursing, 120*(2), 22–33. doi:10.1097/01.NAJ.0000654304.29632.a7
6. Cheng, C. H., Chen, L. R., & Chen, K. H. (2022). Osteoporosis due to hormone imbalance: An overview of the effects of estrogen deficiency and glucocorticoid overuse on bone turnover. *International Journal of Molecular Sciences, 23*(3), 1376. doi:10.3390/ijms23031376
7. Cho, S. T., & Kim, K. H. (2021). Pelvic floor muscle exercise and training for coping with urinary incontinence. *Journal of Exercise Rehabilitation, 17*(6), 379–387. doi:10.12965/jer.2142666.333
8. Craft, N. (1997). Women's health: Life span—Conception to adolescence. *BMJ, 315*, 1227–1230. doi:10.1136/bmj.315.7117.1227
9. Davidson, P. M., McGrath, S. J., Meleis, A. I., Stern, P., Digiacomo, M., Dharmendra, T., & Krassen-Covan, E. (2011). The health of women and girls determines the health and well-being of our modern world: A white paper from the International Council on Women's Health Issues. *Health Care for Women International, 32*(10), 870–886. doi:10.1080/07399332.2011.603872
10. Gold, E. B. (2011). The timing of the age at which natural menopause occurs. *Obstetrics and Gynecology Clinics of North America, 38*(3), 425–440. doi:10.1016/j.ogc.2011.05.002
11. Izetbegovic, S., Alajbegovic, J., Mutevelic, A., Pasagic, A., & Masic, I. (2013). Prevention of diseases in gynecology. *International Journal of Preventive Medicine, 4*(12), 1347–1358.
12. Johnson, O. E. (2019). Awareness and practice of breast self examination among women in different African countries: A 10-year review of literature. *The Nigerian Journal of Medicine, 60*(5), 219–225. doi:10.4103/nmj.NMJ_84_19
13. Kataria, I., Siddiqui, M., Treiman, K., Foley, S., Anand, M., Biswas, S., & Sankaranarayanan, R. (2022). Awareness, perceptions, and choices of physicians pertaining to human papillomavirus (HPV) vaccination in India: A formative research study. *Vaccine X, 12*, 100228. doi:10.1016/j.jvacx.2022.100228
14. Kc, H., Shrestha, M., Pokharel, N., Niraula, S. R., Pyakurel, P., & Parajuli, S. B. (2021). Women's empowerment for abortion and family planning decision making

among marginalized women in Nepal: A mixed method study. *Reproductive Health, 18*(1), 28. doi:10.1186/s12978-021-01087-x

15. Keng, S. L., Smoski, M. J., & Robins, C. J. (2011). Effects of mindfulness on psychological health: A review of empirical studies. *Clinical Psychology Review, 31*(6), 1041–1056. doi:10.1016/j.cpr.2011.04.006
16. Louwers, Y. V., & Laven, J. S. E. (2020). Characteristics of polycystic ovary syndrome throughout life. *Therapeutic Advances in Reproductive Health, 14*, 2633494120911038. doi:10.1177/2633494120911038
17. Maybin, J. A., & Critchley, H. O. (2015). Menstrual physiology: Implications for endometrial pathology and beyond. *Human Reproduction Update, 21*(6), 748–761. doi:10.1093/humupd/dmv038
18. Mindell, J. A., & Williamson, A. A. (2018). Benefits of a bedtime routine in young children: Sleep, development, and beyond. *Sleep Medicine Reviews, 40*, 93–108. doi:10.1016/j.smrv.2017.10.007
19. Mozaffarian, D. (2016). Dietary and policy priorities for cardiovascular disease, diabetes, and obesity: A comprehensive review. *Circulation, 133*(2), 187–225. doi:10.1161/circulationaha.115.018585
20. Nicosia, L., Gnocchi, G., Gorini, I., Venturini, M., Fontana, F., Pesapane, F., Meneghetti, L., Battaglia, O., Pellegrino, G., & Cassano, E. (2023). History of mammography: Analysis of breast imaging diagnostic achievements over the last century. *Healthcare (Basel), 11*(11), 1596. doi:10.3390/healthcare11111596
21. Onarheim, K. H., Iversen, J. H., & Bloom, D. E. (2016). Economic benefits of investing in women's health: A systematic review. *PLoS One, 11*(3), e0150120. doi:10.1371/journal.pone.0150120
22. Onwuachi-Saunders, C., Dang, Q. P., & Murray, J. (2019). Reproductive rights, reproductive justice: Redefining challenges to create optimal health for all women. *Journal of Healthcare, Science and the Humanities, 9*(1), 19–31.
23. Pulvirenti, M., McMillan, J., & Lawn, S. (2014). Empowerment, patient centered care and self-management. *Health Expect, 17*(3), 303–310. doi:10.1111/j.1369-7625.2011.00757.x
24. Roche, O., Chavan, N., Aquilina, J., & Rockall, A. (2012). Radiological appearances of gynaecological emergencies. *Insights Imaging, 3*(3), 265–275. doi:10.1007/s13244-012-0157-0
25. Rostami-Moez, M., Masoumi, S. Z., Otogara, M., Farahani, F., Alimohammadi, S., & Oshvandi, K. (2023). Examining the health-related needs of females during menopause: A systematic review study. *Journal of Menopausal Medicine, 29*(1), 1–20. doi:10.6118/jmm.22033
26. Screening methods for early detection of colorectal cancers and polyps: Summary of evidence-based analyses. (2009). *Ontario Health Technology Assessment Series, 9*(6), 1–65.
27. Soma-Pillay, P., Nelson-Piercy, C., Tolppanen, H., & Mebazaa, A. (2016). Physiological changes in pregnancy. *The Cardiovascular Journal of Africa, 27*(2), 89–94. doi:10.5830/cvja-2016-021
28. Stone, M., Lukaczer, D., D'Adamo, C. R., Dotson, N., Volkov, A., Minich, D., Metti, D., Leary, M., Class, M., Carullo, M., Lundquist, E., Eck, B., Ordovas, J., Lamb, J., & Bland, J. (2023). Lifehouse's functional nutrition examination

(Physical exam, anthropometrics, and selected biomarkers) informs personalized wellness interventions. *Journal of Personalized Medicine, 13*(4), 594. doi:10.3390/jpm13040594

29. Warburton, D. E., Nicol, C. W., & Bredin, S. S. (2006). Health benefits of physical activity: The evidence. *CMAJ, 174*(6), 801–809. doi:10.1503/cmaj.051351

## CHAPTER 15

# Total Quality Management for Female Health

FAISAL SUALEH HAYYAT,* V. GOPINATH,
SHOWKEEN BILAL AHMAD GUL, SAQIB BASHIR,
MOHAMMAD MUZAMIL SHAH, TASLEEMA JAN, SEEHAM JALEEL,
UROOJ NISSAR, and SYED ABEERA ANDRABI

*Corresponding author

## ABSTRACT

This chapter elucidates the principles and practices of total quality management (TQM) as applied to the domain of women's health. It begins by delineating the fundamental concepts of TQM and its relevance in healthcare delivery, emphasizing the importance of continuous improvement, patient-centered care, and stakeholder engagement in optimizing health outcomes for women. The chapter explores the unique challenges and opportunities inherent in implementing TQM principles within the context of female healthcare. It examines strategies for enhancing the quality, safety, and efficiency of women's health services across the continuum of care, encompassing preventive, diagnostic, therapeutic, and rehabilitative interventions. The chapter also addresses the role of leadership, teamwork, and organizational culture in fostering a culture of quality and accountability within healthcare settings catering to women's health needs. Furthermore, the chapter explores the application of evidence-based practices, clinical guidelines, and standards of care in ensuring the delivery of high-quality, evidence-informed services to women across diverse populations and settings. This chapter aims to

Holistic Approaches for Women's Sustainable Health, Volume 1: Foundations, Innovations, Challenges, and Management. Megh R. Goyal, Anamika Chauhan, and Junaid Ahmad Malik (Eds)


DOI: 10.1201/9781779641632-18

equip healthcare professionals, administrators, and policymakers with the knowledge and tools necessary to implement TQM principles effectively in female health.

## 15.1 INTRODUCTION TO TOTAL QUALITY MANAGEMENT

In the pursuit of optimal healthcare outcomes for women, the integration of total quality management (TQM) principles is paramount. TQM represents a holistic approach to quality enhancement that transcends mere product or service inspection. Instead, it encapsulates a philosophy deeply rooted in continuous improvement, customer satisfaction, and organizational excellence. When applied to the domain of female health, TQM becomes not just a methodology but a guiding principle, ensuring that every aspect of healthcare delivery aligns with the unique needs and expectations of women. At its core, TQM underscores the importance of a customer-centric approach. In the context of female health, women themselves are the primary customers of healthcare services. Thus, understanding and addressing their specific healthcare needs, preferences, and concerns becomes imperative.

TQM advocates for the creation of healthcare systems and services that are sensitive to the diverse experiences and requirements of women across various stages of life, from adolescence to menopause and beyond. Furthermore, TQM emphasizes the concept of continuous improvement as a fundamental driver of quality enhancement. Healthcare organizations committed to TQM recognize that achieving excellence is not a destination but a journey. Therefore, they foster a culture of ongoing assessment, reflection, and refinement, constantly seeking opportunities to optimize processes, eliminate inefficiencies, and enhance the overall quality of care delivered to women [9].

Central to the TQM framework is the principle of employee involvement. Healthcare professionals, including physicians, nurses, midwives, and administrative staff, are integral to the quality improvement process. By empowering and engaging these stakeholders, healthcare organizations can harness their collective expertise, insights, and experiences to drive meaningful change and innovation in female health services. Moreover, TQM advocates for the systematic optimization of processes to improve efficiency and effectiveness. From patient intake procedures to treatment protocols and follow-up care, every aspect of healthcare delivery is scrutinized and refined to ensure seamless, patient-centered experiences for women seeking care.

Data-driven decision-making serves as another cornerstone of TQM implementation in female health. By leveraging data analytics and evidence-based practices, healthcare organizations can gain valuable insights into patient outcomes, satisfaction levels, and process performance. These insights inform strategic decision-making, enabling organizations to identify areas for improvement, allocate resources effectively, and monitor progress toward quality enhancement goals. Ultimately, successful implementation of TQM in female health hinges upon leadership commitment and organizational culture. Leaders must champion quality improvement initiatives; allocate resources strategically; and foster a culture of collaboration, transparency, and accountability within their organizations. Through unwavering leadership and a steadfast commitment to excellence, healthcare organizations can realize the full potential of TQM to transform female health outcomes and ensure that women receive the highest standard of care possible [1].

In this chapter, authors delve into the intricacies of TQM as applied to female health. Drawing upon established TQM principles and best practices, authors explore practical strategies, case studies, and real-world examples to illustrate how healthcare organizations can integrate TQM into their operations to enhance the quality, accessibility, and equity of healthcare services for women worldwide. Through this comprehensive review, authors aim to equip healthcare professionals, policymakers, researchers, and advocates with the knowledge and tools necessary to advance the agenda of TQM in female health and ultimately improve the lives of women everywhere.

## 15.2 RELEVANCE OF TQM IN HEALTHCARE

The application of TQM principles in healthcare is of paramount importance due to its potential to revolutionize the delivery of services and improve patient outcomes. TQM, originating from manufacturing industries, has been adapted and adopted in healthcare settings to address the complex challenges faced by healthcare systems worldwide.

First, TQM emphasizes the importance of continuous improvement. Healthcare is a dynamic field, characterized by evolving patient needs, advancements in medical technology, and changes in best practices. By embracing a culture of continuous improvement, healthcare organizations can adapt to these changes swiftly, ensuring that they are always providing the best possible care to patients.

Second, TQM promotes a patient-centric approach to healthcare delivery. Patients are not merely recipients of healthcare services; they are active participants in their care journey. TQM encourages healthcare providers to listen to patients, understand their preferences and concerns, and involve them in decision-making processes. By prioritizing patient satisfaction and engagement, TQM fosters trust and collaboration between patients and healthcare providers, leading to better health outcomes.

Furthermore, TQM emphasizes the importance of evidence-based decision-making. In healthcare, decisions regarding patient care must be guided by scientific evidence and clinical best practices. TQM encourages healthcare providers to collect and analyze data related to patient outcomes, treatment efficacy, and process efficiency. By leveraging data and evidence, healthcare organizations can make informed decisions, identify areas for improvement, and monitor the impact of quality-improvement initiatives over time [15].

Additionally, TQM underscores the significance of teamwork and collaboration. Healthcare delivery is a multidisciplinary endeavor, involving physicians, nurses, pharmacists, allied health professionals, and support staff working together to provide comprehensive care to patients. TQM promotes teamwork, communication, and mutual respect among healthcare team members, leading to enhanced coordination, efficiency, and patient safety. Moreover, TQM advocates for the optimization of healthcare processes. Inefficient workflows, redundant procedures, and communication breakdowns can impede the delivery of timely and effective care.

TQM encourages healthcare organizations to streamline processes, eliminate waste, and standardize practices to improve efficiency and reduce errors. By optimizing processes, healthcare providers can enhance the quality of care, minimize resource utilization, and ultimately improve patient outcomes. In summary, TQM is highly relevant in healthcare due to its focus on continuous improvement, patient-centric care, evidence-based decision-making, teamwork, and process optimization. By embracing TQM principles, healthcare organizations can enhance the quality, safety, and efficiency of healthcare delivery, ultimately leading to better health outcomes for patients [2].

## 15.3 CHALLENGES AND OPPORTUNITIES IN WOMEN'S HEALTH

Women's health encompasses a broad spectrum of physical, mental, and social well-being issues that uniquely affect women throughout their lifespan. While significant progress has been made in advancing women's health globally, several challenges persist, alongside opportunities for improvement and innovation. One of the foremost challenges in women's health is the prevalence of gender disparities in healthcare access and outcomes. Women, particularly those in low-income and marginalized communities, often face barriers to accessing essential healthcare services, including reproductive healthcare, maternal care, and screening for diseases such as breast and cervical cancer. Addressing these disparities requires targeted interventions to improve healthcare access, eliminate financial barriers, and promote gender-sensitive healthcare delivery models. Furthermore, women's health is impacted by a myriad of social determinants, including socioeconomic status, education, employment, and cultural norms. Women who experience poverty, discrimination, or violence may face increased health risks and reduced access to healthcare services. Addressing the social determinants of health is essential for promoting health equity and improving outcomes for women across diverse populations.

Reproductive health remains a significant area of concern in women's health, encompassing issues such as family planning, contraception, pregnancy, childbirth, and postpartum care. While access to reproductive health services has improved in many regions, disparities persist, particularly concerning access to safe abortion services, maternal care, and family planning resources. Ensuring universal access to comprehensive reproductive health services is essential for promoting women's autonomy, reducing maternal mortality, and improving reproductive outcomes [7].

Additionally, women's mental health represents a critical area of concern, with women being disproportionately affected by conditions such as depression, anxiety, and posttraumatic stress disorder. Sociocultural factors, including gender-based violence, stigma, and discrimination, contribute to the elevated prevalence of mental health disorders among women. Promoting mental health literacy, reducing stigma, and expanding access to mental health services are essential strategies for addressing women's mental health needs and improving overall well-being. Moreover, women's health research remains underfunded and underrepresented, leading to gaps in knowledge and understanding of women's health issues. Historically, clinical research has disproportionately focused on male participants, leading to a lack of evidence-based guidelines and treatments tailored to women's specific needs. Increasing investment in women's health research, promoting diversity in clinical trials, and prioritizing sex and gender-based analysis are critical steps toward advancing women's health knowledge and improving clinical care.

Despite these challenges, there are also significant opportunities for progress and innovation in women's health. Advances in technology, including digital health platforms, telemedicine, and wearable devices, hold promise for improving healthcare access, monitoring health outcomes, and empowering women to take control of their health. Additionally, the growing recognition of women's health as a global priority has catalyzed increased investment, advocacy, and policy initiatives aimed at addressing women's health needs and promoting gender equity in healthcare. In conclusion, addressing the challenges and opportunities in women's health requires a multifaceted approach that encompasses healthcare access, social determinants, reproductive health, mental health, research, and innovation. By prioritizing women's health equity, investing in evidence-based interventions, and fostering multisectoral collaboration, we can advance the agenda of women's health and improve outcomes for women worldwide [12].

## 15.4 STRATEGIES FOR QUALITY IMPROVEMENT IN WOMEN'S HEALTH SERVICES

Improving the quality of healthcare services for women requires a multifaceted approach that addresses various dimensions of care delivery, including accessibility, effectiveness, safety, patient-centeredness, and equity [17]. Drawing upon principles of TQM and evidence-based practices, healthcare organizations can implement the following strategies to enhance the quality of women's health services:

- **Promoting accessible and equitable care:** Addressing disparities in healthcare access and outcomes is fundamental to improving women's health. Healthcare organizations should strive to eliminate barriers to care, including financial constraints, geographical disparities, and cultural barriers. This may involve expanding healthcare coverage, implementing outreach programs, providing culturally sensitive care, and leveraging technology to reach underserved populations.
- **Enhancing preventive care and health education:** Prevention is key to promoting women's health and well-being. Healthcare organizations should prioritize preventive care services, including screenings for breast and cervical cancer, vaccinations, and reproductive health counseling. Additionally, health education programs aimed at promoting healthy behaviors, disease prevention, and self-care empower women to make informed decisions about their health.
- **Optimizing maternal and reproductive health services:** Maternal and reproductive health represents critical components of women's health. Healthcare organizations should implement evidence-based practices to improve maternal outcomes, including timely prenatal care, childbirth education, and postpartum support. Moreover, ensuring access to a full range of contraceptive options, family planning services, and comprehensive abortion care is essential for promoting reproductive autonomy and reducing maternal mortality and morbidity.
- **Integrating mental health services:** Mental health is an integral component of women's overall well-being. Healthcare organizations should integrate mental health screening, assessment, and treatment into routine women's health services. Additionally, promoting mental health literacy, reducing stigma, and providing access to counseling and support services can improve mental health outcomes for women experiencing depression, anxiety, trauma, or other mental health disorders.

- **Fostering patient-centered care:** Women-centered care recognizes the unique needs, preferences, and experiences of women and involves them as active partners in their healthcare journey. Healthcare organizations should prioritize patient-centered practices, including shared decision-making, respect for autonomy, clear communication, and compassionate care. Additionally, soliciting feedback from women through patient satisfaction surveys and focus groups can help identify areas for improvement and enhance the patient experience.
- **Investing in healthcare workforce development:** Healthcare professionals play a central role in delivering quality women's health services. Healthcare organizations should invest in workforce development initiatives aimed at enhancing the skills, competencies, and cultural competence of healthcare providers. Training programs on gender-sensitive care, trauma-informed care, and reproductive health counseling can empower healthcare professionals to deliver high-quality, patient-centered care to women.
- **Utilizing technology and innovation:** Leveraging technology and innovation can enhance the quality and efficiency of women's health services. Healthcare organizations should explore opportunities to implement digital health solutions, telemedicine platforms, and electronic health records to improve access to care, streamline communication, and facilitate remote monitoring. Additionally, innovation in medical devices, diagnostics, and treatment modalities can advance the field of women's health and improve health outcomes for women worldwide.

By implementing these strategies, healthcare organizations can enhance the quality, accessibility, and effectiveness of women's health services, ultimately improving health outcomes and advancing the well-being of women globally.

## 15.5 PERFORMANCE MEASUREMENTS AND PROCESS OPTIMIZATION

Ensuring high-quality healthcare delivery for women requires a systematic approach to performance measurement and process optimization. By leveraging data, monitoring key performance indicators, and continuously improving processes, healthcare organizations can enhance the efficiency, effectiveness, and safety of women's health services. Performance measurement serves as a cornerstone of quality improvement efforts in women's health. Healthcare organizations collect and analyze data on various metrics, including clinical outcomes, patient satisfaction, healthcare utilization, and process performance. By tracking these indicators over time, organizations can assess their performance, identify areas for improvement, and monitor the impact of quality improvement initiatives.

Clinical outcomes are among the most critical measures of performance in women's health services. Healthcare organizations monitor outcomes such as maternal mortality rates, infant mortality rates, rates of complications during childbirth, and cancer survival rates to evaluate the effectiveness of clinical care. Additionally, process measures, such as adherence to evidence-based guidelines, timeliness of care delivery, and patient safety indicators, provide insights into the quality and safety of care provided to women. Patient satisfaction is another essential aspect of performance measurement in women's health services. Healthcare organizations utilize patient surveys, feedback mechanisms, and focus groups to assess patients' experiences, preferences, and perceptions of care. By soliciting and incorporating patient feedback, organizations can identify areas for improvement and enhance the patient experience [10].

Furthermore, healthcare utilization metrics, such as appointment attendance rates, follow-up visit rates, and adherence to recommended screenings and vaccinations, provide insights into access to care and healthcare utilization patterns among women. By monitoring healthcare utilization, organizations can identify barriers to access, optimize appointment scheduling, and ensure that women receive timely and appropriate care. Process optimization is integral to enhancing the efficiency and effectiveness of women's health services. Healthcare organizations analyze workflows, identify bottlenecks and streamline processes to minimize delays, reduce errors, and improve resource utilization. This may involve standardizing clinical protocols, implementing electronic health record systems, and utilizing quality improvement methodologies such as Lean or Six Sigma to identify and eliminate waste.

Additionally, healthcare organizations leverage technology and innovation to optimize processes in women's health services. Digital health solutions, telemedicine platforms, and remote monitoring technologies enable providers to deliver care more efficiently, expand access to services, and improve care coordination. Furthermore, predictive analytics and machine learning algorithms can analyze large datasets to identify trends, predict patient outcomes, and optimize resource allocation. In summary, performance measurement and process optimization are essential components of quality improvement efforts in women's health services. By systematically collecting data, monitoring key performance indicators, and continuously optimizing processes, healthcare organizations can enhance the quality, safety, and efficiency of care provided to women, ultimately improving health outcomes and advancing women's health worldwide [18].

## 15.6 QUALITY ASSURANCE AND RISK MANAGEMENT

Quality assurance and risk management are critical components of ensuring the safety, effectiveness, and reliability of women's health services. By implementing rigorous quality assurance processes and robust risk management strategies, healthcare organizations can mitigate potential risks, prevent adverse events, and uphold high standards of care delivery. Quality assurance encompasses a comprehensive set of activities aimed at monitoring and improving the quality of healthcare services. Healthcare organizations establish quality assurance mechanisms, policies, and protocols to ensure that care provided to women meets established standards and guidelines. This may involve conducting regular audits, reviews, and assessments of clinical practices; documentation; and outcomes to identify areas for improvement and ensure compliance with regulatory requirements. Central to quality assurance in women's health services is the implementation of evidence-based clinical guidelines and best practices. Healthcare organizations develop and disseminate clinical protocols, pathways, and guidelines for managing common conditions and procedures related to women's health, such as prenatal care, childbirth, family planning, and cancer screening. By standardizing care delivery based on evidence-based practices, organizations can enhance consistency, reduce variation, and improve the quality and safety of care provided to women [8].

Furthermore, quality assurance in women's health services involves monitoring and managing clinical outcomes and adverse events. Healthcare organizations track key performance indicators, such as maternal mortality rates, cesarean section rates, rates of obstetric complications, and postoperative complications, to assess the effectiveness and safety of care. Additionally, organizations implement systems for reporting; investigating; and mitigating adverse events, errors, and near misses to prevent recurrence and improve patient safety. Risk management is another essential component of ensuring quality and safety in women's health services. Healthcare organizations proactively identify, assess, and manage risks associated with clinical care, processes, and systems to prevent harm to patients and staff. This may involve conducting risk assessments, root cause analyses, and failure mode and effects analyses to identify potential hazards, vulnerabilities, and opportunities for improvement.

Healthcare organizations implement risk mitigation strategies and controls to minimize the likelihood and impact of adverse events. This may include implementing clinical decision support tools, checklists, and protocols to standardize care processes and reduce the risk of errors. Additionally, organizations establish communication channels, reporting systems, and feedback mechanisms to facilitate the timely identification and resolution of safety concerns and near misses. Moreover, healthcare organizations prioritize patient safety culture and promote a culture of transparency, accountability, and continuous learning. Staff members are encouraged to report safety concerns, errors, and near misses without fear of reprisal, and organizations utilize these reports to implement corrective actions and quality improvement initiatives. Additionally, healthcare organizations provide training, education, and support to staff members to enhance their knowledge and skills in quality assurance and risk management practices. In summary, quality assurance and risk management are essential components of ensuring the safety, effectiveness, and reliability of women's health services. By implementing robust quality assurance processes, evidence-based practices, and proactive risk management strategies, healthcare organizations can mitigate risks, prevent adverse events, and uphold high standards of care delivery, ultimately improving health outcomes and advancing women's health [4].

## 15.7 LEADERSHIP AND TEAM DYNAMICS

Effective leadership and cohesive team dynamics are essential for delivering high-quality women's health services. Leadership sets the tone for organizational culture, fosters collaboration, and empowers teams to achieve common goals. Meanwhile, strong team dynamics promote communication, trust, and synergy among healthcare professionals, leading to improved patient outcomes and satisfaction. Leadership in women's health services involves setting a clear vision, fostering a culture of excellence, and providing strategic direction to healthcare teams. Leaders champion the importance of women's health, advocate for resources and support, and prioritize quality improvement initiatives aimed at enhancing the delivery of care. Additionally, leaders create an environment that values diversity, equity, and inclusivity, ensuring that women from all backgrounds receive equitable access to high-quality healthcare services. Transformational leadership, characterized by inspiration, motivation, and empowerment, is particularly effective in driving positive change in women's health services. Transformational leaders inspire and motivate healthcare teams to go above and beyond, fostering a sense of shared purpose and commitment to excellence. By empowering team members to innovate, collaborate, and problem solving, transformational leaders unleash the full potential of their teams and drive continuous improvement in women's healthcare delivery [14].

Moreover, effective leadership in women's health services involves fostering interdisciplinary collaboration and teamwork. Women's health is multidimensional, requiring input and expertise from various healthcare disciplines, including obstetrics, gynecology, primary care, nursing, mental health, and social work. Leaders promote cross-disciplinary collaboration, communication, and mutual respect among team members, recognizing the value of diverse perspectives and skill sets in delivering comprehensive and holistic care to women. Team dynamics play a crucial role in the delivery of women's health services, influencing communication, coordination, and patient outcomes. Effective teams in women's health services are characterized by open communication, mutual respect, and shared accountability. Healthcare professionals collaborate seamlessly, exchanging information, coordinating care plans, and supporting one another to meet the diverse needs of women across the lifespan. Furthermore, high-functioning teams in women's health services prioritize patient-centered care, actively involving women in decision-making processes and respecting their autonomy and preferences.

Team members listen attentively to women's concerns, address their questions and anxieties, and empower them to make informed choices about their health. By fostering a supportive and compassionate care environment, teams in women's health services enhance patient satisfaction and promote positive health outcomes. In summary, effective leadership and cohesive team dynamics are essential for delivering high-quality women's health services. Transformational leaders provide vision, direction, and support, empowering healthcare teams to excel and driving continuous improvement in care delivery. Meanwhile, collaborative and patient-centered teams prioritize communication, mutual respect, and shared accountability, ensuring that women receive comprehensive, holistic, and compassionate care that meets their unique needs and preferences [5].

## 15.8 EVIDENCE-BASED PRACTICE AND CLINICAL GUIDELINES

Evidence-based practice and clinical guidelines serve as essential pillars of high-quality women's health services, guiding healthcare professionals in delivering care that is informed by the best available evidence, clinical expertise, and patient preferences. By integrating evidence-based practices and adhering to established clinical guidelines, healthcare organizations can improve patient outcomes, enhance safety, and promote consistency in care delivery. Evidence-based practice in women's health services involves the conscientious integration of the latest research evidence, clinical expertise, and patient values and preferences in clinical decision-making. Healthcare professionals critically appraise scientific literature, evaluate the strength of evidence, and apply findings to inform their clinical practice. This approach ensures that care provided to women is based on the most up-to-date and credible evidence available, leading to improved health outcomes and patient satisfaction.

Clinical guidelines serve as standardized, evidence-based recommendations for clinical practice, outlining best practices for the diagnosis, treatment, and management of specific health conditions and procedures. Clinical guidelines in women's health cover a wide range of topics, including prenatal care, contraception, screening for breast and cervical cancer, management of menopausal symptoms, and treatment of gynecological conditions. These guidelines are developed by expert panels, professional organizations, and government agencies and are regularly updated to reflect advances in scientific knowledge and changes in clinical practice [11].

Healthcare organizations play a crucial role in promoting evidence-based practice and implementing clinical guidelines in women's health services. Organizations establish processes and protocols for accessing, evaluating, and disseminating evidence-based information to healthcare providers. This may involve providing access to electronic databases, clinical decision support tools, and continuing education resources that enable healthcare professionals to stay informed about the latest research findings and clinical guidelines relevant to women's health. Moreover, healthcare organizations integrate clinical guidelines into clinical practice through the development of standardized care pathways, protocols, and order sets. These tools help standardize care delivery, reduce variation in practice, and ensure that healthcare providers adhere to recommended practices outlined in clinical guidelines.

Additionally, organizations utilize quality improvement initiatives, audit and feedback mechanisms, and performance monitoring to assess adherence to clinical guidelines and identify opportunities for improvement. Furthermore, healthcare organizations engage patients in shared decision-making processes, ensuring that care plans align with patients' values, preferences, and treatment goals. By incorporating patient perspectives into clinical decision-making, healthcare providers can enhance patient satisfaction, improve treatment adherence, and promote patient-centered care delivery. In summary, evidence-based practice and clinical guidelines are essential components of high-quality women's health services. By integrating the latest research evidence and adhering to established clinical guidelines, healthcare organizations can improve patient outcomes, enhance safety, and promote consistency in care delivery. Moreover, engaging patients in shared decision-making processes ensures that care plans are tailored to individual needs and preferences, ultimately leading to improved health outcomes and patient satisfaction in women's health services [6].

## 15.9 PATIENT-CENTERED CARE AND SHARED DECISION-MAKING

Patient-centered care and shared decision-making are foundational principles in the delivery of high-quality women's health services, placing women at the center of their care journey and empowering them to make informed decisions about their health. By prioritizing women's preferences, values, and needs, healthcare providers can enhance the quality of care, promote autonomy, and improve health outcomes. Patient-centered care in women's health services involves actively involving women in all aspects of their care, from treatment planning to decision-making. Healthcare providers take time to listen to women's concerns, understand their preferences and goals, and collaborate with them to develop personalized care plans that align with their individual needs and values.

By fostering a partnership between healthcare providers and women, patient-centered care promotes trust, communication, and mutual respect, leading to improved patient satisfaction and engagement in care. Shared decision-making is a collaborative process in which healthcare providers and women work together to make healthcare decisions that are informed by the best available evidence, women's values, and preferences. Healthcare providers provide women with relevant information about their health condition, treatment options, risks, and benefits, empowering them to actively participate in decision-making. Through open dialogue, exploration of treatment alternatives, and consideration of women's preferences, shared decision-making ensures that care plans are tailored to women's unique circumstances and treatment goals.

Furthermore, patient-centered care and shared decision-making in women's health services encompass a holistic approach to care delivery that addresses women's physical, emotional, and psychosocial needs. Healthcare providers take into account women's life experiences, cultural backgrounds, and socioeconomic factors when developing care plans, recognizing the impact of these factors on health outcomes and treatment adherence. By considering the whole person and providing comprehensive, compassionate care, healthcare providers can improve women's overall well-being and quality of life [17].

Healthcare organizations play a crucial role in promoting patient-centered care and shared decision-making in women's health services. Organizations establish policies, protocols, and training programs that emphasize the importance of patient-centered care and provide healthcare providers with the skills and tools necessary to engage in shared decision-making with women. Additionally, organizations utilize patient feedback mechanisms, satisfaction surveys, and quality improvement initiatives to assess and improve the patient-centeredness of care delivery processes. Moreover, technology plays a significant role in facilitating patient-centered care and shared decision-making in women's health services. Digital health solutions, patient portals, and decision aids empower women to access relevant health information; communicate with healthcare providers; and participate in decision-making from the comfort of their homes. By leveraging technology, healthcare organizations can enhance patient engagement, improve communication, and promote active participation in care among women.

In summary, patient-centered care and shared decision-making are fundamental principles in the delivery of high-quality women's health services. By prioritizing women's preferences, values, and needs, healthcare providers can enhance the quality of care, promote autonomy, and improve health outcomes. Moreover, healthcare organizations play a crucial role in fostering a culture of patient-centeredness and providing healthcare providers with the support and resources necessary to engage in shared decision-making with women. Through collaboration, communication, and mutual respect, patient-centered care and shared decision-making empower women to take an active role in their healthcare journey, ultimately leading to improved health outcomes and greater satisfaction with care in women's health services [10].

## 15.10 CASE STUDIES AND BEST PRACTICES

Case studies and best practices serve as valuable resources for healthcare providers, policymakers, and organizations seeking to improve the quality of women's health services. By examining real-world examples of successful interventions, innovations, and quality improvement initiatives, stakeholders can gain insights into effective strategies and approaches for enhancing women's health outcomes. Case studies in women's health services provide detailed narratives of clinical scenarios, quality improvement projects, and healthcare interventions that highlight challenges, successes, and lessons learned. These case studies offer a window into the complexities of women's health issues and the diverse approaches employed by healthcare organizations to address them. By analyzing case studies, healthcare providers can gain practical knowledge, identify opportunities for improvement, and apply lessons learned to their own clinical practice. Furthermore, case studies offer a platform for sharing innovative approaches and best practices in women's health services. Healthcare organizations showcase successful interventions, programs, and initiatives that have led to improvements in patient outcomes, satisfaction, and quality of care. These best practices may include strategies for improving access to care, enhancing patient engagement, optimizing care coordination, and implementing evidence-based guidelines. By highlighting successful examples, case studies inspire replication and adaptation of effective practices in other healthcare settings [14].

Additionally, case studies provide insights into the importance of interdisciplinary collaboration and teamwork in women's health services. Multidisciplinary teams collaborate to address complex women's health issues, combining expertise from various specialties, including obstetrics, gynecology, primary care, nursing, mental health, and social work. Case studies illustrate how effective communication, shared decision-making, and mutual respect among team members contribute to improved patient outcomes and satisfaction. Moreover, case studies offer a lens into the role of technology and innovation in advancing women's health services. Healthcare organizations leverage digital health solutions, telemedicine platforms, wearable devices, and mobile applications to enhance access to care; facilitate remote monitoring; and empower women to take control of their health. Case studies showcase how technology-driven interventions improve efficiency, effectiveness, and patient engagement in women's health services. Best practices in women's health services encompass a wide range of strategies and approaches aimed at improving quality, safety, and patient satisfaction. These best practices may include initiatives to promote preventive care, optimize maternal and reproductive health services, address social determinants of health, and enhance patient-centered care and shared decision-making. By identifying and disseminating best practices, healthcare organizations contribute to the advancement of women's health and the dissemination of evidence-based care delivery models. In summary, case studies and best practices in women's health services offer valuable insights into effective strategies, interventions, and approaches for improving quality of care and patient outcomes. By examining real-world examples of successful initiatives and learning from the experiences of others, healthcare providers, policymakers, and organizations can identify opportunities for improvement and implement evidence-based practices that enhance women's health services. Through collaboration, innovation, and continuous learning, stakeholders can work together to advance the agenda of women's health and promote better health outcomes for women worldwide [3].

## 15.11 CONCLUSION AND FUTURE DIRECTIONS

Women's health services play a pivotal role in promoting the health and well-being of women across the lifespan. From preventive care and reproductive health services to maternal care and mental health support, women's health encompasses a wide range of clinical, social, and emotional needs that require comprehensive, patient-centered approaches. Throughout this chapter, we have explored various facets of women's health services, including TQM, healthcare delivery models, challenges and opportunities, strategies for quality improvement, leadership and team dynamics, evidence-based practice, patient-centered care, and best practices. By examining these topics in detail, we have gained insights into the complexities of women's health and the diverse approaches employed by healthcare organizations to address them. Looking ahead, there are several key areas for future focus and development in women's health services given as follows:

- **Health equity:** Addressing disparities in healthcare access and outcomes remains a critical priority in women's health. Future efforts should focus on reducing inequities based on race, ethnicity, socio-economic status, geography, and other social determinants of health to ensure that all women have equal access to high-quality care.
- **Innovation and technology:** Embracing innovation and technology holds promise for improving the delivery of women's health services. Future directions include the integration of telemedicine, digital health solutions, wearable devices, and artificial intelligence to enhance access to care; facilitate remote monitoring; and empower women to manage their health more effectively.
- **Interdisciplinary collaboration:** Promoting interdisciplinary collaboration and teamwork is essential for addressing the complex and multifaceted nature of women's health issues. Future initiatives should focus on breaking down silos between healthcare specialties, fostering communication, and enhancing coordination to provide comprehensive, holistic care to women.

- **Preventive care and health promotion:** Investing in preventive care and health promotion is key to improving women's health outcomes and reducing the burden of chronic diseases. Future directions include increasing access to preventive services; promoting healthy behaviors; and addressing modifiable risk factors such as obesity, smoking, and sedentary lifestyle.
- **Mental health support:** By recognizing the importance of mental health in women's overall well-being, future efforts should prioritize the integration of mental health services into women's healthcare delivery models. This includes increasing access to counseling, psychotherapy, and support services, as well as reducing stigma and discrimination surrounding mental health issues.
- **Research and evidence generation:** Continued investment in research and evidence generation is essential for advancing the field of women's health. Future research should focus on filling knowledge gaps, evaluating the effectiveness of interventions, and identifying innovative approaches to improving women's health outcomes.

In conclusion, women's health services play a crucial role in promoting the health, well-being, and empowerment of women worldwide. By prioritizing quality, equity, innovation, and collaboration, healthcare organizations can continue to advance the agenda of women's health and ensure that all women have access to high-quality, patient-centered care that meets their unique needs and preferences.

## 15.12 SUMMARY

In this chapter, we delved into the multifaceted realm of women's health services, exploring various dimensions, including TQM, healthcare delivery models, challenges, and opportunities, as well as strategies for improvement. We highlighted the importance of continuous quality improvement, patient-centered care, evidence-based practice, and interdisciplinary collaboration in providing comprehensive and effective care to women across diverse populations. Throughout the discussion, we emphasized the significance of addressing disparities in healthcare access and outcomes, particularly among marginalized and underserved communities. We explored the role of leadership, teamwork, and innovation in driving positive change and advancing the agenda of women's health. Moreover, we underscored the importance of promoting health equity, leveraging technology, and integrating mental health support into women's health services. By prioritizing preventive care, health promotion, and research, healthcare organizations can improve health outcomes and enhance the well-being of women worldwide. In conclusion, women's health services are essential for promoting the health, dignity, and rights of women. By embracing principles of quality improvement, patient-centered care, and evidence-based practice, we can create a future where every woman receives equitable access to high-quality healthcare that meets her unique needs and empowers her to lead a healthy and fulfilling life.

## KEYWORDS

- **equity**
- **evidence-based practice**
- **innovation**
- **leadership**
- **patient-centered care**
- **quality improvement**
- **women's health**

## REFERENCES

1. Aggarwal, A., Aeran, H., & Rathee, M. (2019). Quality management in healthcare: The pivotal desideratum. *Journal of Oral Biology and Craniofacial Research, 9*(2), 180–182. doi:10.1016/j.jobcr.2018.06.006
2. Babiker, A., El Husseini, M., Al Nemri, A., Al Frayh, A., Al Juryyan, N., Faki, M. O., Assiri, A., Al Saadi, M., Shaikh, F., & Al Zamil, F. (2014). Health care professional development: Working as a team to improve patient care. *Sudanese Journal of Paediatrics, 14*(2), 9–16.

3. Bendowska, A., & Baum, E. (2023). The significance of cooperation in interdisciplinary health care teams as perceived by polish medical students. *International Journal of Environmental Research and Public Health, 20*(2). doi:10.3390/ijerph20020954
4. Boatin, A. A., Ngonzi, J., Ganyaglo, G., Mbaye, M., Wylie, B. J., & Diouf, K. (2021). Cesarean delivery in low- and middle-income countries: A review of quality of care metrics and targets for improvement. *Seminars in Fetal & Neonatal Medicine, 26*(1), 101199. doi:10.1016/j.siny.2021.101199
5. Carnes, M., Morrissey, C., & Geller, S. E. (2008). Women's health and women's leadership in academic medicine: Hitting the same glass ceiling? *Journal of Women's Health (Larchmt), 17*(9), 1453–1462. doi:10.1089/jwh.2007.0688
6. Dagne, A. H., & Beshah, M. H. (2021). Implementation of evidence-based practice: The experience of nurses and midwives. *PLoS One, 16*(8), e0256600. doi:10.1371/journal.pone.0256600
7. Davidson, P. M., McGrath, S. J., Meleis, A. I., Stern, P., Digiacomo, M., Dharmendra, T., Correa-de-Araujo, R., Campbell, J. C., Hochleitner, M., Messias, D. K., Brown, H., Teitelman, A., Sindhu, S., Reesman, K., Richter, S., Sommers, M. S., Schaeffer, D., Stringer, M., Sampselle, C., Anderson, D., & Krassen Covan, E. (2011). The health of women and girls determines the health and well-being of our modern world: A white paper from the International Council on Women's Health Issues. *Health Care for Women International, 32*(10), 870–886. doi:10.1080/07399332.2011.603872
8. Golnik, N., & Pałko, T. (2006). Remarks on risk management and quality assurance in health care. *Polish Journal of Medical Physics and Engineering, 12*, 69–108.
9. Hidayah, N., Arbianingsih, & Ilham. (2022). The impact of integrated quality management-based health services on general hospital quality. *Frontiers in Public Health, 10*, 1011396. doi:10.3389/fpubh.2022.1011396
10. Kruk, M. E., Gage, A. D., Arsenault, C., Jordan, K., Leslie, H. H., Roder-DeWan, S., Adeyi, O., Barker, P., Daelmans, B., Doubova, S. V., English, M., García-Elorrio, E., Guanais, F., Gureje, O., Hirschhorn, L. R., Jiang, L., Kelley, E., Lemango, E. T., Liljestrand, J., Malata, A., & Pate, M. (2018). High-quality health systems in the Sustainable Development Goals era: Time for a revolution. *The Lancet. Global Health, 6*(11), e1196–e1252. doi:10.1016/s2214-109x(18)30386-3
11. Majid, S., Foo, S., Luyt, B., Zhang, X., Theng, Y. L., Chang, Y. K., & Mokhtar, I. A. (2011). Adopting evidence-based practice in clinical decision making: Nurses' perceptions, knowledge, and barriers. *Journal of the Medical Library Association, 99*(3), 229–236. doi:10.3163/1536-5050.99.3.010
12. Malhotra, S., & Shah, R. (2015). Women and mental health in India: An overview. *Indian Journal of Psychiatry, 57*(Suppl 2), S205–S211. doi:10.4103/0019-5545.161479
13. Mogueo, A., Defo, B. K., & Mbanya, J. C. (2022). Healthcare providers' and policymakers' experiences and perspectives on barriers and facilitators to chronic disease self-management for people living with hypertension and diabetes in Cameroon. *BMC Primary Care, 23*(1), 291. doi:10.1186/s12875-022-01892-8
14. Morales-Huamán, H. I., Medina-Valderrama, C. J., Valencia-Arias, A., Vasquez-Coronado, M. H., Valencia, J., & Delgado-Caramutti, J. (2023). Organizational culture and teamwork: A bibliometric perspective on public and private organizations. *Sustainability, 15*(18), 13966.

15. Mosadeghrad, A., & Ferlie, E. (2016). *Total Quality Management in Healthcare*. In: *Management Innovations for Healthcare Organizations: Adopt, Abandon or Adapt*, Routledge (pp. 378–396).
16. Nagineviciute, M., Bartuseviciene, E., & Blazeviciene, A. (2023). Woman-centered care: Standardized outcomes measure. *Medicina (Kaunas), 59*(9), 1537. doi:10.3390/medicina59091537
17. Saha, S., Beach, M. C., & Cooper, L. A. (2008). Patient centeredness, cultural competence and healthcare quality. *Journal of the National Medical Association, 100*(11), 1275–1285. doi:10.1016/s0027-9684(15)31505-4
18. Yu, S. W. Y., Hill, C., Ricks, M. L., Bennet, J., & Oriol, N. E. (2017). The scope and impact of mobile health clinics in the United States: A literature review. *International Journal of Equity Health, 16*(1), 178. doi:10.1186/s12939-017-0671-2

# Index

## F

## G



## H

## N

## S

## T

For Product Safety Concerns and Information please contact our EU representative GPSR@taylorandfrancis.com Taylor & Francis Verlag GmbH, Kaufingerstraße 24, 80331 München, Germany